RADIOGRAPHIC PHOTOGRAPHY

To those whose book this really is:
who gave us the straw for the bricks
and afterwards advised us to remove
some of them.

Radiographic Photography

D. NOREEN CHESNEY
Hon. F.S.R. T.E. S.R.R.

Superintendent Teacher, School of Radiography
Coventry and Warwickshire Hospital

AND

MURIEL O. CHESNEY
F.S.R. T.E. S.R.R.

Teacher Principal, School of Radiography
The United Birmingham Hospitals

THIRD EDITION

BLACKWELL SCIENTIFIC PUBLICATIONS

OXFORD AND EDINBURGH

ISBN 0 632 08370 0

FIRST PUBLISHED 1965
SECOND EDITION 1969
THIRD EDITION 1971

Distributed in the U.S.A. by
F. A. Davis Company, 1915 Arch Street,
Philadelphia, Pennsylvania

Printed in Great Britain by
WILLIAM CLOWES AND SONS LTD
LONDON, BECCLES AND COLCHESTER
and bound by
THE KEMP HALL BINDERY, OXFORD

Contents

List of Plates

Preface to Third Edition

We were surprised and of course pleased to learn from Blackwell Scientific Publications that the 1969 edition of this book had taken itself from the stocks of the publishers to the bookshelves of its readers so speedily that before the end of 1970 some re-issue was necessary. So perhaps this preface should begin where the last one ended with thanks to our readers.

In seeking to make the book useful to those who consult it, we decided this time to include two appendices. Appendix I provides general information on the maintenance of automatic processors, on processing faults and on artefacts. Appendix II is a table which presents certain technical elements in the production of a radiograph and their effects on two important features of the image.

In the first edition on page 1 we were so incautious as to refer to Aristotle's knowledge of pinhole images in 350 B.C. This was later to make Dr George Parker and his friends hunt along a faint trail in quest of a specific reference. We are grateful to them for their interest and enthusiasm and for telling us what they found. In a volume of the Loel Classical Library entitled *Aristotle—Problems Vol. I* there is: *Paragraph 911—when sunlight passes through wickerwork the spots of light are circular, not rectangular. Paragraph 912—it is argued that when the sun shines through a small aperture, the rays form two cones, one between sun and aperture and the other between aperture and screen, the apices being at the hole.*

Reverting to the year 1970, we owe thanks to Mr Peter Higginbotham of Du Pont Company and especially to Mr Peter Ranger of the same firm who interested himself in the book and provided for Appendix I both material and commentary.

D.N.C.

M.O.C.

1971

Preface to Second Edition

At one time it would have seemed unlikely that a textbook on radiographic photography would be out-of-date in any respect three years after its publication. The processing of radiographs seemed a static subject in the Society of Radiographers' syllabus of training and as improbable of further change as human anatomy; perhaps we might say that in every sense it was developed and fixed.

However, during the four years since we wrote the first edition of this book, radiographic photography has moved fast indeed. We welcome the opportunity given by this second edition to try to catch up with it; particularly with rapid cycle processing, which is now widely used, and the implications of automation generally for the planning of processing rooms and the manufacture of emulsions and chemicals appropriate to medical radiography.

In view of the present ascendancy of roller processing machines it has seemed a good idea to give them now a chapter to themselves and to include in this a few further observations on chemistry and suitable emulsions as well as the mechanics of automation. We could not possibly have carried out this project without up-to-date information from film and chemical manufacturers and we are well aware of the debt which this book owes in this respect to two organizations and their expert staff. It is a pleasure to thank particularly Mr L.F.A.Mason of the Ramsden Laboratory, Ilford Ltd, for the interest he took in this and allied parts of the book and for his generosity in giving us a personal communication and more of his time than we had any right to expect. We are grateful also to Mr Donald Bere of May and Baker Ltd for having 'mined out' for us information in the same category.

The duplicating of radiographs is not within the present diploma syllabus of the Society of Radiographers. However, in many X-ray departments radiologists like to obtain copies, for teaching and other purposes, of those of medical interest and radiographers are often involved in executing this work. We have therefore added to the new edition a chapter which includes material on this aspect of radiography.

We make no pretence whatever that this part of the book is a full survey of the subject. Our aim has been to provide as simple an account as possible of not more than one method of duplicating radiographs which is practicable in any X-ray department, using materials and equipment readily to be found or obtained. To the expert no doubt our criteria may contain an element of do-it-yourself handiness and indeed this is the impression we have tried to give. We hope that in this new chapter the accounts of a one-stage duplicating technique and of subtraction will give encouragement and practical help to a radiographer— or even radiologist—who has to undertake either process for the first time.

In the preparation of the new edition no less than of the first we have ourselves been helped by a number of people. It is one of the rewarding aspects of writing a professional textbook to discover the kindness and readiness with which many associated with the profession will make available their own special learning and experience. We are truly grateful to Mr R.F.Farr, Chief Physicist at the United Birmingham Hospitals, for his careful observations on the first edition which have enabled us to improve the second and for allowing us to 'steal' a diagram. We would like again to thank Mr K.W.Goddard and Mr Sydney Marshall of Kodak Ltd who discussed Chapter xix with us and provided for our study a duplicating technique and one for subtraction radiography. Mr C.W.Mead of Watson and Sons (Electro-Medical) Ltd gave us a personal communication related to equipment for recording the intensified fluorescent image and to him, too, we are grateful for continued interest in the book. We welcome the opportunity to express appreciation to Mr V.James of the Oxford School of Radiography for drawing to our attention the work of Dr G.M.Ardran of the Nuffield Institute for Medical Research, in connection with screen/film contact in cassettes; and no less to thank Dr Ardran himself for permitting us to use his material.

Negatives and photographs have been given to us by the Du Pont Company (United Kingdom) Ltd, by Ilford Ltd, by the Pako Corporation, Minneapolis, U.S.A. and by Williamson Manufacturing Co. Ltd; we appreciate their courtesy in permitting us to reproduce their material. We are glad of the opportunity here to voice our thanks for personal help from Mr John Hale, Mr E.W.Lee and Mr Peter Spencer of Ilford Ltd and from Mr Peter Higginbotham of Du Pont Company.

Miss P.M.Kimber of the Wessex Neurological Centre kindly allowed us to reproduce subtraction radiographs made by herself (Plate 19.1) and we are grateful to the Society of Radiographers and *Radiography* for permission to use the blocks of these illustrations.

Extracts from the British Standard Specification for X-ray Film and Cassettes (British Standard 4304 : 1968) on p. 98 are reproduced by kind permission of the British Standards Institution, 2 Park Street, London W1, from whom copies of the complete standard may be obtained.

Finally, we would say 'Thank you' to the readers of the first edition who have made a second one necessary.

D.N.C.
M.O.C.

1968

Preface to First Edition

This book is not about photography; it is about a number of subjects which are grouped together under the title Radiographic Photography in the syllabus of training for the Membership Diploma of the Society of Radiographers. The word camera appears in this book comparatively seldom and those who would seek in its pages for light on their studio lighting must remain perpetually unillumined.

In the first and last analyses, we should recognize that good radiography, though it may depend upon a knowledge of theoretical concepts, in fact is a practical skill. The subjects in their syllabus of training, summarized in the term radiographic photography, are important to radiographers because they are realistic subjects: knowledge and appreciation of them significantly affect the quality of the end-product—the radiograph. It seems strange that no textbook has yet been written for radiographers about radiographic photography and that their teachers must build courses of instruction on manufacturers' pamphlets and photographic manuals in a wider category. The authors hope that this book may fill what appears to be a gap among the aids to those who must learn and the tools of those who must teach.

In attempting to meet the needs of student radiographers, as we believe that they are not scientists and may have only irregular knowledge of chemistry, we have kept to a minimum the appearance of mathematical expressions and have avoided chemical formulae. Of great convenience to those in the know, such shorthand can be only profoundly baffling to those who are not. We hope that we have made to radiographic photography the practical approach which its character deserves.

The syllabus of training for the M.S.R. Diploma has directed the selection of material for this book. While it has been written for the education of student radiographers, we know that in some places greater detail is given than may be required for the M.S.R. course. It seems a proper principle to include in a textbook something more than the minimum demanded by a particular course of study; perhaps especially so in a field of knowledge which is fertile of development. This aspect of the book may attract at least some post-graduate readers who wish to prepare for the Higher Examination of the Society of Radiographers.

From inclusions to an omission. This book has given no space to the reproduction of photographic faults in radiographs. Possibly this may appear a serious defect to its critics. However, it must be evident to radiographers of experience that if the catalogue of such errors is to be usefully extensive, apart from any attempt to make it complete, a large number of illustrations is necessarily required: even then it is certain that someone at some time would be confronted in the viewing room with a bizarre radiographic appearance for which no reference here would enable the radiographer to account. Reproduction on paper of certain classic faults is much less satisfactory than their visualization on original films. We would suggest that for student radiographers a more useful exercise than looking at such copies is always the handling and examination of the real material. Why should they not be permitted some limited experiment from which to form their own library of malpractices in handling radiographs?

No man is an island and, perhaps more than many others, authors of textbooks are dependent on links with certain mainlands of learning and material. We are aware that the substance of this book has been strengthened because a number of people each have given to us generous measures of their knowledge, ability and not least of their time. We are glad of an opportunity to offer to them an expression of our thanks, though the small gesture is incommensurate with the gift received.

We are grateful to Dr D.M.Alexander, consultant radiologist at the Coventry and Warwickshire Hospital, for reading Chapter xiv and discussing it with us; and to Miss A.L.Hebden, medical photographer at the same hospital, who took photographs, with most welcome expedition, of a step-wedge and of parts of the Odelca and Hansen equipment. Dr J.F.K.Hutton, consultant radiologist at the General Hospital, Birmingham, receives our thanks for kindly reading Chapters xii and xiii and giving his comments. Mr. W. Hurt, medical photographer at the Birmingham Children's Hospital, came to our aid at very short notice and provided illustrations to show the appearance of a granular pattern at different degrees of photographic enlargement.

From Mr K.W.Goddard we have had the stimulus of early interest in the project and we appreciate his help in reading the MS of Chapters xi, vi and vii and in mobilizing for us some of the resources of Kodak Ltd who have loaned many illustrations and supplied other material. With

CHAPTER I

The Photographic Process

VISIBLE LIGHT IMAGES

Photography is a record made by means of light. Three separate processes can be distinguished.

(i) The formation of an image. In general photography this is an optical image produced when *divergent* rays coming from a subject are made to *converge* by means of a lens. In radiography it is a shadow image produced when interposed objects attenuate an X-ray beam.

(ii) Recording the image. In the first instance the image exists as a hidden one within the material used for the record; this must be a substance which reacts to light.

(iii) The production of the image in permanent form. This involves the action of a chemical agent to make the hidden image visible. This stage is known as *development*, and it is followed by further chemical processes which fix the image and make it into a permanent record.

Photographic history is the story of discovery of physical and chemical processes by which an image is formed, recorded, and made permanent. It has extended over a long period of time. The science of optics, for example, is a very old one, and the 'pinhole camera' which has pleased many of us in our schooldays is a device by no means new; Aristotle referred to pinhole images as long ago as 350 B.C. Yet it was not until the nineteenth century that real progress was made in obtaining permanent record for photographic images.

In the search for a means by which to make such records, the action of light on certain materials was noticed. That light can produce change is common knowledge to us all. Curtains and carpets fade under the action of sunlight; raw peeled potatoes turn uninvitingly black; some human bodies turn agreeably brown. It is not within the intended scope of this book to recount the evolution of photographic processes, attractive though such by-ways may be. We are concerned at present with the light-sensitive materials encountered by radiographers in their work.

I

These are materials which on exposure to light are found, after chemical development, to have darkened where the light has reached them.

A photographic material recording an image receives more light from the brighter parts of the subject. If the material reacts to light by becoming *darker*, it follows that in the developed result those parts of the subject which were bright to the eye are dark in the recorded image. Those parts of the subject which are dark to the eye are light in the recorded image. This image with reversed tones constitutes a *photographic negative* (Fig. 1.1).

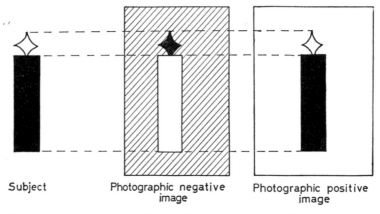

Subject   Photographic negative   Photographic positive
image   image

FIG. 1.1. The bright parts of the subject (e.g. the candle-flame) in the first photographic image (a negative one) are dark. From the negative, a positive can be made. The dark parts of the negative transmit less light, and in the positive these parts correspond in tone to the bright parts of the original subject.

From this negative another positive image can be made quite simply. If the negative image is on a transparent film or glass base, it will allow light to pass. Obviously the dark parts of the image will allow less light to pass than do the light parts of the image. The procedure then is to pass light through the negative image on to another piece of photographic material which, like the first, responds to light by becoming black after development. The two photographic materials may be in contact with each other, or the image may be projected from the one to the other. The light parts of the negative transmit more light to blacken the second piece of material than do the dark parts of the negative. The second image is therefore dark in areas corresponding to the dark parts of the subject, and light in areas corresponding to the light areas of the subject. The recorded image is therefore in the same tones (or it may be expressed that the record is in the same sense) as the original. This type of photographic image is called a *positive*.

IMAGES PRODUCED BY X RADIATION

Radiography is the making of images by means of X rays. The light-sensitive materials used in photography respond to X radiation as they do to light. Given exposure to X rays and then developed, they are seen to have darkened where the radiation reached them.

When an X-ray beam passes through a body, some of the radiation is absorbed and some is transmitted. The subject will transmit the beam to a varying amount depending on the penetrating power of the radiation, and upon the atomic number and density and upon the thickness of the material traversed. When the subject consists of tissues which are of different atomic numbers, there is difference of absorption. The emergent radiation shows this difference, and a pattern of varying amounts of radiation reaches the film (Fig. 1.2).

This is closely analogous to the varying amounts of light reflected from a subject in ordinary photography. Some parts of the radiographic subject transmit more radiation and correspond to the bright parts of a photographic subject. Some parts of a radiographic subject transmit less radiation or no radiation, and they therefore correspond to the dark parts of a photographic subject. The radiographic image appearing on X-ray films, with the partially radio-opaque bony structures appearing white and the radioparent gas-filled organs appearing black, is considered to be a negative image (Plate 1.1, following p. 94).

This negative image can be used to make a positive image with reversed tones in precisely the same way as a photographic negative can be used. Radiographic reproductions in the positive image are sometimes used to illustrate textbooks. The student should note that the image seen on a fluorescent screen during fluoroscopy is a *positive* one (Plate 1.2, following p. 94). This is because the response of the screen to radiation is the opposite response of a photographic material; the screen becomes *bright* when radiation falls on it, the photographic material becomes *dark*. Thus the radiolucent parts of the subject are light upon the screen, dark up the film, and the radio-opaque parts are dark upon the screen, light upon the film.

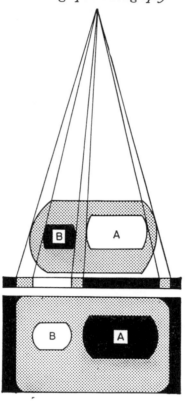

Fig. 1.2. B represents a bone which is relatively opaque to X rays and therefore allows least radiation to reach the film. The film is light underneath it. A represents a hollow gas-filled organ which is radiolucent and allows most radiation to reach the film. The film is dark underneath it. The bone and the organ are surrounded by soft-tissue allowing some radiation to reach the film, which is therefore an intermediate tone. At the edges of the film there is nothing in the way of the radiation. The radiographic image is a pattern of varying amounts of radiation transmitted through the subject to the film.

LIGHT-SENSITIVE PHOTOGRAPHIC MATERIALS

Radiography is a highly specialized application of the photographic process and, as has been seen, certain fundamentals are common both to the wider science and to this special branch. One of these fundamentals is the general character of the light-sensitive materials used.

The group of elements known as the halogens—bromine, chlorine, and iodine—combine with silver to form salts, which are silver bromide, silver chloride, and silver iodide. These salts undergo a change when exposed to light or X rays which enables them to form a photographic image.

Photographic materials may be divided into those which are intended to produce negatives (this group includes X-ray films), and those which are intended to produce positive images (for example the paper on to which holiday 'snapshots' are printed). Virtually all negative materials use silver bromide as the light-sensitive salt. Silver iodide is never used alone, but in combination with silver bromide; the iodide is added to the bromide as a very small proportion of the order of 2–3 per cent. Certain positive materials use silver chloride (which has low sensitivity) or silver bromide, or a combination of the two, according to the type of response which is required.

PHOTOGRAPHIC EMULSIONS

In order to use any silver halide in a photographic material, it is necessary to prepare it in a form which can be coated upon a support; this support is called a *base*. It may be a transparent base such as glass or film, or it may be paper. The form the silver halide takes for this purpose is a suspension of tiny crystals of the salt in a suitable binding agent. This suspension, as it should properly be called, is termed in photography a *photographic emulsion*.

Characteristics of Sensitive Emulsions

Any photographic material has certain characteristics which are important to the photographer who is to use it. One of these is the *speed* of the material; this determines whether the material needs more or less exposure to light in comparison with another material in order to produce a similar picture.

Another important characteristic is *contrast*; this refers to the way in which the material reacts to a range of different exposures. These characteristics—speed and contrast—are determined when the photographic emulsion is made. Speed depends on the size of the silver halide crystals (which are called 'grains'), the preparation of the emulsion, the nature of the radiation used for the exposure, and the development given. Contrast depends on the distribution of size and sensitivity of the grains, and on development.

In any given emulsion the grains are of various sizes. If all the grains in an emulsion are small, the sensitive material is then said to be of fine grain, and it is usually of high contrast and low speed. Photographic materials which are of high speed are of large grain size, and are of relatively lower contrast.

Making a Photographic Emulsion

It has been explained that the emulsion consists of silver halide crystals or grains suspended in a suitable agent. This agent is extremely important. The one chosen is gelatin, and it has certain valuable characteristics as a suspending and binding agent for the silver halide grains.

(i) It is a suitable medium in which to form the silver halide crystals. These are produced in a chemical reaction between solutions of silver nitrate and alkaline halides, as a result of which the insoluble silver halide crystals are formed; they remain suspended in the gelatin, finely dispersed.

(ii) It maintains the silver halide crystals evenly distributed within the suspension.

(iii) When warmed, the gelatin forms a solution which will flow over the base on to which it is to be coated.

(iv) When cooled it forms a firm jelly which sets on the base. It can then be dried, when it has some resistance to moderate mechanical stress, such as abrasion.

(v) It allows solutions to penetrate the emulsion when, at a subsequent stage in its life, the material is chemically processed after photographic or radiographic exposure.

(vi) Some of the constituents of gelatin act on the silver halides as sensitizers and influence the speed of the emulsion. Others act as restrainers and reduce fog.

(vii) On exposure to light, change takes place in the silver halide grains. It is believed that gelatin helps to prevent any reversal of this change, which would of course reduce the effect of the exposure.

Manufacturers producing photographic materials choose the gelatin very carefully and test it stringently. The making of an emulsion is a complex process, carried out with close control of the materials, and of each stage of the procedures involved. The characteristics of the emulsion are precisely regulated. Today there is a great range of photographic materials available of various speeds and different contrast. That this should be so, and that all these diverse materials should be consistent in performance and physical character are indications of the advances which have been achieved, and of the fine control in the processes of manufacture.

The making of an emulsion can be considered in four stages. These are (i) precipitation, (ii) ripening, (iii) digestion or after-ripening, and (iv) finishing.

PRECIPITATION

This process produces the emulsion by combining silver nitrate, an alkali halide, and gelatin. This can be done by a single-jet process in which the silver nitrate solution is run into the alkali halide and gelatin at a controlled rate. Another method involves a double jet by means of which a silver nitrate solution and an alkali halide solution are run into gelatin through two jets. The chemical reactions which occur result in insoluble silver halide grains being dispersed through the gelatin. This process, and subsequent ones during manufacture, must be undertaken in special lighting conditions or in complete darkness.

RIPENING

In this process the emulsion is kept at a raised temperature for a fixed period of time. The silver halide crystals increase in size, the small ones being redissolved and the larger ones growing. The emulsion is then set, shredded, and washed.

DIGESTION OR AFTER-RIPENING

In this process the shreds are remelted, and then again held at raised temperature for a certain time. During this period there is considerable effect on the sensitivity of the grains, and the formation of sensitivity specks within them is encouraged. These sensitivity specks are important in forming the hidden photographic image produced by exposure of the material to light. They are more fully explained in Chapter vi.

FINISHING

Final additions to the emulsion are made at this stage to aid coating and to modify the properties of the material.

When it is ready, the emulsion is coated upon its glass, film, or paper base. Emulsions for materials to make negatives are usually coated upon film or glass, and positive emulsions are usually coated upon film, glass, or paper. When coated, the material is chilled to set the emulsion, and it is then dried.

Since light-sensitive materials are affected by such factors as moisture, temperature, presence of impurities, exposure to certain gases, airborne fluff and dust, static electricity, and by mechanical stress, it is clear that the difficulties of manufacture are great. A very high standard of control and general cleanliness must be vigilantly maintained.

THE PHOTOGRAPHIC LATENT IMAGE

It has been seen that the basis of photography is a sensitive emulsion containing silver halide which undergoes change when exposed to light (or to X radiation). This change is the decomposition of the silver halide into its two constituents. These are metallic silver and whichever halogen (chlorine, bromine, or iodine) has been in combination with the metal. This metallic silver is in a finely divided state, and it is black in colour. Its presence accounts for the darkened appearance of the photographic material on development after exposure to light.

The light-initiated change, which is a minute one, is amplified many million times by the chemical developer. This acts rapidly on the silver halide grains which have received exposure, and produces a visible image. The exposed grains and the change existing in them before development constitute the *photographic latent image*; this and the action of the developer are considered fully in Chapter vi of this book.

POSITIVE PROCESSES

The Negative–Positive Process

It will be understood from the opening section of this chapter that the first stage in making a photograph yields an image in which the tones of the original are reversed, and this is described as a photographic negative. Only in certain special applications are negative images accepted as an end in themselves. We know that they are so accepted in radiography, and the practice also applies in some types of document copying.

However, every student will realize from previous common experience that pictorial records in which the tones are reversed are not acceptable at all. Even the brunettes among us who yearn to be blondes would hardly care for portraits which totally reversed the tones of skin and hair, and a landscape with ashen trees and jet sky does not impress us as realistic. In general therefore negatives exist as the first stage towards obtaining a positive image in which the tones correspond to those of the original subject. As was indicated previously, in order to obtain a positive two stages may be necessary—(i) obtaining the negative image, and (ii) using this negative to make a positive image. This process of making a negative first and using it to make a positive is known as the *negative–positive process*.

Colour photography involves specialized work beyond the intended scope of this book. In black-and-white photography the positives used are of two main types.

(i) Positive images on transparent bases, known as *transparencies* or *diapositives*. They may be projected. This group includes lantern slides, film strips, and cine films.

(ii) Positive images on paper base are called *reflection positives*, but to most of us the term *paper prints* is more familiar. They are viewed by reflected light.

Although the necessity for two stages may seem to add to the difficulty of the negative–positive process, at the same time it has certain practical advantages for the general amateur and professional user. For example, many prints can be made easily from a single negative, which can be used repeatedly at different times. Furthermore, the second stage of the process gives opportunity for closer control of the result; this is important to the pictorial photographer who aims for a beautiful and striking picture. Many of his finest effects would be denied him without the opportunity given at the stage of making a positive print from the first negative. Those who have tried it know how much time can be spent at this stage in varying the control to give different results, and the varieties of result to be obtained can be seen on the walls of photographic exhibitions.

However, the reader may feel that it is time to come back to the X-ray department. It seems reasonable that the student should have some understanding of the negative-positive process as it applies to radiographs.

A radiograph is a negative image. If the radiograph is used, as a photographic negative is used, to print another image on to a paper base, the result is a *positive print*. If it is used to print on to a transparent base, the result is a *positive transparency*. The positive print on paper and the positive transparency, it is clear, are both second-stage results from the radiograhic negative.

The positive print may be used to illustrate a book, but often authors prefer their radiographic illustrations to be negatives, that is in the same sense as the originals; or it may be that what is wanted is a *copy* of the original radiograph, that is a negative image on a transparent base. In using the negative–positive process to obtain either of these, it is necessary to proceed to a *third* stage. The *positive transparency* must now be used as the negative was used, and a print must be made from it on to a paper or film material. If the print is made on a paper material, the result is a *negative image print* with the tones of the original radiograph; if the print is made on a film material, the result is a *negative image transparency* just as the original radiograph was, and it is in fact a copy or facsimile of the first.

Other Positive Processes

Procedures have been devised which give positive images in a single operation, eliminating the two stages of the negative–positive process, but they are not so generally useful as might be thought. It is unnecessary to consider them in detail here, but the main differences of method may be mentioned since it is possible for radiographers to encounter some of them in certain applications within the X-ray department.

DIRECT POSITIVE MATERIALS

These are materials which yield a positive instead of a negative image. Use is made of a specially prepared emulsion. If this film is chemically developed in the ordinary way, it emerges from the developer a uniform black from a deposit of metallic silver. If it is given a photographic exposure before development, the blackening *decreases* with increased exposure—exactly the reverse of the normal photographic process. The resultant image is therefore a positive one.

Film material of this type, although too slow for ordinary photographic purposes, can be used to make copies in the same sense directly from original radiographs, eliminating the tedious and time-consuming stage of the intermediate positive transparency. Some manufacturers are supplying such material to X-ray departments for this purpose, and radiographers who are asked to copy radiographs find it a valuable aid. Some details of a copying technique are given in Chapter xix. To sum up, this method consists of special material given ordinary development.

REVERSAL DEVELOPMENT

An ordinary photographic emulsion can be used to obtain a positive result instead of a negative one if it is given special processing. This technique is called *reversal processing*. It is used in some forms of cinematography and also in colour photography to obtain a positive image directly from negative material exposed in the camera, the result in both cases being a positive transparency. To sum up, this method consists of ordinary material given special development.

IMAGE TRANSFER SYSTEM

The image transfer system is called the diffusion transfer reversal process, which is a long but reasonable name; it is reasonable because the system involves a diffusion process, it achieves the transference of an image from one piece of sensitive material to another, and it gives reversal of the image.

The two pieces of material involved are one which is sensitive to light (photo-sensitive) and one which is sensitive not to light but to chemicals. A negative image is produced in the photo-sensitive material in the ordinary way by exposure to light. At the time of development, the sheet of photo-sensitive material is put in close contact with the chemically sensitive one, which is known as the transfer or receiving paper.

At this stage therefore three things are brought together:
(i) The photo-sensitive material with a latent image in it;
(ii) the developer;
(iii) the receiving material which is chemically sensitive.

The latent image in the photo-sensitive material is acted upon by the developer and the exposed silver halide is reduced to black silver, giving a negative image in the usual way. At the same time the special developing agents also act upon the unexposed silver halide and free silver atoms in it. These silver atoms in the unexposed parts are free to diffuse into the receiving layer (while those in the exposed parts are not free), and they form a black deposit on the receiving material, attaching themselves to minute silver particles which are already there. Fig. 1.3 is a diagram indicating how the process takes place in the different parts of the image.

The result is a positive image developing in the receiving layer at the same time as the negative image is developing in the photo-sensitive layer.

This transfer method has been used in various ways for document copying. It is the basis of the Polaroid-Land camera; this is a specially designed hand-camera providing a finished picture in the positive image 10 seconds after the exposure is made. In this camera, the sensitive paper and the receiving paper are both in rolls and the chemical agents for the processing are in plastic pods. After the exposure, both papers are brought out together through rollers which keep them in contact, break the pods, and spread the chemicals between the papers.

By means of a special cassette and processor, this system has been adapted for radiography. The cassette is loaded with a special pack containing the sensitive material and the receiving paper; between the

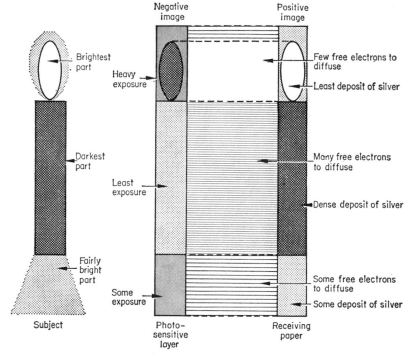

FIG. 1.3. Diffusion transfer reversal process.

surfaces of these two papers are pods containing the developing gel. After exposure in the ordinary way, the cassette is put into the processor. Pressure on a button initiates processing. The photo-sensitive paper and the receiving paper are withdrawn from the cassette together through motor-driven rollers which break the pods containing the developing chemicals. The final radiographic print (a positive) is delivered in 10 seconds, and when the layer of sensitive material which formed the negative has been peeled away, it is ready for viewing. The image can be given greater permanence by being coated with a colourless varnish within one hour of being processed.

There are obvious advantages in the Polaroid system for radiography. No darkroom and no wet processing are needed and the radiographic result is available very quickly—within a minute after the exposure has been made. These advantages make the technique applicable to radiography undertaken during the course of surgical procedures, and the saving in time suggests its use for 'scout films' in pneumoencephalography, angiocardiography and other examinations.

The disadvantages of the system include cost and its lack of similarity to conventional radiographic techniques. The picture is a positive image on paper viewed by reflected light, and is not the familiar negative image viewed by transmitted light. The radiographer must remember that the results in the image of underexposure and overexposure are the reverse of the usual ones—that is a *darkening* of the picture is the result of *underexposure* and a pale image is the result of *overexposure*.

CHAPTER II

Film Materials

Chapter 1 described the preparation of a photographic material by coating a sensitive emulsion on to a suitable base. The construction of a film is not quite so simple as this, and it will now be considered in more detail. The structure of an X-ray film will be taken first, and later it will be seen how a film used for conventional photography may differ from it.

THE STRUCTURE OF AN X-RAY FILM

The structure is built up in layers upon the base which provides a support. The base will therefore be considered first.

The Base

Film base is made of substances derived from cellulose. Cellulose can be treated with acids to form cellulose salts, which are called cellulose esters, and for many years cellulose nitrate was used as film base. This is the cellulose ester produced by treating cellulose with nitric acid. It was in wide use as a film base, but had certain marked disadvantages, one of which was its readiness to burn. Not only did it burn very freely, giving off noxious gases as it did so, but it was liable to spontaneous combustion. It also disintegrated on prolonged storage.

Cellulose nitrate has for a long time been superseded by base made of cellulose acetate, cellulose triacetate, or similar related materials. These keep well and provide what is known as *safety base* that burns slowly if ignited and is not liable to spontaneous combustion. This safety base was used for X-ray film by Eastman in 1924, and following this it came into use for all types of film. In the last few years certain other bases have been tested and introduced for special applications of photography and for radiography. At the present time manufacturers can offer X-ray films on a new synthetic base called 'polyester base'. It is made from polyethylene terephthalate resin. This base is flexible and so strong that it can be considered untearable. It is impermeable to water and processing solutions, and this makes it easier to transport through automatic processors as it remains firm when wet. An important advantage from the manufacturer's point of view is that this base can be made with hardly any risk of contamination from air-borne radioactive particles which eventually cause black spots of fog in an emulsion coating. The base presents a very clear appearance which is said to come from the degree of chemical purity which is maintained during its manufacture.

The fact that a polyester base does not tear easily is an advantage in manual processing when the tension-type of hanger is used because the film does not tear away from the clips at the four corners of the hanger. But the very strong base can be a nuisance if films become jammed in an automatic film changer and it can make their removal very difficult indeed. Another problem is that a corner-cutter used to trim the edges of films on polyester base, if the manufacturer does not supply them with corners already rounded, very soon becomes blunt.

The thickness of film base depends on the use for which the finished product is designed. The base constitutes the thickest layer of the complete film. X-ray film has a base which is 8/1000 in. thick if it is acetate and 7/1000 in. thick if it is polyester base.

The physical characteristics of the base are important and in recent years have tended to increase in importance for X-ray films because of the precise requirements of automatic processing. The base must be entirely free from any defect or blemish and must be uniform in its thickness, since lack of uniformity here will lead to variations in the depth of the emulsion layer.

Since the base is required to transmit light, it must be uniform in its ability to do this. X-ray film base (whether cellulose acetate or polyester) is given a blue tone and is then described as *blue base film*. This blue tone inevitably diminishes to some extent the ability of the base to transmit light, but modern blue base film transmits about 85 per cent of the light falling on it. The blue tone is required to be uniform in colour, should show batch-to-batch consistency in colour, and should not change in colour with time. The blue tone gives intermediate densities in the image a more pleasing appearance and radiologists in the United Kingdom tend to object to its absence. In fact it has no effect on the properties of emulsion coated on to the base and it does nothing to improve the visibility of detail in the image. There seems little reason for its continuing use other than the maintenance of a tradition.

Film base must be sufficiently rigid to avoid kinking (which could occur very readily in the large film sizes if the base were not stiff enough), and yet it must not be too thick.

The Substratum Layer

Before emulsion is coated upon it, film base must be prepared so that the emulsion will adhere to it well. The emulsion and its base do not behave in the same way when they become wet and are dried; the gelatin of the emulsion swells with moisture and contracts when dry to a degree that the base does not. There would therefore be a tendency in these conditions for the two to part from each other unless the base was specially prepared. This preparation consists of putting upon the base a very thin layer of a solution of cellulose ester and gelatin in water and acetone. The process eventually leaves on the surface of the base a deposit mainly of gelatin which constitutes the *substratum layer*. The technique of applying the substratum layer to the base is more elaborate for polyester than for acetate base. With a polyester base it may involve the use of coatings made of other synthetic resins. For an X-ray film this substratum layer is coated upon both sides of the base.

The Sensitive Emulsion Layer

The sensitive emulsion, coated upon the substratum on *both* sides of the base, constitutes the next layers of the film. As has been explained in Chapter 1, the sensitive emulsion consists of silver halide crystals suspended in gelatin. These undergo change under the action of light or X rays. The characteristics of the film material depend on the size of these silver halide grains, their size range, and their sensitivity range. The two emulsion layers on each side of the X-ray film base are each 1/2000 in. thick and the film is said to be *double sided*.

Advantages of Two Emulsion Layers

Increase in Sensitivity. Since there is a sensitive emulsion on both sides of the film base, there are in fact two images formed one on each side of the base, each emulsion being exposed simultaneously with the other. These two images are viewed by light transmitted through the film, and are thus seen as a single image formed by the two superimposed upon each other. The degree of blackness of each silver image is therefore added to that of the other one. The two sides together consequently give an image which has twice the silver deposit obtained if a single-sided material were used. The efficiency of the process is about double what it would be with the use of a single-sided film. This enables much shorter exposures to be used, with less risk of blurring from the movement of parts being radiographed, and with markedly less radiation dose to the patient.

Increase in contrast. Contrast in the image is difference between the degree of blackness of various regions. The blackness differences are greater for double-sided than for single-sided materials.

Another factor to be considered is the reduction in radiographic contrast that results from an increase in the X-ray tube voltage. As the radiation becomes more penetrating, the absorption differences in the various tissues of the subject become levelled. The result is an image of less contrast, and this effect would be very marked if a single-sided film were used. Double-sided film allows higher tube voltages to be employed without a deterioration in contrast beyond acceptable limits.

Production of an image in two layers. For X-ray film exposed in a cassette, the production of an image is achieved partly by X radiation but mainly by visible light produced by an intensifying screen within the cassette. The fact that sensitive emulsion is coated on both sides of the base allows the film to be sandwiched between *two* screens, each screen producing an image on the emulsion surface nearer to it. This practice clearly doubles the efficiency of the process, and allows use of shorter exposures and reduction in radiation dose.

If a cassette and screens are not being used and the film is of the envelope-wrapped type to be exposed directly to X rays, then in this case the image is obviously produced by X radiation only. However, it is still possible to have the advantage of image formation in two layers at once. The X radiation penetrates the base. Very little of the X-ray beam is absorbed in the first layer (depending on kilovoltage). Hence the exposure of the second layer is nearly (but not quite) the same as that received by the first layer.

The fact that the single image viewed actually consists of two superimposed images adds an element of unsharpness to the result, as will be noted later. This effect is increased by increased thickness of the base, which results in the two images being further apart. It is one reason why the film base must not be too thick.

CHARACTERISTICS OF THE EMULSION LAYER

The emulsion layer must be sufficiently flexible to allow the film to bend. Some bending will be required of it in use—for example in curved cassettes, in some types of film changer for angiography and in some automatic processing units.

When the film is processed there must be rapid and uniform dispersion of chemicals through the emulsion, so wetting agents are included in its manufacture. Chrome alum is added to harden the emulsion, for adequate hardness is important. This is particularly so in view of the widespread use of automatic processing. Soft emulsions absorb more water and will take longer to dry, so that quick drying in the unit becomes difficult. If the processing unit has rollers to transport the film, their grip on a soft emulsion may remove the gelatin with disastrous results, the unhardened emulsion being warmed by the high temperature at which the developer solution is used. At the other extreme too much hardening will impede dispersion of chemicals through the emulsion.

The Supercoating

The silver halide grains in a sensitive emulsion can be made developable by light pressure or abrasion. This results in such damaged areas appearing as dark spots or patches in the image. Since film has to be handled at many stages both in manufacture and in use, it is important that the sensitive emulsion should be protected as much as possible from this type of harm.

A thin layer of gelatin is therefore applied over it, and this protective gelatin is known as the *supercoat*, nonstress supercoat, or anti-abrasion layer. Since X-ray film has emulsion on both sides of the base, supercoating is applied to both emulsion layers.

The supercoat provides a shiny surface for the film which improves both its appearance and its durability. It must not be too shiny or the film cannot be marked with a pencil or white ink, methods of identification which may be used still in some departments. Furthermore radiologists are apt to find objectionable a highly glossed surface. Certain types of film changer for angiography require a slippery supercoat to the film to prevent its jamming as it is moved through the changer. To achieve this additives are in the supercoats for X-ray film.

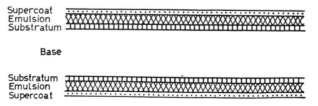

FIG. 2.1. Diagram of an X-ray film in cross-section. The base is about 8/1000 in. in thickness.

The diagram in Fig. 2.1 shows all these layers built up, to form the complete X-ray film in cross section.

THE STRUCTURE OF FILMS FOR GENERAL PHOTOGRAPHY

The Base, The Emulsion Layer, The Supercoat

What has been said of film base in relation to X-ray film applies also to materials used for general photographic purposes, there being some difference in the thickness of the base according to the type of film being made. Films to be used flat generally have thicker base than roll film. The base is prepared to receive the emulsion by the addition of a substratum layer, as already described, to ensure adhesion between the sensitive emulsion and the base. The distinguishing feature here between X-ray film and general photographic materials is that in the case of film to be used for ordinary photography the sensitive emulsion is coated upon *one side only* of the base.

This emulsion layer may consist of one layer of a slow emulsion with another layer of very fast emulsion coated upon it. This is a common practice with modern fast negative materials, and such material may be said to be double coated, with the meaning that there are two emulsions coated upon one side of the base. There is thus room for confusion in the use of this term, since in the case of X-ray film 'double coating' expresses for some people the fact that there is an identical layer of emulsion on each side of the base. Radiographers and photographers may believe they are speaking the same language when in fact they are not. The emulsion layer on one side of the base of photographic film is covered with a protective layer of gelatin as previously described for X-ray film.

The Non-curl Backing

It has been explained that photographic film has its emulsion layer coated upon one side only of the base. When this layer dries after processing there is a tendency for it to shrink, and this tendency results in the film curling, emulsion side inwards. In the case of X-ray film this tendency to curl does not exist, since the emulsion layers on both sides of the base shrink equally.

The curl on photographic film can be prevented if the other side is given a tendency either to curl in the opposite direction or to shrink.

Base for flat and roll films is given a tendency to curl the other way by being coated with a layer of gelatin of the same thickness as the emulsion layer. This anti-curl layer can be made to serve another purpose also, as will be seen in the next section. In order to ensure adhesion of this anti-curl layer, the base is given a substratum coating on this side just as if it were being prepared to receive emulsion.

In the case of 35 mm film for miniature cameras and cine film the problem of curl is solved in another way by giving the base a tendency to shrink. This can be done by treating it with solvents on the side opposite to the emulsion.

The Anti-halo Backing

Before it can be understood why this is required it is necessary to appreciate the results of light falling upon film. The emulsion layer is made of grains of silver halide, and when light strikes these grains there is some inter-reflection between them. This results in light being scattered sideways within the emulsion, an effect which is called *irradiation*. This scattered light does not form the image proper; it is a sideways spread of light beyond the boundaries of the image, and it is a source of unsharpness in the image. Thicker emulsion layers allow more irradiation than do thin ones of fine grain.

Some of the light falling on the film will pass through the emulsion layer and reach the base, being scattered into the base. According to the angle at which it strikes the base-air surface at the back of the film, it may either pass out of the base or be totally reflected back towards the emulsion (Fig. 2.2).

The light which is reflected back towards the emulsion produces another image separated from the proper image; this second image is known as *halation*. If the object being photographed is a small bright one such as a candle flame or naked light, halation takes the form of a ring or halo encircling the image and is then most readily observed. It can also be present with large areas of considerable brightness (Plate 2.1, following p. 94).

Halation is most noticeable when the base is thick, as for example in a glass plate as opposed to film, since then the second image is at a greater distance from the primary image point and the 'halo' may not fuse with the true image but be entirely separated from it. Both halation and irradiation are most marked with bright images, such as naked light sources. This is because both effects show most in areas where the image is heavily exposed (that is, when plenty of light is reaching the film from

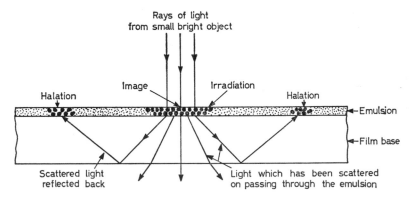

(a) Unbacked film

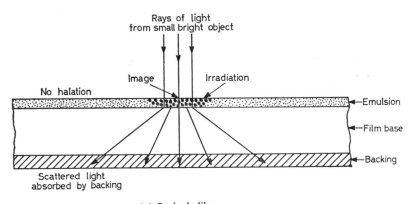

(b) Backed film

FIG. 2.2. Irradiation and halation. *By courtesy of Ilford Ltd.*

the subject). Irradiation is least in emulsions which are thin. Where there is least irradiation there is also least risk of halation.

Halation can be prevented by adding a suitable dye to the gelatin of the non-curl backing on flat and roll films. Scattered light therefore passes into the gelatin where it is absorbed by the dye. Thus the non-curl backing becomes anti-halo backing as well.

The dyes require to be carefully chosen for they must have no damaging effect on the emulsion and they must be removable during processing. If the film remained with a coloured back it would be difficult to use the negative for the production of prints. So dyes are used which will be bleached by processing solutions, and thus they disappear.

Cine films and 35 mm film for use in miniature cameras have no layer of gelatin as a non-curl back (Fig. 2.3) so in these cases a different answer must be found to the problem of halation. In these instances the dye is put into the film base itself, and the base is grey in colour. This dye cannot be removed in processing. Its density must therefore be selected so that it will prevent halation adequately without making it difficult to use the negative in producing a print. This dye within the base does not *prevent* reflection of light from the base-air surface at the back, but it absorbs light as it goes through the base towards the back *and* as it comes back through the base towards the emulsion. The intensity of light is thus reduced and halation is prevented.

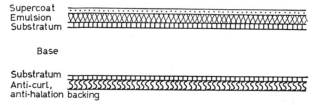

Supercoat
Emulsion
Substratum

Base

Substratum
Anti-curl,
anti-halation backing

FIG. 2.3. Diagram of a photographic film in cross-section. The thickness of the base depends on whether it is flat film (8/1000 in.), roll film (3/1000 in.), or cine film (5/1000 in.).

PHOTOGRAPHIC FILM IN RADIOGRAPHY

Films used for photography of fluorescent screen images (fluorography) are essentially photographic film materials and are not 'X-ray films' as used for direct radiography, with or without intensifying screens. As with other photographic materials, those for fluorography have their emulsion coated on one side only of the base. The base is thinner than that of X-ray film and measures are taken to prevent halation as previously described. More is said in Chapters xvii and xviii of films used for fluorography.

THE RESOLVING POWER OF FILM MATERIALS

Resolving power is related to the ability of a photographic emulsion to record fine details. In making tests of the resolving power of film material it is usual to photograph a test object which consists of a number of lines—often white lines on a black background so that the negative to be studied shows black lines on a white ground. A material of high resolving power is able to show these lines as separate entities even when they are very close together. If the image of each separate line spreads to occupy the intervening space then the images of the lines are not resolved. Resolving power is expressed as the number of lines per milli-metre which can be distinguished in the image as separate entities.

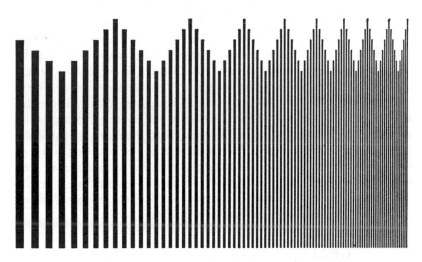

FIG. 2.4. A typical resolving power test chart. *By courtesy of Ilford Ltd.*

A chart for testing resolving power (Fig. 2.4) may consist of parallel lines separated by a space equal in width to the lines, the lines being arranged in groups of diminishing width. This is photographed with reduction in size and the image is then studied with magnification. The finest group of lines which is just resolved gives the resolving power of the emulsion.

The resolving power of an emulsion depends upon various factors such as grain size, contrast and the extent to which the emulsion absorbs and scatters light. The results of tests for resolving power of any given emulsion are influenced by such factors as the arrangement of the lines on the chart, the contrast between the tone of the lines and the tone of their background, the wavelength of the light used to make the exposure, the exposure and development given to the film. The tests are made with specified standardization of these conditions using a camera lens of high resolving power. The resolving power of any photographic system as a whole is limited by the resolving power of the lens as well as that of the material; so these tests are made with a lens of resolving power much higher than that of the material being used.

Fast negative materials can resolve about 40–50 lines per millimetre, medium speed film about 70–100 lines per millimetre, and very slow emulsions designed for maximum resolution of detail may resolve over 1,000 lines per millimetre. In certain technical applications of photography the ability to resolve fine detail is most important.

The case of the resolving power of materials used for radiography is somewhat different. Here there are various factors which influence the resolving power of the system as a whole. Later in this book (Chapter XII), the features of the radiographic image will be considered more closely and it will be seen that there are many causes of image blur. These and not the resolving power of film materials are limiting factors in the resolution of the image. Cine radiography and fluorography entail the photography of an image on a fluorescent screen. The resolving power of the screen is very much less than that of the film materials used. The resolving power of the films used in radiography is therefore generally not a stringent consideration in the resolution of the images obtained although it may assume importance in cinefluorography.

GRAININESS OF FILM MATERIALS

If a photographic negative is viewed under sufficient magnification, the individual grains of silver which form the image can be seen by the eye. These grains are unevenly distributed through the emulsion. At lesser degrees of magnification the eye cannot resolve individual grains and the grains appear to be clumped together in colonies. This clumping gives rise to unevenness in density or a variation in photographic tone. The result is an impression of a granular pattern. This is known as *graininess* in the material (Plate 2.2, following p. 94; and Plate 2.3(a), (b), (c), following p. 94.

Graininess in photographic negatives is influenced by various factors, the most important one being the grain size of the film material used. If it is a fast emulsion with large average grain size, graininess will be more apparent than in the case of slower emulsions with small average grain size. Another important consideration is the type of developing solution used. It is possible to obtain fine grain developers which act to reduce graininess in the image. Exposure and degree of development also have some effect.

Graininess is insignificant in negatives which it is not intended to enlarge, for it is not apparent until some magnification has been given to the image. It may, however, be troublesome if the negative is to be projected as a slide or used to make an enlarged print, for the magnification thus given may be sufficient to reveal the grainy structure to an objectionable degree.

SPECTRAL SENSITIVITY OF FILM MATERIALS

This term refers to the colour sensitivity of photographic films. It is important to realize that such materials are sensitive to colours in a different way from the human eye.

Spectral Sensitivity of Film and the Eye

If white light is passed through a glass prism the various colours of which it is composed are separated. The human eye sees a spectrum of colours ranging from violet-blue through green, yellow and orange to red. The green-yellow part in the middle of this spectrum looks brighter

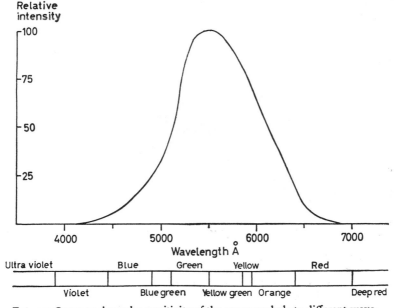

FIG. 2.5. Curve to show the sensitivity of the eye as a whole to different wavelengths.

than the violet-blue colours of the short-wavelength region and the red colour of the long-wavelength region at the ends of the spectrum. This is because the human eye is most sensitive to the green-yellow part of the spectrum. A sensitivity curve can be made for the eye in its response to the visible spectrum, and the curve will illustrate this fact (Fig. 2.5).

The response of photographic film to the colours of the visible spectrum is quite different. Untreated silver halide emulsions are very sensitive to the blue-violet parts of the spectrum but to none of the longer wavelengths, so that in this direction their sensitivity stops considerably short of that of the human eye. At the same time film materials are very sensitive to parts of the light spectrum in the short-wavelength range to which the eye is relatively insensitive. The photographic emulsion responds to ultra-violet light which the eye cannot see, and is sensitive to even shorter wavelengths (for example X rays) in the electro-magnetic spectrum of which the visible light spectrum is but a short part.

This explains the fact that X rays and gamma rays can be used for radiography. The photographic emulsion can in effect 'see' these radiations which the eye cannot.

If a sensitivity curve is drawn for the response of a photographic film to the same spectrum as given in the previous diagram, the difference between it and the eye can be shown (Fig. 2.6A).

It can be seen that the maximum sensitivity of the photographic emulsion is in the blue part of the spectrum. The response of the emulsion does not fall to nothing at the short ultra-violet end of the spectrum but

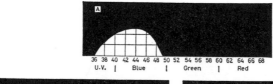

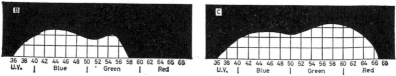

Fig. 2.6. (A) Curve to show the colour sensitivity of a non-colour-sensitive photographic emulsion.

(B) Curve to show the colour sensitivity of an orthochromatic photographic emulsion.

(C) Curve to show the colour sensitivity of a panchromatic photographic emulsion. *By courtesy of Kodak Ltd.*

will continue into regions of the electro-magnetic spectrum which are much shorter in wavelength than visible light (and are not included in the range of wavelengths shown in this curve).

The Importance of Spectral Sensitivity in Photography

The sensitivity of photographic materials to blue light and (unless specially treated as below) their lack of sensitivity to other colours mean that they will not record an image as the eye sees it. A girl in a yellow dress standing against a 'royal blue' curtain impresses the eye as a light figure against a dark ground, for the eye is very sensitive to the green-yellow part of the spectrum and much less sensitive to the blue region. In a black-and-white photograph of this subject the eye will expect to see a light-toned dress against a dark-toned ground.

The photographic film, however, is markedly sensitive to blue and renders this as a light tone in the black-and-white photographic print. It is completely insensitive to yellow, so that in the photographic print this colour is rendered as a dark tone. The photograph therefore shows a girl in a dark dress standing against a light ground, and this cannot be accepted by the eye as a faithful reproduction of the original.

To make photographic film satisfactory from this point of view its colour sensitivity is extended into regions of the visible spectrum of wavelengths longer than the violet-blue range. This is done by adding suitable dyes to the emulsion, and the terms *dye sensitizing, optical sensitizing* or *colour sensitizing* are given to the process. This sensitizing extends the response of the emulsion to the longer wavelengths of the spectrum, while leaving unimpaired its original sensitivity to the short-wavelength regions—to blue, violet, and ultra-violet light and to the shorter wavelengths of X rays and gamma radiation beyond them. The high sensitivity to blue and the short end of the spectrum remains as an inherent characteristic of silver halide emulsions.

Photographic materials can be divided into four main groups according to whether this colour sensitizing has been done and (if it has been done) to which part of the spectrum the sensitivity of the emulsion has been extended. These groups are listed and considered below.

Blue-sensitive Film

Some film materials do not have any further sensitizing. They are used quite satisfactorily without response to wavelengths longer than the blue parts of the visible spectrum, and they are known as *blue-sensitive, ordinary,* or *non-colour sensitive* materials.

These films are used successfully for reproducing black-and-white subjects—for example documents, line drawings and diagrams—and even some coloured subjects where the colours are subdued and diluted. Films used in radiography are ordinary blue-sensitive materials except in certain special cases which are discussed in Chapter xvii and in Chapter xviii.

Orthochromatic Film

This class of material has its sensitivity extended into the green part of the spectrum, and modern orthochromatic film is sometimes described as being 'fully orthochromatic'. These words like many others do not really mean what they seem to say. *Ortho* means 'correct, proper', and *chromatic* relates to colour, so the term implies that this material renders colours correctly. This is untrue, for it is still insensitive to the red part of the spectrum and will reproduce unsatisfactorily subjects in which there are many red tones. However, in photographic terminology the term orthochromatic film is fully understood to mean one which has had its sensitivity extended to the green part of the spectrum but no further (Fig. 2.6B). Photographers are neither deceived nor troubled by the exaggeration implicit in this name.

Panchromatic Film

This type of film has its sensitivity extended to include the whole of the visible spectrum, and it responds to red as well as to green light. The name *panchromatic* implies sensitivity to all colours (Fig. 2.6C). If it is wished to reproduce a coloured subject in black-and-white so that there is correct representation of the various tones, panchromatic film must be used.

Photographers frequently modify colour rendering in black-and-white photography with the use of coloured light filters over the camera lens. These, together with panchromatic film, provide full control of the result and enable the photographers to achieve in black-and-white a faithful rendering of coloured subjects.

Infra-red Film

This film has its sensitivity extended further than the red portion of the visible light spectrum, and its response includes reaction to wavelengths of the infra-red range. Such material is used with a colour filter over the lens of the camera which prevents any ultra-violet and blue light from reaching the film. It is not intended for general photography in which the aim is to produce a faithful rendering of original tones, although infra-red film can be used in pictorial work for striking effects in certain cases. It has technical applications in aerial photography where the longer wavelength radiation used to make the picture penetrates haze, and a medical application in which use is made of the ability of infra-red rays to penetrate superficial tissue (Fig. 2.7, and Plate 2.4 following p. 94).

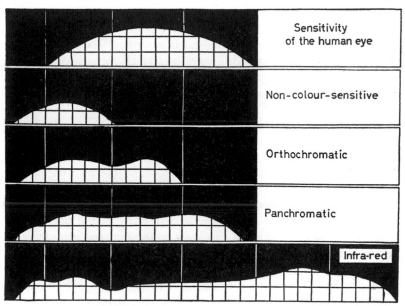

FIG. 2.7. Curves to show the spectral sensitivity of the human eye, and of various types of photographic material. It is shown that all the photographic materials respond to short wavelengths in the ultra-violet region to which the eye is insensitive. Radiations of the electromagnetic spectrum of shorter wavelength than the ultra-violet range (such as X rays and gamma rays) are not included in the curves; photographic materials are of course sensitive to them and the eye is not.

SPEED AND CONTRAST OF PHOTOGRAPHIC MATERIALS

These characteristics were mentioned in Chapter I as being significant to the photographer. They will be considered in more detail in Chapter III for it is important that these topics should be understood.

Sensitometry

Before consideration is given to various types of available X-ray film, certain aspects of photographic materials must first be discussed. It has been said previously that such materials have characteristics which are significant to the photographer who is to use them. Clearly it is possible to undertake some photography with a limited appreciation of the processes involved, but full understanding of the response of his materials to light is required of the photographer who is to use them most knowledgeably. Radiographers, using the photographic process in a technical application must be included within the group recognized as knowledgeable and they too should understand the response of films to radiation—both visible light and X rays.

The study of this response is known as *sensitometry*. The name suggests that it is a measurement of the sensitivity of the film. This is determined by giving known exposures to the film and measuring the results of the exposures when the film is developed.

For the sake of clarity this topic will be discussed in terms relating to photography. At the present stage it is unnecessary to differentiate between radiographic and photographic negative images, because we are concerned with the response of the film. This may be considered now to be the same both to visible light and to X radiation; in both cases the effect of the exposure is to deposit on the film black metallic silver when the film is chemically developed.

PHOTOGRAPHIC DENSITY

When a negative is held up to be viewed by the light passing through, it is obvious that the deposit of silver prevents the light passing to an extent which may be only partial or may appear to the eye to be complete. The deposit of silver may be said to have a light-stopping effect or a degree of blackness; this varies with the amount of silver present, which in turn varies with the exposure.

There are several ways in which this degree of blackness may be numerically expressed. All are based upon the fact that the intensity of the light falling on the film (the incident light) and the intensity of the light passing through a particular area of blackness (the transmitted light) can both be measured (Fig. 3.1).

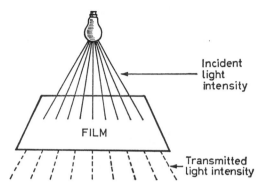

FIG. 3.1. Incident and transmitted light. *By courtesy of Kodak Ltd.*

Obviously greater blackening of the film allows less light to be transmitted. Thus the relationship between the separate intensities of incident light and transmitted light alters with the degree of blackness, and can be used as a measure of it. The relationship between the incident light (L_i) and the transmitted light (L_t) can be expressed in several ways, of which three will be considered now.

(i) Transmission

This is the ratio of the transmitted light to the incident light. Thus:

$$\frac{\text{Transmitted light}}{\text{Incident light}} = \frac{L_t}{L_i} = \text{transmission ratio}$$

It is often expressed as a percentage:

$$\frac{100 L_t}{L_i}$$

If 100 units of light fall on the film and 10 are transmitted, the transmission ratio is 10/100, and transmission is 10 per cent.

Since the incident light is bound to be greater than the transmitted light even for a slight deposit of silver, this value must always be a fraction less than unity and a percentage less than 100. This, together with the fact that transmission decreases with exposure, make the expression less useful than those which now follow.

4

(ii) Opacity

This is the ratio of the incident light to the transmitted light; it is the reciprocal of the transmission. Thus:

$$\frac{\text{Incident light}}{\text{Transmitted light}} = \frac{L_i}{L_t} = \text{opacity}$$

The film considered in the previous paragraph which has a transmission of 10/100, has an opacity of 100/10 — that is 10.

It can be appreciated that the opacity always has value greater than unity and that it increases with exposure. As sensitometry is concerned with measuring the results of exposure when the film is developed, this form of expression for the blackening of the film would seem to be a sensible one to use.

(iii) Density

This is the common logarithm of the opacity. Thus:

$$\text{Log}_{10} \frac{L_i}{L_t} = \text{density}$$

To take the film previously considered with a transmission of 10/100 and opacity 100/10, its density would be

$$\text{Log} \frac{100}{10} = \text{Log } 10 = 1$$

To give this some practical reality for the student radiographer, the range of densities most commonly encountered in the diagnostic areas of medical radiographs is 0·25–2·0. A radiograph of a chest has densities between 0·3 and 1·5 in those parts of the film where the rays have been absorbed by the subject. Areas of the film not covered by the subject have much greater densities, the range being of the order of 2·0–3·0. This looks to the eye so black that it is difficult to detect any difference between, say, 2·5 and 3, but a wide range of density differences can be measured by an instrument such as a densitometer. This device uses a photo-electric cell to measure the light intensity which falls on the density to be measured and the light intensity which is transmitted through it.

It can be appreciated from the foregoing description of these three terms that a density of 1 means a 10 per cent transmission; and a density of 2 (being a logarithmic value) means an opacity which is greater by 10 times, giving a 1 per cent transmission. A density of 3 is 0·1 per cent transmission, so it is hardly surprising that it seems completely opaque to the human eye, unless it is illuminated from behind by a very intense light and precautions are taken to prevent glare.

It has been explained that these three expressions—transmission, opacity, and density—give a numerical value to the degree of blackness in various parts of the exposed and processed negative. The last one—density—is most widely used in sensitometry, and is the most useful and important of the three. There are some reasons for this.

(i) Density increases with exposure.

(ii) Density is proportional to the amount of silver present. A density of 2 has twice the amount of silver present compared with a density of 1. These are approximate relationships.

(iii) In calculating the results of placing upon each other two areas of certain light-transmitting power, it is much simpler to add their densities (which are logarithmic values) than to multiply their percentage transmissions. This is obvious if the arithmetic required in both processes is considered for the following figures: $D = 0.5$ gives a per cent transmission of 32, $D = 0.9$ gives a per cent transmission of 12.5, $D = 1.2$ gives a per cent transmission of 6.3.

(iv) The eye seems to respond to differing tones in a way which is approximately logarithmic. If presented with a series in which density increases by equal steps, the eye accepts the increasing blackness as occurring in equal stages.

(v) The easiest way to appreciate the relationship between exposures and the results of the exposures is to make a graph. It is found that the most useful graph is obtained by plotting logarithmic values on both axes. Density, a logarithmic value as has been shown, is plotted on the vertical axis (the ordinate), and the logarithm of the exposure is plotted on the horizontal axis (the abscissa). Logarithmic scales enable a much wider range of values to be appreciated with understanding; also equal increments have the same ratio. The sensitometric graph which results is called a *characteristic curve* and will be considered now.

CHARACTERISTIC CURVES

A characteristic curve can be made for any photographic material. Here it will be considered in terms of negative material, since radiographers deal with X-ray film coming within this group. Such a curve is not characteristic of the material under every condition but is characteristic of the material under certain conditions of exposure and processing. The curve is a diagram which shows the results of exposure on the material, given certain conditions of exposure and processing; with these factors standardized, two different materials may be compared by study of their characteristic curves.

To make a curve a strip of the material to be tested is given a series of exposures which progress in steps. This could be done by adding a constant amount to the exposure as each section is exposed, or by multiplying the exposure by a constant factor for each step. A constant factor of multiplication is useful in practice: for example, the exposures might increase from step to step by a factor of × 2. Each step of the strip naturally has a different density as each receives a different exposure, and the series of densities can then be measured with a densitometer.

A graph is then made in which the densities are plotted on the vertical axis against *log* exposure values on the horizontal axis. The resultant curve has the same general shape for all photographic materials, and a typical one is seen on page 38 in Fig. 3.3. Such curves may be called Hurter and Driffield curves (sometimes abbreviated to H and D) after two pioneers in sensitometry; and sometimes D log E curves for the obvious reason that these are the values plotted on the axes.

Making a Characteristic Curve for X-ray Film

Characteristic curves can be made for X-ray films, and can be used for the comparison of different films. Strips, one for each film, are exposed together in a series of steps in such a way that each step receives twice the exposure of the previous one. If it is wished to compare the performance of films used with intensifying screens, all the strips to be tested can be placed side by side in one cassette. If no screens are to be used, the films can be exposed together in one light-tight paper envelope. It may be wished to make a comparison between two films both without and with screens. This could be done by arranging screens and films together in one cassette as indicated in Fig. 3.2.

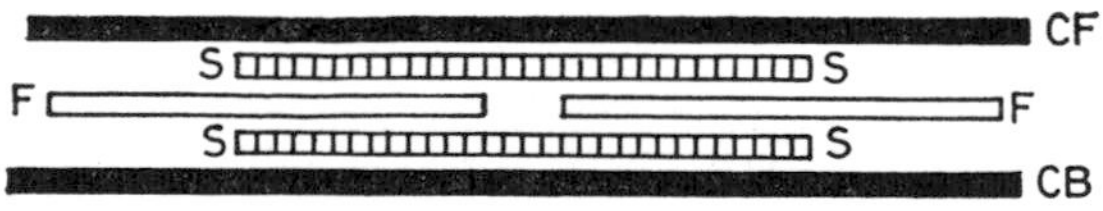

Fig. 3.2. Screen and film combination for sensitometry.
CF   cassette front
S   intensifying screens
F   films
CB   cassette back

With constant kilovoltage and tube-film distance for all steps, there are two ways of varying the exposure (which is calculated as the product of the X-ray intensity and the time). These are (i) by varying the intensity and (ii) by varying the time.

VARIATION IN TIME (TIME-SCALE SENSITOMETERS)
A method using variation in time can be extremely simple. The film strips are put side by side into a light-tight container, and this is put into a lead tunnel which masks the whole length of the film strips. The X-ray set is switched on, and the container of the film strips is pulled out of the tunnel by a cord or wire so that it proceeds through the X-ray beam. The first step out of the tunnel receives the longest exposure, and by timing the pulls on the cord it can be arranged for each step to receive half the exposure of its predecessor. Scattered radiation from the table must be prevented from reaching the films. There are certain practical limitations to this method; manual advance of the films requires that the shortest exposure is long enough to make timing easy and small errors insignificant, and some attention must be paid to securing a smooth advance.

Another method uses a rotating lead disc which masks the films so that radiation reaches them through windows cut in the disc. These windows are arcs of circles especially arranged so that exposures through them have a known relationship to each other. The disc is rotated at a uniform speed by a synchronous motor.

The student may perhaps be wondering why alterations in time could not be achieved simply by giving a series of exposure intervals timed by the timer of the X-ray unit, but in practice this would not be a satisfactory way of doing it. Possible inaccuracies and variations in timing on short exposures could invalidate the result, and if exposures long enough to make these errors unimportant were to be used, as they increased by a factor of 2 they would soon extend beyond the scale of the timer.

VARIATION IN INTENSITY (INTENSITY-SCALE SENSITOMETERS)
Radiographers are eventually interested in the reaction of a film to the various intensities of radiation reaching it through the subject, so if tests are done with variation in exposure by variation in intensity, the experimental conditions are closer to those of practice.

Perhaps the student radiographer will think first of varying the X-ray tube current as a way of varying intensity, since this is so familiar in radiographic practice. It is not satisfactory for sensitometric tests since alterations in tube current alter the current flowing through the secondary winding of the high-tension transformer, and therefore alter transformer losses. Unless these are accurately compensated in the X-ray set, there will be some alteration in tube voltage when the tube current is altered. Since alteration in tube voltage makes its own contribution to the intensity of the beam, the intensity in these circumstances is not truly proportional to the tube current, and the result would thereby be invalidated.

Another way to vary the intensity is to use the inverse square law and arrange to expose simultaneously pieces of film at different distances from the X-ray tube. There are difficulties connected with this: the location of the focal spot must be exactly known, the distances must be measured carefully (especially if they are very short), and pieces of film near the tube must not overshadow those at a greater distance. There is also the inconvenience of having as many separate pieces of film as there are exposures, instead of having one continuous strip of film which contains all the exposures given for that particular piece of material.

The most common method is to vary the intensity by giving one exposure through a stepped wedge of a material such as aluminium. This in effect looks like a flight of metal stairs (Plate 3.1, following p. 94). Clearly it allows varying amounts of radiation to reach the film resulting in a series of exposures with variation in intensity; this variation is from the least amount of radiation which is transmitted through the top step of the staircase to the greatest amount which is transmitted through the bottom step of the staircase. Step-wedges are made of aluminium or plastic if the beam of radiation is soft, and of steel if harder radiation is being used.

It must be realized, however, that there is an alteration in the quality of the radiation as it is filtered by the different steps of aluminium or other metal. If the steps have a constant increase in thickness going up the stairs, the intensity changes in the beam do not also proceed in a constant relationship; the change in intensity per step will be greater at the thin end of the wedge than at the thick end where the beam is more heavily filtered. This difficulty can be overcome by adjusting the thickness of the steps at the thin end of the wedge so that there is a constant change in intensity per step throughout the wedge. The addition of a thin copper filter at the underside of the wedge has been of help.

In testing the response of X-ray films to the fluorescence of intensifying screens it is of course possible to avoid the use of X rays. The films can be exposed to a series of light intensities which are equivalent in spectral distribution (i.e. colour) to the light from the screens; it is arranged for correct relative exposures to be made on various parts of a test strip of film. This method is commonly used by manufacturers of screen-type film as one of many tests undertaken to control the quality of their products.

In practice radiographers in hospital X-ray departments do not make D log E curves; such departments may doubtless easily possess themselves of step-wedges and graph paper, but it is rare indeed to find densitometers among departmental equipment. Without a means to measure density, D log E curves cannot be made. However simple step-wedge tests *can* be undertaken on different types of film and different types of screen. These can be visually compared, the densities under each step of the wedge on one strip of film being matched with the corresponding ones of the other. Thus it is possible to make approximate assessment of relative speed and contrast.

The making of D log E curves may be left to film manufacturers, but an understanding of the main features of these curves is required of the radiographer. They are considered and explained in the following sections.

FEATURES OF THE CHARACTERISTIC CURVE

Fig. 3.3 shows a typical characteristic curve. It can be seen that the exposures are plotted logarithmically as relative exposures and not as absolute values of exposure. This is common practice and it does not alter the shape of the curve. Only when a curve is required to give information on absolute values of film speed is it necessary to plot logarithmically as abscissa an absolute exposure scale.

The three main regions of the curve commonly described are:

(i) The toe.
(ii) The straight-line part.
(iii) The shoulder.

These three parts have also been described as regions of (i) underexposure (ii) correct exposure and (iii) overexposure.

In the *toe* of the curve it can be seen that density has a small value, even although there has been no exposure or only a very small exposure. This density is produced by the development of silver halide grains which have not been exposed, or have received from the exposure such a small amount of energy that no latent image is produced. This low density is

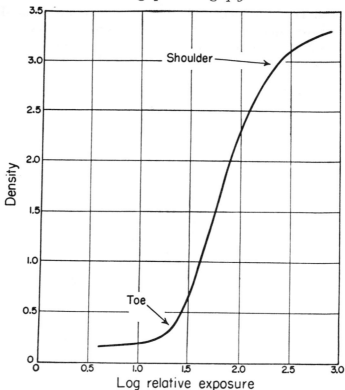

Fɪɢ. 3.3. Characteristic curve of a typical medical X-ray film, exposed with calcium tungstate intensifying screens. *By courtesy of X-ray Sales Division, Eastman Kodak Co., Rochester, New York.*

called *fog*. All film materials have some fog, and this will tend to increase with age. It is also a function of the developer since failure by the developer to differentiate between exposed and unexposed grains (i.e. any tendency to treat unexposed grains as if they were exposed ones) results in fog. Fresh film materials and fresh developer correctly used should produce very low fog. The toe of the characteristic curve shows the fog value of the film material being tested under the particular conditions used.

The point where the curve begins to turn up from the toe and the line of the graph ceases to be parallel to the horizontal axis is called the *threshold*. The density at this point is the first perceptible density above fog, and it represents the first reaction of the material to the exposure.

The *shoulder* of the curve depicts the state where increasing exposure leads to decreasing differences in density. A horizontal line extended from the uppermost part of the curve at this point to cut the density axis as in Fig. 3.4 gives the maximum value of density which the material achieves in response to the exposure in the given development conditions. This maximum density is known as D max.

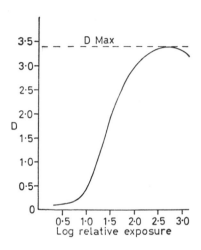

Fig. 3.4. A typical curve, showing D Max.

It can be seen from the bend of the graph in Fig. 3.4 that beyond D max. there is a part where increase in exposure results in decrease in density. This means that the material will become lighter as the exposure increases. Since this is a reversal of the normal response to light there will be as a result reversal of the image.

This region of reversal is known as the *region of solarization*, and different materials vary in the extent to which they can be solarized; the effect also varies with development. Exposures required to produce solarization are of the order of several thousand times greater than those in the region of correct exposure.

On page 10 in Chapter 1 a specially prepared emulsion was described to be used for obtaining positive images instead of negative ones. The material provided by the manufacturers has been previously solarized. On being developed without exposure it gives maximum density. On being photographically exposed before being developed it uses the solarization region of the characteristic curve, and yields a positive image from a positive subject, or (as described in Chapter 1) it results in a negative image copy from the negative image radiograph without need of an intermediate positive.

This is useful application of the reversal effect. Less happily radiographers can find themselves using solarized film unintentionally. If a film is accidentally fogged in the X-ray room or in the darkroom before or after being used for a radiographic exposure, partial or complete reversal of the image may result (Plate 3.2, following p. 94).

The *straight-line* part of the curve has been called the region of correct exposure. In this part of the graph, since it is a straight line, the resultant densities increase linearly with the logarithms of the exposures causing them. One of the qualities on which this part of the curve provides information is the average contrast of the film material used.

Contrast and the Characteristic Curve

It was said in Chapter 1 that contrast is the way in which a material reacts to a certain exposure range. This can be considered in terms of photography by imagining a scene which contains both highlights and shadows—for example a white-sailed boat at a lakeside bordered with trees. The range of exposures to be accommodated on the film is between the small exposure reaching the film from the tree shade (the shadows of the image) to the relatively much greater exposure reaching the film from the white boat-sail (the highlights of the image). In the negative the highlights will be dark and the shadows light. A film material of high contrast will render the highlights black and the shadows white; a film material of low contrast renders both as tones of grey. The film material of higher contrast gives a greater density difference between the lightest and the darkest tones than does the one of low contrast.

This can be translated to radiographic terms by considering a subject such as a posteroanterior view of the chest. Here the range of exposures to be accommodated on the film is between the relatively little radiation transmitted to expose the film through the heart and the regions below the diaphragm; the much greater amount of radiation transmitted to expose the film through the air-containing lungs; and the maximum amount of radiation reaching the upper part of the film above the patient's shoulders, where his body has not been interposed as an absorber. Film material of high contrast will give maximum density differences in the radiograph from these radiation differences, which constitute exposure differences analogous to those of visible-light photography.

Radiographers require from their material much higher contrast than is needed in that used for conventional photography. It is important that small radiation differences should produce appreciable density differences in the image if various bodily structures are to be well seen. For this, high contrast in the film emulsion is required.

In a characteristic curve of any film material it has been seen that density on the vertical axis is plotted against log exposure on the horizontal axis. The film material of high contrast mentioned earlier (recording a white boat-sail and the shade of trees) will have a bigger density rise from shadow to highlight than the film of low contrast, though the range of exposures is the same in each case. It is clear that in the straight-line part of the characteristic curve a material with a bigger density (vertical) rise for the same excursion along the horizontal axis *must* have a steeper slope to the straight line. This can be seen in Fig. 3.5.

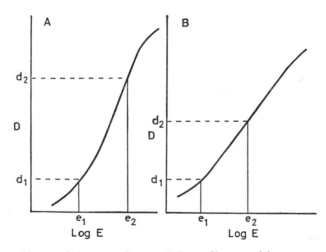

Fig. 3.5. Characteristic curves for two different film materials.
$e_1 e_2$ exposure range
$d_1 d_2$ density range
The curve under A shows higher gamma than the curve under B.

The contrast of the material can therefore be measured by the slope of the straight-line part of the curve, high contrast material showing a steeper slope. This slope of the straight line is called the *gamma* of the material; gamma is the third letter of the Greek alphabet and corresponds to our C.

Gamma can be measured and given a numerical value in this way: the straight-line part of the curve is continued until it intercepts the log E axis as in Fig. 3.6.

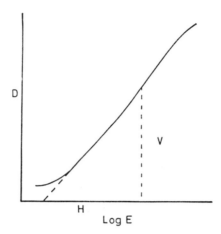

FIG. 3.6. Gamma = V/H.

A vertical line is now raised from any point on the log E axis (within the straight-line part of the graph) until it intersects the straight-line portion of the curve. The ratio of the vertical rise (V) to the horizontal distance (H) gives gamma.

$$\text{Gamma} = \frac{V}{H}$$

The numerical value of V/H is fixed by the angle which the straight-line part of the curve makes with the horizontal axis, and it will be the same at whatever point the vertical is raised as long as it remains within the straight-line portion of the graph. It can be appreciated that V/H is a trigonometrical function, being the tangent of the angle between the straight-line extension and the horizontal axis. Gamma is therefore the tangent of this angle and takes its value from the angle.

To the photographer gamma is important because it measures contrast and it tells him how truthfully the negative will reproduce the various tones of the original subject. If gamma is less than unity, the tones of the subject are compressed in the negative and the image will be 'flatter' than the original. If gamma is greater than unity, the image contrast is greater than that of the subject. Radiographic materials have gamma greater than unity so that small variations in the radiation transmitted through various parts of the subject may produce appreciable contrast in the image tones; the radiation contrasts (or differences in radio-opacity) in the subject require to be amplified in the image. Although radiographers may not be concerned with values of gamma, an understanding of the significance of the steepness of slope of the straight-line part of the graph enables them to make comparison between the curves of different film materials.

Speed and the Characteristic Curve

In general the term *speed* in relation to a photographic material refers to whether it requires more or less exposure in relation to another material in order to produce a comparable negative. The material which requires more exposure is said to have less speed than the other or to be not so fast.

In regard to the characteristic curve it can be said simply that the speed of the material determines the location of the curve along the D log E axis. In Fig. 3.7 are shown characteristic curves of two materials—Film C and Film D. From the curves it can be seen that Film C requires less exposure than Film D to produce say, a density of 1. Film C has therefore greater speed than Film D. Faster materials thus have their curves located further to the left along the horizontal axis since exposure increases to the right along this axis.

Expressing the speed of photographic materials in numerical values raises many problems, and the situation, like some of the systems, is complex. There are various methods in use today for the numerical expression of speed and their detailed examination is beyond the intended scope of this book. Interested students may pursue them in textbooks on general photography.

It may be said briefly that three important systems have been in use; (i) B.S. degrees, (ii) D.I.N. degrees, (iii) A.S.A. numbers. The first two are logarithmic scales, an increase of 3 deg. meaning an increase in speed by × 2. The third is arithmetical, so a doubling of the number means an increase in speed by × 2.

For X-ray film a numerical expression of speed is not used. The use of speed rating systems in photography involves the ability to measure the intensity of visible light employed to make the exposure. Comparable systems for radiography would involve measurement of the intensity of radiation reaching the film. It would require radiographers to express and compute exposures in terms of milliroentgens reaching the film.

Modern automatic exposure devices are concerned with film dose.

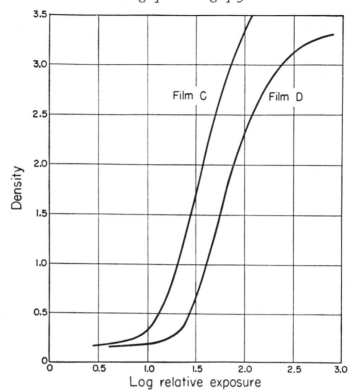

FIG. 3.7. Characteristic curves of two typical medical X-ray films, one (C) being faster than the other (D). Exposures made with calcium tungstate intensifying screens. *By courtesy of X-ray Sales Division, Eastman Kodak Company, Rochester, New York.*

Perhaps increasing use of automation and dosimetry in the diagnostic X-ray department could lead one day to numerical expressions for the speed of X-ray films. In the photographic world, however, it has been questioned whether it is in fact possible to express absolute speed of materials under all conditions and many difficulties have been encountered in trying to do this.

A present practice for X-ray films is to assess them in terms of relative speed. This means that the speed of a film is expressed in comparison with that of another taken as its control—Film A may be described as being twice as fast as Film B. Their relative speed values can be obtained from characteristic curves in terms of the exposure required to give a certain density as was done in considering Fig. 3.7 previously. This might be a density of 1, since the densities within areas of diagnostic importance in medical radiographs usually lie between 0.25 and 2.0. This system of relative speeds has been satisfactory to radiographers in the past, and perhaps there is no reason to change it. It is very often based in a simple and practical manner on a comparison of the exposures required by different emulsions to produce radiographs which seem to the observer to be comparable. This is a purely visual assessment made without reference to characteristic curves, and it must vary between observers and for the same observer in different conditions of judgment. It is of course a subjective and not a mathematical evaluation.

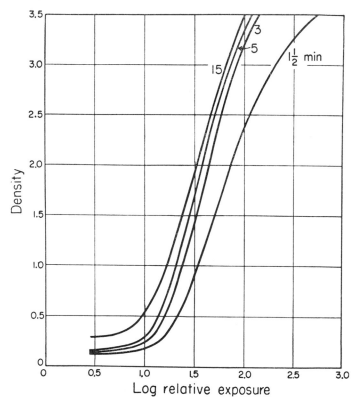

FIG. 3.8. Characteristic curves of a typical screen-type X-ray film, developed for a series of times at 68°F. *By courtesy of X-ray Sales Division, Eastman Kodak Company, Rochester, New York.*

VARIATIONS IN THE CHARACTERISTIC CURVE
WITH DEVELOPMENT

It was said earlier that a characteristic curve is not characteristic of an emulsion in every condition, and it is affected by conditions of exposure and processing. The curve alters with degree of development. This effect can be seen if a family of characteristic curves is made for one emulsion, the development time being varied and other conditions remaining constant. The result is seen in Fig. 3.8.

It can be appreciated from this that the slope of the straight line becomes steeper as developing time is increased; that is, the gamma or contrast of the emulsion is increasing. This increase in the angle of slope does not take place equally with equal increases in development time. Eventually the increase in gamma with development time will cease.

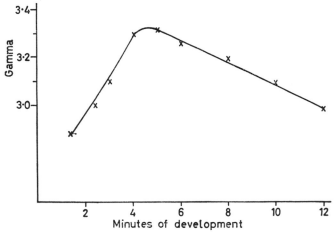

Fig. 3.9. A hypothetical gamma-time curve.

It is possible to make from this family of curves a new curve in which the development times are plotted as abscissa with the resultant values of gamma (the slope of the straight-line part of the curve) plotted as ordinate. This curve is known as a gamma-time curve and one is shown in Fig. 3.9.

It can be seen from this that gamma increases very rapidly in the early stages of development. After that it increases more gradually until eventually further development results in no increase in gamma. The value of gamma achieved at this point is known as *gamma infinity*.

With prolonged development the developer begins to act on the unexposed as well as the exposed silver halide grains; it therefore increases fog. This means that there is reduction in contrast as a result, and the gamma-time curve falls off from gamma infinity if the graph is continued.

Gamma infinity will vary for different photographic emulsions. High contrast material has high gamma infinity. High speed materials are usually lower in contrast and have low gamma infinity. For the photographer, gamma-time curves are useful in providing information on the behaviour of any given material. They can be used also to compare the performance of photographic developers, since separate curves will result for the same material processed in differing developer solutions.

It can be seen from the family of curves for differing development times shown in Fig. 3.8 that, in addition to a change in slope of the curve, there is shift of the curve to the left as development time is increased. This corresponds to an increase in speed of the material, and as can be seen it does not take place at a uniform rate, being greatest in the early stages of development.

It should not be thought that prolonging the development time is a useful technique in radiographic processing in order to increase both the contrast and speed of the film used. The standard time for manual processing is usually 4 minutes at 68°F (20°C). The material should reach maximum contrast and, if it has been correctly exposed, maximum usable density in that time. Development prolonged beyond this may be of *some* assistance if the film has been somewhat underexposed, but the resultant image is not likely to be of the highest quality.

COMPARISONS OF EMULSIONS BY THEIR CHARACTERISTIC CURVES

In Fig. 3.10 are shown the characteristic curves of two emulsions used for radiography. With an understanding of the features of the graphs certain comparisons can be made between the emulsions from study of these curves. The conclusions to be drawn are:

(i) Film C is faster than Film D since the whole of its curve is further to the left on the horizontal axis. The amount of their separation is a measure of the speed difference between the emulsions.

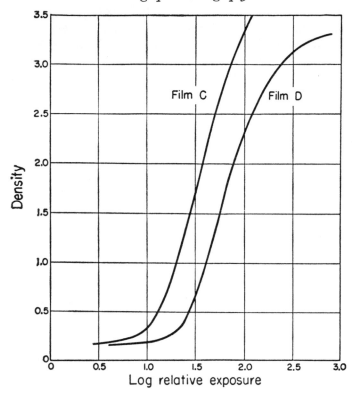

FIG. 3.10. Characteristic curves of two typical medical X-ray films, one (C) being faster than the other (D). Exposures made with calcium tungstate intensifying screens. *By courtesy of X-ray Sales Division, Eastman Kodak Company, Rochester, New York.*

(ii) Film C begins to react to the exposure before Film D, since the threshold (the point where the graph begins to turn upwards) of C is further to the left on the horizontal axis.

(iii) Their gamma is not markedly different over the range of densities 0·25—2·0 (commonly encountered in diagnostic fields). This is deduced since the slope of the straight-line parts of the two curves looks the same.

(iv) Film C has slightly greater fog level than Film D since the toe of its curve is placed slightly higher on the vertical axis.

(v) Film D has a lower shoulder than Film C. The maximum density achieved by Film C is not accommodated within the range shown on the vertical axis. (It reaches its maximum density above a density of 3·5.)

The curves of two emulsions may show a different relationship to each other, as shown in Fig. 3.11.

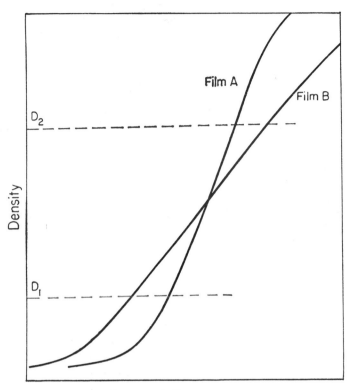

Log relative exposure

Fig. 3.11. Characteristic curves of a hypothetical high contrast film (A) and a low contrast film (B). The relative speeds of the two films depend upon the density at which they are measured. *By courtesy of X-ray Sales Division, Eastman Kodak Company, Rochester, New York.*

Here it can be seen that:

(i) The curves intersect and cross over. This means that in the lower range of exposures and densities (D_1) Film B is faster than Film A. At the exposure and the density represented by the point of intersection, the two films are of equal speed. At the exposures and density ranges beyond this (D_2) Film A is faster than Film B. This is why on page 43, in stating the relative speeds of films from their characteristic curves, it was necessary to consider the density level at which the speeds were being compared.

(ii) The gamma of Film A is higher than that of Film B since the straight-line part of A's curve has the steeper slope. This steeper slope means that Film A will show more clearly small differences in radiation transmitted through the subject. At the same time this steeper slope indicates that exposure selection when using Film A must be more precise; this aspect will now be considered and further explained.

It has been said that the range of densities to be encountered in medical radiographs within areas of diagnostic interest is likely to be between 0·25 and 2·0. This refers to regions of the film covered by the subject. Regions not covered by the subject (for instance above the shoulders in posteroanterior views of the chest) are not within the range of diagnostic interest and reach much higher densities.

The reasons why densities greater than 2·0 are not useful in medical radiographs is that most X-ray illuminators are not bright enough for viewing higher densities; even if they were to be made bright enough, the eye would be so dazzled by the light transmitted by regions of low density (behind the heart in a posteroanterior view of the chest), that it could not perceive details in the high density range. The student should keep in mind the meaning of density 2; 1/100 part of the light falling on this density is transmitted through it.

The range of densities 0·25 to 2·0 may be described as the *useful density range*. In Fig. 3.12 horizontal lines have been drawn from the vertical density axis at the extremes of the useful density range. From the points at which they meet the curves, verticals are dropped to meet the log E axis.

It can be seen that in the case of Film B these verticals occur further apart on the log E axis than they do for Film A. Film B is therefore said to have greater *latitude* than Film A (latitude being defined as the exposure range covered within the useful density range).

It is clear that films with curves of lower slope must always show more latitude than films with curves of steeper slope; high contrast material always has less film latitude than low contrast material. The importance of film latitude to the radiographer is this: a wider range of exposures can be accepted by Film B and the resultant densities will be within the useful density range and the radiograph will be acceptable for viewing. This wider range of usable exposures means that for a given kilovoltage the radiographer can select over a wider milliamperesecond range and still achieve an acceptable result. The selection of exposure

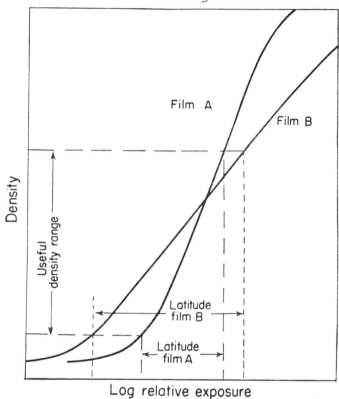

FIG. 3.12. Characteristic curves of two hypothetical radiographic films. (A, high contrast film; B, low contrast film). The range of exposures that can be covered within the useful density range (i.e. the latitude of the film) depends upon the average gradient. *By courtesy of X-ray Sales Division, Eastman Kodak Company, Rochester, New York.*

conditions must be more precise when using high contrast material with little film latitude if the range of densities in the resultant radiograph is to be placed within the useful range acceptable for viewing.

Latitude may be considered also in relation to another range of exposures—those produced by the different radiation intensities transmitted through the subject being radiographed. Some subjects transmit a long scale of radiation intensities. Examples are the dorsal spine in an anteroposterior view, and the pregnant abdomen in a lateral projection. The region of the upper thoracic spine transmits very much more radiation than that of the lower, where the overlying heart and diaphragm absorb X rays heavily. In the pregnant abdomen there is a marked difference in absorption of the beam by the region of the posterior uterine wall close to the spine, where absorption is heavy, and by the region of the anterior uterine wall, where transmission is much greater. Some subjects—for example the fifth lumbar vertebra in a coned view—transmit a short scale of radiation intensities.

If a long scale of intensities (or exposures to the film) is to be recorded and the resultant densities are all placed within the useful density range, a film material with little latitude requires this range of exposures to be most precisely placed on the log E axis: this requires careful selection of exposure factors by the radiographer. If the latitude is too small in extent it may be in fact impossible to place the range of exposures or intensities so that *all* the resultant densities come within the useful density range. A film material with extensive latitude will record a long scale of radiation intensities, and allows this long scale to be moved about on the log E axis (or less precise selection of exposure factors by the radiographer) without placing the resultant densities outside the useful density range.

It can therefore further be said of the two emulsions in Fig. 3.11 that: (iii) Film B will transmit a longer scale of radiation differences than Film A and will allow greater range for exposure choice. If correctly exposed, Film A will show the radiation differences more clearly as it has the higher gamma, and it will therefore render more distinct from each other structures which show little difference in radio-opacity. The maximum differentiation of detail will be obtained in the ideal condition when the log E range is adjusted so that the whole of the useful density range is utilized. The exposure, however, would need to be accurately determined.

Information from the Characteristic Curve

It may be useful to sum up the characteristic curve simply with a list of the points on which it can provide information about a film material.
(i) Fog level—from the toe of the curve.
(ii) Contrast—from the slope of the straight-line portion (gamma).
(iii) Extent of film latitude—by consideration of the useful density range and the corresponding range on the log E axis.
(iv) The maximum density which the material will give in the conditions of exposure and development used to make the curve—from the shoulder of the curve.

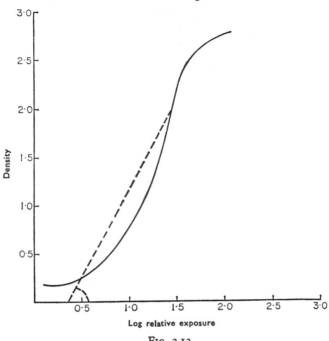

Log relative exposure

Fig. 3.13.

(v) The solarization region (if the material will solarize)—from the region of the curve beyond D max.

(vi) The speed of the material—from the location of the curve on the horizontal axis.

(vii) The comparative performances of different emulsions over the same exposure and density range in the same conditions of development.

In radiography characteristic curves can be used for:

(a) The comparison of films.

(b) The comparison of intensifying screens.

(c) The determination of the added speed gained by the use of intensifying screens.

(d) The testing of developer solutions to check their performance.

Modern Emulsions and their Characteristic Curves

Throughout the chapter characteristic curves have been discussed in terms of the classic curve, with its toe, its straight-line portion and a region of solarization. However, many X-ray films and films used for fluorography have a shape like a flattened, elongated 'S' and the straight-

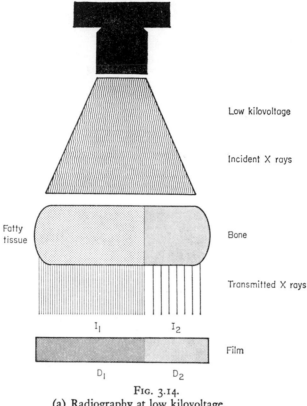

FIG. 3.14.
(a) Radiography at low kilovoltage.
Radiation contrast in the subject $= I_1/I_2$.
Radiographic contrast in the image $= D_1 - D_2$.

line portion is not really a straight line at all, even though to the casual glance it may look very like one. The curve shown in Fig. 3.13 is an example.

Where there is no true straight-line part of the characteristic curve, gamma (the slope of the straight-line part of the characteristic curve) ceases to be useful as a number to indicate the contrast of the film material. Another consideration which makes gamma not very useful is that when films are being employed for radiography the densities may not fall within the straight-line parts of characteristic curves. The reader should remember that the useful range of densities in a medical radiograph is between 0·25–2·0. To look at Fig. 3.13 with this in mind is to see that this range of densities relates to parts of the curve which are at

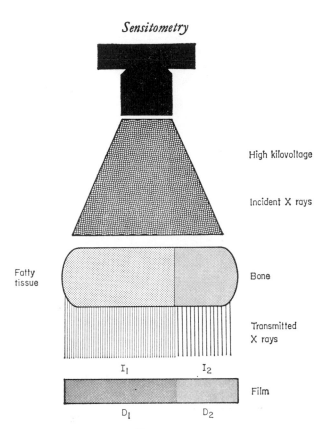

FIG. 3.14.
(b) Radiography at higher kilovoltage.
Radiation contrast in the subject $= I_1/I_2$.
Radiographic contrast in the image $= D_1 - D_2$.

different slopes. The minimum end of the range is on the toe of the curve and not on the straight-line part at all; the maximum end of the range comes on a portion of the curve which is approaching the shoulder. In this case gamma as a statement of the contrast of the material would not tell us anything about the contrast in some parts of the curve which were in fact being used.

There remains a need for a number to indicate the contrast of the material, and the number used in this case is the *average gradient*. This is the slope of a straight line joining two points of density on the characteristic curve. In Fig. 3.13, the two points $D = 0.25$ and $D = 2.0$ have been joined by a dotted line; these two points are the minimum

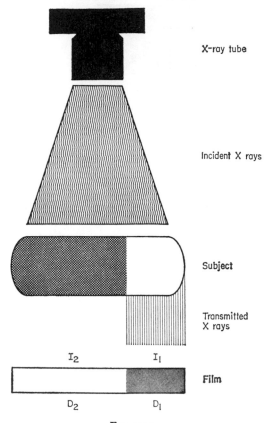

X-ray tube

Incident X rays

Subject

Transmitted
X rays

I_2 I_1

Film

D_2 D_1

FIG. 3.15.
(a) Radiation contrast in a barium meal.
Radiation contrast in the subject $= I_1/I_2$.
Radiographic contrast in the image $= D_1 - D_2$.

and maximum densities occurring in general radiographic use and it is
usual to take two such points in order to specify average gradient. The
slope of the dotted line joining these points is the average gradient of the
parts of the curve being used. The useful numerical value for contrast is
the tangent of the angle which this line makes with the exposure axis
when it is extended to intersect the exposure axis of the graph.

RADIOGRAPHIC CONTRAST

In order to assist the student to appreciate the qualities required in

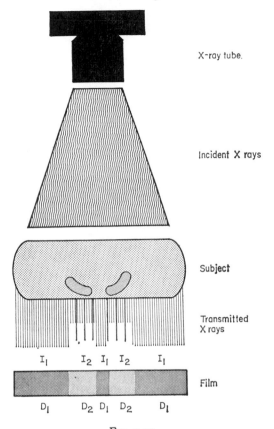

X-ray tube.

Incident X rays

Subject

Transmitted
X rays

I_1 I_2 I_1 I_2 I_1

Film

D_1 D_2 D_1 D_2 D_1

FIG. 3.15.

(b) Radiation contrast between the kidneys and their surrounding soft tissues.

Radiation contrast in the subject = I_1/I_2.

Radiographic contrast in the image = $D_1 - D_2$.

emulsions used for radiography, it may be helpful to consider further the term *contrast.*

There are three elements here:

(i) The radiation contrast of the subject.

(ii) The film contrast.

(iii) The radiographic contrast of the resultant image.

Radiation Contrast of the Subject

This is the result of the differential absorption of the radiation by

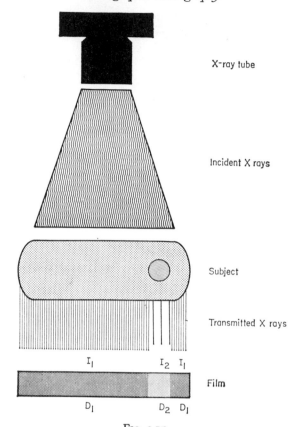

X-ray tube

Incident X rays

Subject

Transmitted X rays

I_1 I_2 I_1

Film

D_1 D_2 D_1

Fig. 3.15.
(c) Radiation contrast in a cholecystogram.
Radiation contrast in the subject $= I_1/I_2$.
Radiographic contrast in the image $= D_1 - D_2$.

different parts of the subject. This differential absorption in tissues—for example bone and fat—leads to different intensities of radiation being transmitted to the film through different parts of the subject. These intensities will have a range for a given subject from a certain minimum to a certain maximum. If I_1 is the greatest and I_2 is the least intensity transmitted, the subject contrast can be expressed as the ratio I_1/I_2. It can be expressed logarithmically as the difference between the logarithms of these intensities.

For any given subject this ratio is reduced by increasing the tube kilo-voltage. Fig. 3.14(a) depicts two structures, one composed of fatty tissue and the other of bone, irradiated by means of a beam produced at a relatively low kilovoltage. The fatty tissue does not absorb the radiation very much and a high intensity (I_1) is transmitted through this part of the subject; beneath this area the film is black. The bone absorbs the radiation very heavily and a low intensity (I_2) is transmitted through this part of the subject; beneath the area the film is white-grey. There is a big difference between I_1 and I_2 and the ratio I_1/I_2 is high.

In Fig. 3.14(b) the fatty tissue and the bone are irradiated by means of a beam produced at a higher kilovoltage. The fatty tissue again transmits a high intensity (I_1) and the film beneath this part of the subject is black. The more penetrating radiation produced at the higher kilovoltage is now absorbed less heavily by the bone than the previous radiation was. So more radiation is transmitted through the bony structure (I_2) than before; the film beneath this part of the subject is black-grey. I_1 and I_2 have come closer together and the ratio I_1/I_2 is reduced.

In the image the contrast is obviously reduced since the difference in density is in (a) between black and white-grey and in (b) between black and black-grey.

Higher kilovoltage thus 'levels out' differential absorption and makes different tissues transmit intensities which are more nearly the same. So the radiation contrast of the subject depends on the kilovoltage.

It also depends on the nature of the tissue traversed.

For example in a barium meal study taken erect the barium-filled stomach will absorb radiation heavily and transmit none; the 'gas bubble' in the stomach will transmit a great deal. Thus the ratio I_1/I_2 is high. In a plain radiograph of the abdomen there will be little difference between the intensities transmitted by each kidney and its surroundings, and the radiation contrast ratio (I_1/I_2) will be low. In the absence of a contrast agent, there will be no difference in the intensity of radiation transmitted by the normal gall bladder and its surroundings; no image of the gall bladder is obtained. If, however, the gall bladder is filled with contrast agent, there will be an appreciable difference in the transmitted intensities from the organ and from its surrounding tissue and the ratio I_1/I_2 will be relatively higher. Fig. 3.15(a) (b) and (c) indicates these differences.

Film Contrast

This has been already explained in terms of the characteristic curve and gamma. It depends on the type of film and the conditions of exposure and development.

Radiographic Contrast

This is a function of the previous two. Radiographic contrast is altered by (i) altering the gamma of the film and (ii) altering radiation contrast in the subject as shown in Figs. 3.14 and 3.15. In practice film gamma is not altered by the radiographer, since gamma is an inherent characteristic of the material in given conditions of exposure and development. The radiation contrast of the subject can be altered by the radiographer in selection of tube kilovoltage, being for a given subject greater at low kilovoltages than at high. From what has been said, it can be understood that the use of contrast agents in radiography is designed to extend the radiation contrast of various body parts beyond that given them by nature in order to make them demonstrable upon film.

The gamma of the material, it is clear, is in the knowledgeable hands of the manufacturer. The radiation contrasts of the subject (which in many cases may be slight) require to be amplified by the film. It is found that satisfactory results may be obtained when the gamma of the material can give a radiographic contrast which rather more than doubles the radiation contrast of most subjects. Radiographic contrast is discussed again in Chapter xii.

CHAPTER IV

X-ray Materials and their Storage

X-RAY FILMS

The student realizes early during practical radiographic training that X-ray films are exposed in two different ways. One way is to expose the film in a light-tight paper envelope as it is supplied by the manufacturer. The other way is to expose the film in a specially designed container known as a *cassette*. The cassette contains two *intensifying screens*, one at the back of the cassette known as the back screen, and one at the front of the cassette known as the front screen, the film lying between the two at the time of exposure. The action of the screens is to fluoresce when activated by X rays, producing ultra-violet, violet, and blue light to which the film responds. When intensifying screens are used, the latent image in the film is formed mainly by the light from the screens rather than by X radiation.

X-ray films can therefore be classified first into two distinct categories of material:

(i) Film for direct exposure to X rays.

(ii) Film for indirect exposure by means of intensifying screens.

Film for Direct Exposure to X rays

This is usually known as non-screen film and, even less sensibly, by the descriptions envelope-wrapped or double-wrapped film. All these terms are in common use in X-ray departments, but the significant feature about this class of film is that it is used for exposure directly to X rays. From this it follows that the most pointed description would be 'direct exposure film', but it does not seem to be called that in practice.

For material of this type the emulsion layer is comparatively thicker than for film to be used in visible-light exposure. X radiation has the ability to penetrate the emulsion layer, and the image can thus be produced at a depth in the emulsion that would be impossible with visible light. Obviously a thicker emulsion layer results in a greater density or degree of blackening from a given exposure, and the film will

61

therefore be effectively faster. The limit to the thickness of the layer is usually set by the amount which can be coated on the base or by the cost.

Since this type of film is used for exposure by X radiation and not by light, its sensitivity to any part of the visible light spectrum is not important. Its sensitivity to X rays is the significant feature and it should give high speed and high contrast when exposed to this radiation. The emulsion has a greater weight of silver than is used in material for exposure between screens.

The characteristic curve of such material differs somewhat from the typical shape previously considered—it has a sweeping toe, a less obvious straight-line part and usually no apparent shoulder. The shoulder of the characteristic curve of this type of material occurs at densities much higher than those used in medical radiography—usually at densities 10–12.

Since the emulsion layer in direct-exposure film is thicker and contains a greater weight of silver in comparison with the emulsion layers of other films used for radiography, direct-exposure film must be allowed a longer period for fixation during the processing cycle. For this reason some types of automatic processing unit cannot be used to process these films. This is a disadvantage. One firm, however, has surmounted the difficulty by producing a direct-exposure film which can be fixed in the same period of time as screen-type film. The characteristic curve of this material has a lower shoulder but the straight-line part of the curve has not altered in slope and the contrast of the emulsion is not less than that of other direct-exposure film, although at first it may appear so by reason of the paler background to the image. Nor is there any alteration in the useful density range which can be accommodated on the straight-line part of the curve.

Direct exposure film is used for radiography of relatively thin body parts. It requires several times more exposure than a screen and film combination. This fact makes it unsuitable for the larger body parts, from considerations both of radiation dose and of risk of movement (especially the involuntary movement of viscera) during the longer exposure times that would be needed.

The use of intensifying screens adds to the unsharpness in the image; the student may care to experiment by radiographing a specimen bone on direct-exposure film and on a screen-film combination and comparing the results. Direct-exposure film is therefore very useful in radiographic examination of the extremities to give excellent bone detail: this is of particular value in radiographs taken to exclude the presence of hair-line fractures and slight bone changes. The availability today of such material which is much faster than the early examples, and of X-ray sets giving high radiographic output, led to the occasional practice of using direct-exposure film for thicker parts of the body in examination of bony structures where the risk of movement might be considered minimal. Such practice gives increased radiation dosage to the patient that is probably not justified by the gain in radiographic quality.

It is the practice in some departments to use direct-exposure film for examinations for suspected foreign body in the eye. Here it has the advantage of removing all element of doubt as to whether a certain opacity is or is not an artefact in the intensifying screens. Screens *should* be entirely free from artefacts, but let us admit that in general departmental practice few of us achieve the standard of having all our screens all the time so absolutely free from defects that this troublesome doubt in these cases does not arise.

Direct-exposure films are made by the principal manufacturers under various trade names.

Film for Exposure with Intensifying Screens

It has been said previously that for radiographs made with film-screen combinations in a cassette the image is produced almost entirely by light emitted by the screens when they are activated by X rays. Some direct radiation of course reaches the film, but the exposure from direct X rays is only about 2–7 per cent of the total exposure, the remainder being a visible-light exposure.

It follows from this that the most important characteristic of the film is its response to the ultra-violet, violet, and blue light emitted by the screens, and not its sensitivity to X radiation. Since the image is produced mainly by visible light acting on the surface of the emulsion with very little penetration to a depth within it, there would be no gain in having an emulsion layer as thick as it is for direct-exposure film. X-ray film for use with intensifying screens is generally known as screen-type film or screen film, and it has an emulsion layer with a lower silver halide content than film in the other category.

Screen-type film can be exposed without intensifying screens, but it is not usual practice to do this as the film would be slow in comparison with one designed for direct exposure. Characteristic curves have nevertheless been made to show the performance of screen film when it is used (a) with intensifying screens, and (b) without them. The usual result ob-

6

tained is similar to that shown in Fig. 5.2 on page 82. Here the curve AA₁ is for a screen-type emulsion exposed between screens, and the curve BB₁ is for the same emulsion exposed without screens. The two curves should be compared for difference in shape. It can be seen that when exposed between screens the film has a steeper central portion, indicating that contrast is greater in these conditions; this is attributable to difference in response of the film to a light source and to X rays.

Curve BB₁ has a sweeping toe and less apparent shoulder than curve AA₁ and in these features it is similar to the characteristic curves of film materials for direct exposure to X rays. The two curves may be taken as typical of those resulting when any screen film is tested with the two different conditions of exposure—direct exposure to X rays and exposure to the fluorescent light from intensifying screens. The two curves are separated from each other, since the film used with screens is effectively very much faster than when used without them. Curve AA₁ is thus much further to the left along the exposure axis than curve BB₁, their separation being a measure of the added speed gained by the use of screens in the particular conditions used to make the curves.

Screen-type films are available from the principal manufacturers in different grades of speed under trade names such as Kodak Standard, Kodak Blue Brand, and Kodak Royal Blue, Ilford Standard, Ilford Red Seal, Ilford Gold Seal, and others. The grades of speed are differentiated by the manufacturers as a high contrast material (relatively slower), a fast material, and a very fast material.

Film Sizes and Film Packs

The student doubtless has appreciated long ago that the manufacturers provide X-ray films in various sizes. These are not internationally standardized, and vary in different countries where the film originates and is used.

In Great Britain the dimensions are given in inches and the sizes most generally used are:

$$4\tfrac{3}{4} \times 6\tfrac{1}{2}$$
$$6\tfrac{1}{2} \times 8\tfrac{1}{2}$$
$$8 \times 10$$
$$10 \times 12$$
$$12 \times 15$$
$$14 \times 14$$
$$14 \times 17$$

In the U.S.A. inches are used and common sizes are:

5 × 7
6½ × 8½
7 × 7
8 × 10
12 × 10
14 × 17
14 × 36

In Europe centimetres are used and sizes are:

9 × 12
13 × 18
15 × 30
15 × 40
18 × 24
20 × 40
24 × 30
30 × 30
30 × 40

The packing of X-ray film is no casual process. It is given much attention by the manufacturer who naturally is anxious that his product should reach the user in the best possible condition, and should remain in that condition until it is used. The paper used for packing is stringently tested; if this paper is lacking in certain qualities it can cause deterioration in the film which it wraps. The whole process of manufacture of the wrappings is strictly controlled. Doubtless as we discard these wrappings so casually we give no thought to the care and time which have been spent in their production, but it is nevertheless essential that the manufacturer should do this in order to preserve in good condition the photographic materials which he has so carefully made.

Screen-type films are supplied 'folder-wrapped'. This means that they are inserted in a sheet of paper folded to make two sheets which cover each side of the film; this arrangement is of course not light-tight. Twenty-five films in their individual folders are put together into a pack in a closed paper wrap. These packs of twenty-five, separated by stiff card, are put together in boxes of up to seventy-five films. These boxes must be opened in the darkroom under safe-light conditions as recommended by the manufacturer. Another form of packaging which has been introduced does away with the folder wraps. The films are put up without interleaving paper in packs of 100 films and these are assembled to make boxes of 300 and 500 films. This saves money in packaging films and space in storing them, for the packs take up much less room than would be needed for a comparable number of films which were folder-wrapped. A point to be kept in mind is that film material stored in a darkroom hopper without any interleaving paper to give it protection must be particularly secure from any leakage of light into the hopper.

Direct-exposure films may be 'envelope-wrapped', and are then sometimes said to be 'double-wrapped'. Each film is initially folder-wrapped like the screen-type film, and is then enclosed in a light-tight paper envelope with a piece of firm card for backing; in this sealed light-tight envelope it is used for exposure. Twenty-five films each in its sealed envelope are packed in a box, from which they can be taken in white light and exposed to X rays in their envelopes, the envelopes then being opened in the darkroom where the films are processed.

This direct-exposure film is also supplied folder-wrapped exactly as the screen-type, and it is then taken from its packings in the darkroom and loaded into an exposure-holder. This is a light-tight cardboard holder, usually with lead backing, which is reloaded with fresh film for each exposure. Film is cheaper to buy folder-wrapped than envelope-wrapped, so the use of these holders may be considered as an economy. They are, however, difficult to keep clean. This is particularly disadvantageous in traumatic units where direct-exposure film is most likely to be used for the examination of extremities recently injured. The holders need frequent renewal.

Film for Dental Radiography

Dental films are usually available in two sizes. The larger is $1\frac{1}{4} \times 1\frac{5}{8}$ inches, and this is in general use for most intra-oral radiography. The smaller is approximately $1 \times 1\frac{3}{4}$ inches and is suitable for use in the mouths of children, and of adults with narrow dental arches where the larger films might prove difficult to use satisfactorily.

Some manufacturers provide dental films of different speed and contrast. These are usually differentiated as (i) a film of high speed, and (ii) a film of much lower speed, probably requiring at least twice the exposure but giving higher contrast. The higher contrast results in the different densities of the image being amplified, but the longer exposures require more sustained immobility in the patient, whose unreserved co-operation it is not always easy for the radiographer to secure despite the best of intentions on both sides.

Dental films may be packed singly or in pairs. Each film or pair of films is between two pieces of black paper, and on the side which in use will be remote from the X-ray tube is placed a sheet of lead foil. This protects the film from radiation scattered back towards it in the patient's mouth and improves the contrast of the final image. One manufacturer marks a pattern of lines on this foil; if the film is inadvertently used with the wrong aspect towards the X-ray tube, this pattern is usefully reproduced upon it and makes clear the nature of the error which has occurred.

The film (or films) in paper and the foil are enclosed in a light-tight packet of non-absorbent paper. Both the films and their wrappings have rounded corners which may make them slightly less unacceptable in the patient's mouth. The aspect of the pack which must be nearer the X-ray tube is clearly indicated on the outside. The films are usually available in boxes of fifty, or 150 singles or pairs.

It is important to be able to identify positively the tube aspect of the film once it has been removed from the pack. To this end an embossed dot is set near one corner on one of the long edges of the film. Its position is also apparent on the external surface of the pack, either by an emboss-ment on the tube side of the wrapping, or by a star printed on the opposing side. On one film surface this dot is concave or a 'dimple'; on the other it is convex or a 'pimple'. The convex surface of the dot is on the side of the film nearer to the X-ray tube during the exposure.

OCCLUSAL FILMS

These films are for intra-oral radiography with the film placed in the occlusal plane, and their size is $2\frac{1}{4} \times 3$ inches (6×7.5 cm.). They are packed similarly to the dental films in singles or in pairs, wrapped in the same manner, with an embossed dot on one of the long edges. Like the dental films, they have rounded corners. They are available in boxes of 25 singles or pairs. They may be used for direct exposure to X rays or for exposure between intensifying screens in a special intra-oral cassette. For the latter technique they are provided sometimes folder-wrapped in the same way as other screen-type film: if the occlusal film is to be removed from its wrapping and loaded into a cassette in the darkroom, it is clearly not necessary to give it the special light-tight foil-backed pack required for its use in direct exposure techniques.

There is, however, no difference in the emulsion. Some manufacturers make their occlusal films of screen-type material for exposure with or without the intra-oral cassette; some manufacturers make their occlusal films of direct-exposure material for use with or without the intra-oral cassette.

Films for Radiation Monitoring

The student is doubtless familiar with the use of small films for measuring dose received by staff exposed to ionizing radiations. Externally these look very like dental films for they are the same size as the larger ones, have rounded corners and are in a similar pack. No lead foil is enclosed to back the film—it is simply between two pieces of paper in the pack—and there is no embossed dot as such a device for identification of the tube aspect of the film is not required.

The response of photographic film to radiation depends upon wavelength, and a dose of one rad delivered by radiation produced at 80 kVp results in greater film density than the same dose delivered by radiation produced at 200 kVp. An emulsion which gives an adequate range of measurable densities for small doses of radiation in the 50–100 kVp range might be unsuitable for recording doses of very high energy radiation as the densities produced would be very much lower. One manufacturer provides for personnel monitoring films in three different emulsion speeds. Two of these are relatively much faster than the third, the characteristics of the emulsions being adjusted so that these two give a markedly greater density for small film doses when used for measurements in the high-energy range of radiations.

Another firm makes film for radiation monitoring which has a more sensitive emulsion coated upon the front and a less sensitive emulsion coated upon the back of the base. It can record a wide range of doses, avoiding the use of several films differing in sensitivity. The fast emulsion can be removed and the slow emulsion used alone for assessment of very large doses.

Films for Kidney Surgery

Sometimes a surgeon may request X-ray examination of a kidney exposed during operation for removal of renal stones. This check enables him to see whether or not he has removed the last vestiges of calculus before he retraces his surgical steps out of the patient's abdomen. A fast film especially for examination of the exposed kidney is on the market.

It is enclosed in a flexible light-tight polythene packet and is about 4 × 5 inches in size. The shape is so designed that the film can readily be put under the kidney, there being a curved indentation along one of its edges to allow for the ureter and other vessels at the hilum of the kidney.

The pack is not sterile when it comes to the user, but it can be sterilized by a suitable dry method—for example by the use of paraform tablets. These tablets liberate formaldehyde; this is one of the substances to which photographic film is sensitive, but as the film is enclosed by an impervious plastic pack it is undamaged by this method of sterilization.

Industrial X-ray Films

Some film materials designed for industrial radiography are used in the medical field particularly for mammography. These films for industrial use are slower than the direct-exposure films for medical work and have smaller grain size (with inanimate subjects, the problem of motion does not occupy the industrial radiographer's mind in the way that it does for his medical colleagues). These films give images with good detail and require more exposure.

Industrial X-ray films are often used for mammography enclosed with a medical direct-exposure film in a single film-holder which contains one medical film and one or more industrial films (each with a different speed). The films are exposed simultaneously in the one holder and on development they show images of different densities since the films are of different speeds. This technique is of help in recording with one exposure the different tissue thicknesses of the breast.

X-ray Negative Paper

X-ray paper is a sensitive material used for radiography in the conventional manner, exposed either directly to X rays or in a cassette with one intensifying screen. The emulsion is coated not upon a transparent film base but on a smooth photographic paper base of the weight of thin card. This paper is coated upon one side only, not upon both sides as in the case of film materials. The emulsion is a screen-type X-ray emulsion and there is a supercoating similar to that used for X-ray films. Since the base is not transparent, the image cannot be viewed by transmitted light but must be viewed by reflected light just as ordinary photographs are seen. No image on paper seen by reflected light can be as high in contrast as an image on a transparent base viewed by transmission. Radiographic images on paper are therefore lacking in contrast and density range as compared with their film counterparts.

X-ray paper, which is less costly than X-ray film, may have a limited use for examinations where this loss of contrast and the necessity for longer exposures are immaterial—for example demonstration of bone alignment after the reduction of fractures. It can be said that in the medical field the United Kingdom uses little or none of the X-ray paper which is manufactured but there is some market for it in other parts of the world. It finds industrial use for the radiography of light-weight assemblies (for example, electrical fuses in ceramic holders) which may require examination in large numbers.

STORAGE OF UNPROCESSED X-RAY FILMS

It has been said already that photographic materials are very sensitive and require to be made and handled with care if they are to remain in the first class condition for which the manufacturer aims in production. It follows that when these materials reach the user they must be stored with the same degree of attention if all the previous care is not to be in vain. Even in the best conditions of storage, material will deteriorate inevitably with keeping, and the period for which it may safely be kept before use has been called its 'shelf-life'. Fast film materials have shorter shelf-life than slow ones.

Much care, time, and money are spent by the manufacturer in devising film wrappings, and these clearly cannot be bettered by the less knowledgeable. Films should be stored therefore in their original wrappings intact for as great a part of the keeping period as is possible; only when it is close to the time of use should they be taken to the darkroom and unwrapped. Screen-type film kept in the darkroom hopper for immediate use is best left with each film in its loose folder of black or yellow paper. This separates the films, and makes easy the removal of each one for loading into a cassette. The folder and film can be taken from the hopper and the film slid from its folder into the cassette as the folder is withdrawn. The film itself is thus not touched at any stage with the hands, and finger marks can be avoided.

When ordering film stocks for their departments, radiographers should adjust the intake to the rate of use and keep a stock sufficient to meet week-to-week needs without a large reserve supply. In this way no batch of films need stay too long upon the shelf, and spoil simply with keeping. When the boxes of film reach the department they should be checked to see that they are sound, and they should be date-stamped on arrival so that the oldest stock can be detected. The boxes should be stored so that they can be used readily in order of arrival, the oldest first.

The boxes should stand vertically upon the shelves not laid horizontally like a pile of pancakes. X-ray film in quantity is not light, and the lower boxes in such a pile would be under pressure liable to produce artefacts upon the films. A further reason for vertical storage is that it is more easily arranged to enable the oldest stock to be used first.

Dampness and high temperatures have a most damaging effect on photographic materials, and probably moisture is the more severely ravaging and the more difficult to exclude. The ideal store is one in which the temperature is in the region of 50°F (10°C) and does not rise above 65°F (18°C), the relative humidity being in the region of 50 per cent. Rooms with damp walls and floor, and rooms prone to sudden changes of temperature and the probability of condensation are to be avoided.

The store should be well ventilated, and the storage shelves arranged with adequate air-space above and below them. They should not run past heating pipes or any pipes from which water may leak. Films must be stored away from the effects of ionizing radiations, and this will be no problem if the store is at sufficient distance from diagnostic and treatment rooms. If it should be close at hand then it may be necessary to pay special attention to this aspect, and ascertain that walls, ceiling, and floor as may be necessary have full protection incorporated in them. It is the practice for some manufacturers to include in film boxes a strip of lead foil running round the upper part of each box. If the film should be fogged by radiation while in the box an image of the strip on the films gives the clue to what has happened.

As well as being sensitive to heat, moisture, light, and other actinic radiations, film material can be damaged by various chemical fumes, and even by emanations from some paint. The best possible storage conditions are therefore not easy to achieve or maintain, and storage has such an influence on the length of time a material will satisfactorily keep that no manufacturer will commit himself and say dogmatically that a certain film will keep for so long. All materials begin to deteriorate from the time of manufacture, and poor storage hastens this. With good storage, deterioration is not noticeable before use. Film has given reasonable results in some single cases after a very long period of time.

On keeping film *after* exposure and *before* processing, it can be said that this seldom comes within the practice of the radiographer since it is usual to process radiographs almost immediately after they are exposed. It is a fact, however, that the latent image regresses if the film is kept for a long time before being developed. This process is more rapid than the loss of sensitivity shown by unexposed materials during the time they are kept, although there have been instances of film successfully developed years after it had been exposed.

CHAPTER V

Intensifying Screens and Cassettes

When X rays fall upon certain substances light is emitted. The physical principles involved in this phenomenon should be familiar to the student radiographer and are outside the scope of the present work. They are summarized in the statement that energy changes have occurred in the irradiated material which result in the production of characteristic radiation of wavelengths within the visible spectrum.

The emission of light from a substance bombarded by radiation is termed *luminescence*. This includes two effects, *fluorescence* and *phosphorescence*. The first means that luminescence is excited only during the period of irradiation and will die upon termination of the X-ray exposure. Phosphorescence is afterglow; that is the irradiated material continues to emit light for a time after cessation of exposure. Both these phenomena are important radiographically, though from rather different aspects.

It can be said that the property of X rays of exciting luminescence played a part in their discovery. It was the fluorescence of a card coated with barium platino-cyanide for some other purpose which drew Röntgen's attention to the presence of this invisible penetrating radiation.

The luminescent effect is used radiologically in two ways.

(1) To obtain on a fluorescent screen an image which may be observed directly by the eye, as in the procedure of fluoroscopy, or may be recorded by a camera, as in mass radiography of the chest (fluorography).

(2) To increase the photographic response of a silver halide emulsion. In this case the fluorescing material in a practical form is referred to as an *intensifying screen* and is placed in direct contact with the film during exposure. Its function is to reinforce the action of X rays by subjecting the sensitive emulsion to the effects of light as well as X radiation.

In this chapter we are concerned with intensifying screens rather than with those designed for fluoroscopy or fluorography.

CONSTRUCTION OF AN INTENSIFYING SCREEN

It has been established that a silver halide emulsion changes on exposure to X rays in a manner similar to its reaction when exposed to light. However, when such an emulsion is exposed to X rays it absorbs very little of the incident radiation. An intensifying screen exposed to the same radiation absorbs the beam much more heavily and the effects of this absorption are seen in the emission of light. The use of the intensifying screen provides a method of converting X rays to another actinic radiation to which the photographic emulsion is responsive and thus obtaining after processing a comparable degree of blackening for a shorter interval of exposure or at a reduced level of intensity.

In practice an intensifying screen consists of a base which may be card or polyester or cellulose acetate. This base must be radioparent and chemically inert. It must combine characteristics of toughness and flexibility and should not either curl or discolour with age. The base is coated first with a smooth white pigment and then with a uniform homogeneous layer of the fluorescent material. This in turn receives a thin transparent supercoat. The purpose of the latter is protective but for reasons explained later it must be very thin and care is always required in handling intensifying screens to avoid any kind of abrasion.

In some instances the flexibility of the material is especially significant in order to allow the screen to be bent in a small radius without fear of cracking. In this case the fluorescent material is necessarily mounted on the other bases described, rather than on card. An intensifying screen of this type of structure would be required in situations where the film must be adapted to a curved surface, for example in some projections of the knee and shoulder joints.

Since X-ray films are coated on both sides intensifying screens are commonly employed in pairs. Each emulsion surface is placed in close contact with the effective surface of one intensifying screen. When this sandwich of screen-film-screen is exposed to X rays both screens fluoresce, the light from each activating the emulsion surface which is its immediate neighbour.

Though used as a pair the intensifying screens may not in fact be twins. It is accepted practice to try to obtain equal blackening on both emulsion surfaces of the film as theoretically this arrangement results in maximum speed. Radiation which has passed successively through the first screen, the first emulsion, the film base and the second emulsion is necessarily attenuated. The lessened intensity of radiation in turn produces decreased fluorescence in the second screen. It is clear that this sequence of events will result in unequal blackening of the two film surfaces, that remote from the X-ray tube being lighter than the one proximal to it.

To overcome this, the two screens are not identical in structure. The first or front screen is only thinly coated with fluorescent material, since a deep layer will increase the attenuation of the X-ray beam. The second screen is more thickly coated; increasing the density of the luminescent substance leads to greater fluorescence if stimuli are equal and here operates to maintain the same level of brightness from a diminished stimulus. There is naturally an optimum thickness for both screens, in which the need to match the blackening of the two emulsions is not the only factor. There is also the consideration that light produced in the deep layers of a thick screen may fail to reach the film because of absorption in the superficial layers and thus will be ineffective. This aspect is significant in the design of screens for fluoroscopy: increasing the thickness of the screen beyond a certain limit is not efficacious in brightening the luminescence to the eye any more than to the film.

The difference in thickness of such paired intensifying screens makes it important not to interchange them in their relationship to the X-ray source. If the thicker screen faces the tube aspect of the film and thus functions as a front screen considerable attenuation of the beam will occur from absorption. The thinly coated, less active front screen—now behind the film—no doubt will fluoresce from the action of such X rays as reach it but the intensifying effect from a practical point of view will be plainly inadequate. Due to both factors the resultant radiograph is found to be seriously underexposed.

In practice this source of underexposure can be troublesome to determine as other agents are usually blamed first: the X-ray tube current is thought to fluctuate mysteriously, no one having observed the behaviour of the milliampere meter, or processing techniques become suspect. Care should be exercised in the use of unequally-coated intensifying screens to ensure that this error does not occur.

Not all intensifying screens are thus differentiated, however. At present many manufacturers put equal coating weights on both of a pair of screens and either screen can be used in the front or the back position in a cassette. The economic advantages of this and the elimination of errors outweigh the very slight gains in obtaining equal blackening of both emulsions.

THE CHOICE OF FLUORESCENT MATERIAL

Materials which convert invisible radiation into luminous radiation are known as phosphors. A number of such substances exist though we are concerned in radiography with only one or two of them. They are used in crystalline form, since their luminescent characteristics are virtually absent in any other, and their correct chemical preparation is a delicate and exacting procedure. Even small traces of impurity—of the order in some instances of one part in a million—will diminish the efficiency of many phosphors. Such imperfections can be considered as minute islands of inactive material and in the case of intensifying screens will lead to an appearance of mottle on the film. It is obvious that the standards of purity and cleanliness required for the manufacture of these phosphors are extremely high and could scarcely be more demanding even in a laboratory employed in bacteriology. Perhaps it is not surprising that intensifying screens are quite expensive pieces of equipment: they deserve respectful handling.

The Colour of Luminescence

All phosphors do not luminesce with the same colour. This is clearly of importance in their radiographic applications. The colour of light emitted by a fluoroscopic screen should be that to which the human eye is most readily receptive: in fact this is in the yellow-green region of the spectrum. On the other hand the fluorescent colour of phosphors employed for the manufacture of intensifying screens or of those designed for fluorography has an obvious relation to the spectral sensitivity of the film with which they will be used. A screen which is emitting green light can be effective only if the associated film is either orthochromatic or panchromatic. (Chapter ii.)

In many phosphors the production of any appreciable luminescence requires the presence of an *activator*, a small quantity of some foreign element. This activator is significant not only in increasing the fluorescent powers of the material but because it affects the colour of the resultant light.

The spectral range of screens used for fluorography and its influence on film emulsions designed for this radiographic procedure will be considered again (Chapter xviii). In the manufacture of intensifying screens for direct medical radiography virtually only one phosphor is employed at the present time in the United Kingdom. This is calcium tungstate.

Properties of Calcium Tungstate

Calcium tungstate appears to have been the first substance used in the preparation of intensifying screens. Its early defects in manufacture were considerable. The crystals tended to vary in size and sensitivity, with resultant mottling of the film. Probably a worse nuisance was the proneness of the screens to phosphorescence or afterglow. As explained earlier this means that their luminescence was prolonged after termination of the X-ray exposure. It necessitated the lapse of a considerable interval of time before the same pair of screens could be re-loaded and used for a second radiograph.

We can now see that in radiography afterglow is a property of phosphors which is important from a negative aspect. If it is prolonged more than a fraction of a second its presence is impermissible in a fluoroscopic screen since it will blur the detail of moving images.

Afterglow may be accepted in a very minor degree in the case of intensifying screens. For practical purposes it is absent from the modern calcium tungstate screen and improved processes of manufacture have long resulted in crystals of uniform size and fluorescence. These screens now are of a high order of efficiency.

The presence of prolonged afterglow could be determined by the simple procedure of reloading the cassette in question immediately after exposure. During this exposure some part of the film should be masked with lead in order to have a standard of comparison. Subsequent processing of the second film will reveal reproduction of the original exposed area if marked afterglow exists. However, it is an academic experiment unlikely to be positive with the calcium tungstate screens of the present day.

A more stringent test would be to put the screens under examination in a rapid film changer, such as the AOT changer employed for angiography. Films could then be passed through the changer, for instance at a rate of six per second. The centre of the films should be masked with lead for some of the time. Even under these conditions it is unlikely that any evidence of afterglow would be found in current calcium tungstate screens.

The spectrum of the fluorescence of calcium tungstate is within the range 3,500 A.U. to 5,800 A.U.; that is, it extends from the ultra-violet to the yellow-green bands of the spectrum. However, the region of maximum fluorescence is about 4,200 A.U., i.e. the colour of the emitted light is violet or violet-blue. The student radiographer may easily prove this by exposing an open cassette to a beam of X rays. The demonstration will be the more impressive if the room lighting can be temporarily subdued, in which case the violet-blue luminescence of the screens appears very brilliant and is certainly easily memorable. The experiment, if repeated at a different value of tube currents, will also show that the brightness of luminescence is dependent on the intensity of radiation reaching the screen surface.

Under present day conditions the colour of fluorescence produced by a calcium tungstate screen is independent in practice of the wavelength (i.e. kilovoltage) of the exciting radiation, at least over a very wide range of tube tensions. The blue fluorescence of these screens results in a maximum photographic response, since X-ray film is most sensitive to this region and also to ultra-violet light which comes within the luminescent spectrum of calcium tungstate. This means that comparable blackening of the film is produced for much shorter intervals of exposure or at markedly reduced levels of radiation output. We can say that the screens have a pronounced intensifying ability and we may refer to and analyse this as the *intensification factor*.

Their intensifying effect—and consequently the reduction in radiographic exposure to which they lead—are the main reasons for employing salt screens in medical radiography. Minor side effects occur which are advantageous:

(1) the use of screens increases contrasts between low densities in the radiograph;

(2) in a small way the screens protect the radiograph from the effects of scattered radiation. This is partly because the screens themselves absorb 'soft' scatter and partly because they do not intensify radiation of long wavelength to the same extent as the more energetic primary beam.

However, by far the most important aspect of the use of salt screens is the reduction in exposure time which they allow and we shall now consider this intensifying effect in greater detail. Before doing so, brief reference must be made to the applications in medical radiography of screens constructed of metal.

Metal Intensifying Screens

Metal intensifying screens have been for a long time predominant in industrial radiography for use at tube tensions over about 120 kVp or with gamma radiation. They have a marked filtering action and consequently are not appropriate to most medical work.

In recent years, however, a significant exception has developed in the practice of making a radiographic check of treatment fields in radiotherapy. This is done by means of the therapy unit itself as the source of exposure and in these circumstances radiation of extremely short wavelength activates the film. The emulsion used is that sold for industrial purposes. Diagnostic student radiographers should visit the radiotherapy department to see for themselves the type of radiograph produced when a medical subject is submitted to this particular combination of film, screen and highly penetrating radiation. It is informative, for example, to compare the appearances of the larynx as seen in this and in conventional diagnostic radiographic techniques.

Like salt screens, metal screens are employed in pairs, usually in a cardboard film holder of the type described in the previous chapter. In fact their function is dual.

(1) They preferentially absorb scattered radiation and therefore improve film contrast in the same way as a secondary radiation grid.

(2) They have a relatively limited intensifying effect which arises from the photographic action of secondary electrons ejected from the metal by X or other radiation of short wavelength. The student should note that this is *not* luminescence.

Both the absorption of scattered radiation and the emission of secondary electrons become greater in materials of high atomic number. For these reasons lead is a very suitable metal. It has also the advantage of being malleable and can be rolled to any desired thickness. In practice these metal screens take the form of a thin sheet of foil. The front screen might have a thickness of 0·004 in. and the back screen 0·006 in. The lead is alloyed with a smaller percentage of other metals to make it harder and the screens in consequence more durable. There is no kind of supercoat on these screens and the film is placed in immediate contact with the surface of the metal.

THE INTENSIFICATION FACTOR

The intensification factor of a pair of screens can be simply stated. It is the figure by which we should have to multiply the exposure if we were to use the film without intensifying screens. Putting it differently, we can say that it is the ratio of the energy (which we will express in milliampere seconds) necessary to produce a certain blackening on a film exposed alone, relative to that required by the *same* film in conjunction with intensifying screens.

Referring to an imaginary numerical example, we might know that a certain pair of screens has an intensification factor of 15. If 3 sec., 50 mA and 60 kVp were technical factors applicable to a certain subject without the use of screens, then we could alter these to 0·2 sec. (3 divided by 15), 50 mA and 60 kVp if we used the same film with the screens in question.

However, closer examination of the intensification factor makes plain that the matter is considerably less simple than it appears. Looking again at the example given above it must occur to the student that in radiographic practice film emulsions designed for direct exposure are not usually employed with intensifying screens. Yet the intensification factor must be derived from the performance of the *same* film under the two conditions of either absence or presence of the screens. It is a justifiable inference that this factor is not a realistic figure for the radiographer, being indeed virtually irrelevant in practice. Other considerations tend to produce the same conclusion.

In assessing the intensifying effect of any particular pair of screens, it will be found that the intensification factor is not an absolute but depends upon a number of variables. The more important of these are discussed below.

Duration of Exposure

The variation of the intensification factor of a pair of screens with the duration of the X-ray exposure is not an inherent feature of the screens themselves. It is due to reciprocity failure (p. 294) of the film emulsion when it is affected by light. The operation of this phenomenon results in the intensifying effect being less than its predicted value at low levels of intensity for prolonged exposure; it is also reduced when very high values of tube current activate the film during a brief interval of time. This is unlikely to be of practical significance to the medical radiographer, except conceivably in the course of millisecond exposures from a constant potential unit. However the variation which can be shown to occur under either of these conditions means that the intensification factor cannot correctly be stated as a single absolute value. It is considered to be maximum for exposure times of the order of 0·1 seconds.

Quality of Radiation

It can be shown that the intensification factor of a pair of screens is not constant over a wide range of kilovoltages. In the case of calcium tungstate it becomes greater as the wavelength of the exciting radiation decreases. This is true of the voltages employed in diagnostic medical radiography, though at very high tube tensions, of the order of 500 kVp or more, there is evidence that the intensifying effect of salt screens in fact becomes less for radiation of very short wavelength.

If we consider for a moment only the relevant wavelengths of diagnostic radiology it must be recognized that in fact it is not the general practice of radiographers to make an allowance for variation in the intensification factor of calcium tungstate screens when any change in tube voltage is considered. Students may find an exception to this observation if there are in use in their departments screens of another material; barium lead sulphate. This phosphor is no longer popular in the United Kingdom for the manufacture of intensifying screens but it is used in the U.S.A. for certain high speed screens.

The fluorescence of barium lead sulphate, while visibly less than that of calcium tungstate, extends well into the ultra-violet region of the spectrum. Figure 5.1 shows that the intensification factor for barium lead sulphate is rather higher than for calcium tungstate at 50–60 kVp and becomes very much higher at peak tensions of 90–100 kVp.

In using these screens radiographers normally allowed for the variation in the intensification factor by the assumption that at 90 kVp they were approximately twice as fast as they were at 60 kVp. We shall examine this assumption more closely in due course.

Despite its more intense luminescence throughout the diagnostic range of wavelengths, barium lead sulphate has disadvantages as a phosphor for intensifying screens which have discouraged its use in the United Kingdom at the present time.

Referring again to Fig. 5.1 we see that in the screens considered the intensification factor for calcium tungstate is about 23 at 50 kVp and about 35 at 100 kVp. This of course is a considerable variation but in practice radiographers need make little allowance for it, since changes made in kilovoltage are generally not great. It is extremely doubtful if a radiographer who alters certain exposure factors by adding or subtracting 10 kVp consciously thinks of any accompanying variation in the intensification factor of the screens, nor can we realistically state that the omission of this consideration is apparent on observation of the resultant radiograph. The point is clearly of theoretical interest rather than practical significance.

Zinc sulphide is another phosphor which is used in the U.S.A. for the manufacture of certain intensifying screens, although its employment

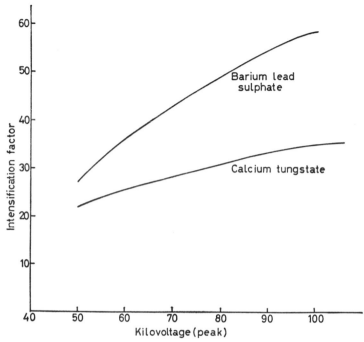

FIG. 5.1. Comparison of the intensification factor of barium lead sulphate with that of calcium tungstate over a kilovoltage range between 50 and 100 kVp. The increasing speed of barium lead sulphate with mounting kilovoltage is shown. *By courtesy of RADIOGRAPHY, The Journal of the Society of Radiographers.*

has been discontinued in the United Kingdom. It is characteristic of zinc sulphide screens that their intensifying effect is maximum in the low kilovoltage range. Above 60–65 kVp the intensification curve flattens and the screens are no faster than a pair of standard or medium speed. However, this feature of zinc sulphide makes the screens suitable for use in situations where only low powered apparatus is available. In hospital perhaps such situations are becoming more rare owing to the development and increasing use of mobile X-ray units of high output; but in domiciliary practice high-powered equipment is not appropriate and zinc sulphide screens might well be favoured for reasons of their speed at low kilovoltages.

It should be remembered that when we discuss variation in the intensification factor with applied tube kilovoltage we really speak of the influence upon the factor of radiation quality and that there are other elements in this: the waveform of the apparatus, the filtration of the X-ray tube and not least the filtering action of the subject itself. These variables, too, have an influence on the value of the figure obtained.

The Photographic Density

When intensifying screens are used film contrast is greater than when the same emulsion is exposed without screens, unless the densities compared are very high. This is due to a more rapid increase in blackening for the same exposure interval.

As a result of this effect the intensification factor of any particular pair of screens will vary in value depending upon the density at which 'screened' and 'unscreened' exposures are compared. When the two radiographs are matched at a low density the intensification factor is

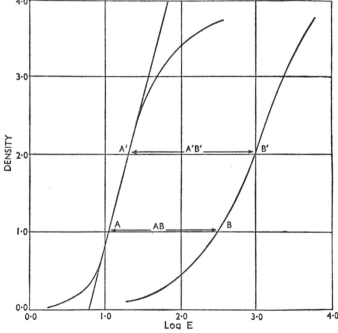

Fig. 5.2. Characteristic curves for a screen-type emulsion exposed between screens AA$_1$, and without screens BB$_1$. The intensification factor, which is related to the horizontal distances between the curves, is seen to be greater at density 2 than at density 1. *By courtesy of RADIOGRAPHY, The Journal of the Society of Radiographers.*

found to be less than when they are balanced at a high one. The characteristic curves in Fig. 5.2 prove this point. Both curves relate to the same screen-type emulsion.

The left hand curve A is what happens when the film is exposed between intensifying screens: curve B represents exposures without the screens. We see that A has a steeper slope than B, so we know that the contrast of the first radiograph is higher (Chapter III). This is particularly noticeable at low densities: study the respective slopes of the two lines between zero density and a density of 1 on the graph.

Though the student radiographer is not required to know this derivation, it can be shown that the intensification factor is related to the horizontal distance between the curves, increasing as this increases. If we look at the line A^1B^1 at density 2 we can easily appreciate that it is longer than the line AB at density 1. We will thus obtain a different value for the intensification factor of these screens, depending upon the density at which we balance the radiographs.

The Degree of Development

To understand how the degree of development influences the intensification factor we must consider two points in the production of the latent image. When it is formed by X rays alone it is distributed uniformly, or nearly so, throughout the depth of the emulsion. When light is the activating radiation the image tends to be concentrated in the superficial layers of the emulsion and this of course is the situation when intensifying screens are used: here about 95 per cent of the image density is due to fluorescence and only the small remainder to the energy of the X-ray beam.

During processing the developing agents must act first upon the surface layers of the emulsion before penetrating to the deeper levels. Thus a short period of development is productive of greater density if the image has been made by light than if X rays alone have entered into its formation. In the latter case relatively little of the latent image will be developed in the same interval of time. If we compare 'screened' and 'unscreened' exposures following a short period of development the intensification factor may be found to be high. Prolonging the time of development will decrease the intensification factor of the screens, as then the density of the latent X-ray image has opportunity to 'catch up' with the one formed by fluorescent light.

Summarizing, we can say that there are at least four main variables upon which the intensification factor depends:

(1) the intensity of radiation;
(2) the quality of radiation;
(3) the radiographic density at which comparison is made;
(4) the time of development.

From this we can appreciate how difficult it is to give to the intensification factor a numerical value which has either reality or significance for the practising radiographer. It is doubtful if any of us know or have ever been told such a figure for any of the screens we habitually employ.

Nevertheless, the student radiographer will commonly hear in the X-ray department comments or instructions to the effect that a certain pair of screens is 'slow' or that another pair will need 50 per cent less exposure because the screens are 'fast'.

Let us think what these statements really mean. We may ask ourselves, if these screens require a reduction to half the normal exposure, with what are they being compared? The answer then is obvious. We are certainly not talking about the intensification factor which relates the screens to the performance of the same film without screens. Instead we are balancing the effect of the 'fast' screens against the same film and some other pair of screens which we regard as requiring 'normal' exposure. Indeed the radiographer who took the speed of the former barium lead sulphate screens to be twice as great at 90 kVp as at 60 kVp was really acting from the knowledge that at the lower tension barium lead sulphate and calcium tungstate have an approximately equivalent intensifying effect (at least for practical purposes), and that at high values of kilovoltage the first becomes twice as active as the other.

Manufacturers' data may sometimes refer to the intensification factor of a new pair of screens but it is recognized that this is not a particularly useful figure and where given is for general guidance only. It is much more likely that the information provided will relate the performance of the new screens to some standard type already familiar in radiographic practice. Exposure ratios between different varieties of intensifying screen are frequently stated in technical publications and are used by radiographers as a realistic and helpful assessment of the intensifying effect.

DETAIL SHARPNESS AND SPEED

In an earlier chapter (Chapter 11) the resolving power of film materials was explained and discussed and we saw that when we speak of the resolution of a photographic system we refer to its ability to render the separate parts of an image distinguishable by the eye; that is, to show fine details of structure. It was said that the capacity of an emulsion to resolve detail was influenced by grain size, contrast and the extent to which it may absorb or scatter light.

In the crystalline form of calcium tungstate or other salt intensifying screen we have a composition analogous to the silver halide grains of a film emulsion. It must be evident that when such an intensifying screen is used in medical radiography the same features of crystal size and dispersion of light are significant in the production of resolution. Indeed the resolving power of the intensifying screens may be the limiting factor in the production of detail by a radiographic system.

In theory we cannot record radiographically details of the subject which are smaller than the salt particles composing the screen. However, in medical radiography this is not a practical consideration. The dimensions of these crystals are expressed in microns, a micron being a thousandth part of a millimetre: even the smallest lesion which could be observed on a radiograph is many, many times larger and its size is normally expressed in terms of one millimetre or more.

In a later chapter (Chapter xii) the several sources of unsharpness in a radiograph will be further discussed, particularly their relationships to each other and their combined effect upon the X-ray image. They are of three kinds.

(1) Geometric unsharpness, dependent upon the size of tube focus and anode-film and subject-film distances.

(2) Motional unsharpness which arises from voluntary or involuntary movements of the subject during the exposure.

(3) Intrinsic or photographic unsharpness due to the characteristic structure of the luminescent screen and film material.

All of them are important. They cannot be added together arithmetically and in any particular case the one which makes the largest contribution will dominate the radiograph, however the others may be diminished. Consequently it is ineffectual technique to attempt to reduce any of these factors at the marked expense of another.

At the present time it is only intrinsic unsharpness which we shall consider. The presence of intensifying screens increases intrinsic unsharpness in the radiographic image, although not necessarily to an unacceptable level. We can appreciate that it does so if we compare the radiograph of an extremity taken on direct exposure film with another for which intensifying screens were used.

The explanation of the unsharpness inherent in all intensifying screens is to be found in the fact that light diverges.

Diffusion of Light

From simple experience we are all familiar with the fact that light spreads outwards in all directions from its source. We may visualize the fluorescing particles of an intensifying screen as a number of sources of light.

Theoretically if there were no divergence of the radiant beam there would be no spread of image detail in the radiograph. In practice this state of affairs cannot exist. Even from crystals considered to be in contact with the film there would be a spread of light in other directions and this light could be bent towards the film by remote crystals: even crystals at the surface of the screen are not in contact with the film owing to the supercoat and this is a reason why the transparent supercoat is made as thin as possible. The further away is each source of fluorescence from the film the greater will be the degree of image spread and the worse the obtainable radiographic definition.

Speed

Reference has been made earlier to differences in the speed of intensifying screens. It was stated that increasing the density of the phosphor, that is the thickness of the fluorescent layer, must increase also the amount of light activating the film. Consequently a thick screen has a greater intensifying effect and it is said to be faster than a thin one of the same material.

However, if the screen is thick the average distance between its particles and the photographic emulsion must be greater. We have already seen that this means that radiographic resolution will be worse because of wider divergence of the light.

The speed of an intensifying screen can be increased if the size of the calcium tungstate crystals is large because this again leads to a higher emission. However, large flat crystals provide an unrestricted pathway for light travelling obliquely through them. This situation is depicted diagramatically in Fig. 5.3 in which the lines L_1, L_2 and L_3 represent variously diverging rays of light.

When light is spread in this way over a wide area, radiographic sharpness inevitably is poor. These effects can be overcome on the principle of providing 'obstacles' which hinder the passage of the light. In Fig. 5.3 the rays represented by L_2 and L_3 are more influenced by the presence of obstructing devices than are the rays L_1 because their track

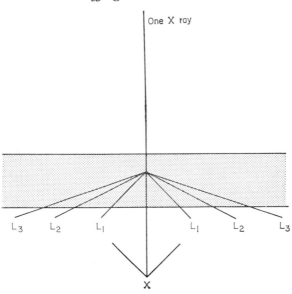

FIG. 5.3. Diagram to illustrate how light spreads over a wide area from an X-ray beam passing through an intensifying screen composed of large flat crystals. This effect deteriorates image sharpness.

to the film is longer. In this way the cone of light reaching the film is made narrow and detail sharpness in the image improved.

In the manufacture of intensifying screens two methods are available for obstructing the sideways spread of light.

(1) The use of crystal powder which causes light to be scattered by the surfaces of the many small crystals in its path.

(2) The use of dyes—usually yellow or red—in the fluorescent layer to absorb light. Both these measures—because they decrease the quantity of actinic radiation reaching the film—also reduce the speed of the intensifying screen; while at the same time, they improve detail because of their greater effect on obliquely travelling light. These characteristics are irreconcilable: intensifying screens which have a fine crystal structure give sharp images but lack speed; those which are composed of large crystals have greater speed but their use results in poorer detail.

Speed in an intensifying screen is very desirable in medical radiographic practice since shorter exposure times can then be used. This will reduce patient dosage and decrease the likelihood of movement unsharpness. However it is obvious that speed can be gained only at the expense of radiographic resolution.

At the present time manufacturers supply intensifying screens in three grades of speed. These may be described as (i) standard or regular, (ii) fast or high speed and (iii) high definition or fine grain. In the case of those of British manufacture these screens are all calcium tungstate. The difference between the first two is one of size in the calcium tungstate crystals; the fast screen has about twice the speed of the other. Critical laboratory tests show that the definition obtained with the fast screen is not as good as that given by the standard one but for medical work this is not usually detectable in practice. In the U.S.A. barium lead sulphate is popular for high speed screens.

In general one may say that the fast screens are intended for use on subjects where the contribution from motional unsharpness may become dominant over intrinsic unsharpness if the exposure time is long; for example, in gastro-intestinal work where the potential exists for both respiratory and peristaltic movement. These screens might also be appropriate in circumstances where it is necessary to keep exposure values to a minimum for other reasons, perhaps in a high speed angiographic series.

In the high definition screens the fluorescent layer is dyed and they require about 50 per cent more exposure than the standard type. They would be used in some circumstances to obtain fine bone detail, assuming that radiation output were of subordinate importance and immobilization of the subject no problem. The resolving power of high definition screens for a subject of low contrast has been stated as approximately 10 lines per millimetre and of standard screens at about 8 lines per millimetre.

Measurement of Unsharpness

The unsharpness introduced into a radiograph by the use of intensifying screens is difficult to measure. It must be separated from other sources of blur which are present and the results obtained vary with the experimental conditions, for example with the kilovoltage and type of film employed. Assessments of this kind do not come within the experience of the medical radiographer and no doubt are outside the scope of this book.

The detail attainable in a radiograph can be recorded in the form of an *unsharpness curve*. The required measurements are made in the following manner. A radiograph is taken of a sharp metal edge. This must be placed close to the film and accurately aligned to the central ray, the beam being perpendicular to its surface. The subject-film separation is negligible and the anode-film distance should be such that the geometric unsharpness is less than the expected value of the blur attributed to the film/screen combination. Motional unsharpness of course is nil.

When a radiograph obtained in this way is examined with a microdensitometer it is seen that the high density along the edge of the specimen does not change sharply and immediately to an area of no density. There is in fact a band of density change which can be defined as radiographic unsharpness. The density variation across the image is measured and a curve of density—or rather light intensity—against distance is obtained: this is known as the unsharpness curve. An example of such a curve is shown in Plate 5.1, following p. 94. From it experimental values of blur can be derived. Typical figures might be 0·2 mm for a pair of high definition screens and 0·3 mm for a standard pair.

However, numerical quantities which profess to state the resolving power of intensifying screens and the unsharpness attributable to them should be accepted cautiously. They are of value only when the conditions of measurement are fully specified and in any case have little practical meaning or relevance for the radiographer using the screens for clinical work.

Consideration of the number of absorbed X-ray quanta at different stages has been of value in calculating the minimum size of detail observable with fluoroscopic and image intensifier systems. It has been suggested that this approach, in terms of the number of quanta absorbed per unit area of the film during the exposure time, might prove rewarding for the assessment of the performance of X-ray sensitive materials.

Random fluctuations in the number of absorbed quanta are recorded on the film as fluctuations in density, giving a clumped or mottled effect. Of this appearance the term *quantum mottle* is used. It is easier to understand how quantum mottle occurs if we imagine that the area irradiated—that is, the intensifying screen or in some cases the film directly—is divided up into a number of much smaller areas, just as a large paved court is composed of many individual paving stones. We may think of a thin shower of rain just beginning to fall on this court. If we were to examine several separate paving stones we should not find the same number of rain drops on each. The raindrops' fall is random: on some stones there will be fewer drops than on others and—because the raindrops are not yet very numerous—there is an appearance of mottle over the whole paved area.

In the same way the number of quanta falling upon and being absorbed by many little areas of the intensifying screen is not consistent. The number varies between one place and another and the magnitude of the variation increases as the number of quanta becomes smaller. When exposures (intensity × time) are small, then quanta of radiation are also few in number. The trend to use faster screens, faster films and thus shorter exposure times is one which also increases the possibility of the appearance of quantum mottle upon radiographs. We can say that a situation favouring the production of quantum mottle is that in which high energy radiation is incident on the film for an exposure period of very short duration.

The student should recognize that quantum mottle is a totally different entity from the mottle apparent in some intensifying screens which is of a structural nature and influenced by the size and packing of the grains. Lack of uniformity in these produces variations in the light output of the screen. Quantum mottle can be seen on fast calcium tungstate screens.

CASSETTE DESIGN

A cassette by definition is a small flat box used for transporting a film —but it is doubtful if anyone who has carried a couple having dimensions 14 × 17 in., from the department to a distant ward in order to X-ray a patient's chest, would consider that 'small' is an operative term.

The general appearance of an X-ray cassette is no doubt quite familiar to student radiographers once they have begun to give practical assistance in a radiological department (Plate 5.2, following p. 94). Cassettes are used in association with intensifying screens and they have three related purposes.

(1) To maintain the film in close uniform contact with each of the screens during exposure.

(2) To exclude light.

(3) To protect the intensifying screens from physical damage.

In fact the structure of a cassette suggests perhaps a book rather than a box, as it consists of two flat rectangular plates hinged at one long edge. It is conventional to describe one of these as the front of the cassette; that is, it is that aspect which will face the X-ray tube. The other is the back of the cassette; it is the side turned away from the X-ray tube during the exposure.

The front of the cassette consists usually of a sturdy metal frame into which is fixed a sheet of either some lighter metal such as aluminium, or very often some plastic material: the critical point is that it must be transparent to X rays. This and the frame constitute a shallow container into which can be placed a thin intensifying screen and a film.

The back of the cassette is usually of some strong metal. It is customary to spray the internal surface with lead paint of which the purpose is to absorb secondary radiation otherwise scattered back on to the film from the table or other surface. However, there is not sufficient filtering effect to absorb primary radiation totally, as anyone knows who has ever inadvertently positioned a cassette with the wrong aspect facing the tube during exposure—usually in the operating theatre when the cassette is surgically draped. Some curious radiographic appearances are thereby produced.

Whether or not it is lead protected the back of the cassette certainly will possess a felt pad. The back intensifying screen lies on this, usually fastened to it, and its function is to maintain this screen, the film and its fellow screen all in uniform, firm contact. The back and front of the cassette are held tightly together, usually by spring clips on the long edge opposite to the hinge or by means of pivoted resilient metal bars on the back of the cassette which can be slid into grooves in the frame. Very often also on the back are such refinements as a name plate and a small leather tag to facilitate opening the cassette. The general appearance of a typical X-ray cassette is shown in Plate 5.2, following p. 94.

Cassettes are available from a number of manufacturers with minor variations in design. Criteria of a good practical cassette should relate to the following points.

(1) Weight. It should not be so heavy as to be a constant source of distress in handling.

(2) Robust structure. Cassettes are in continuous daily use and even assuming that no one actually drops one—this is to be avoided for the sake of the cassette and the radiographer's toes—nevertheless, thrust into darkroom hatches, loaded into serial changers or edged under heavy patients, they are subject to considerable stress and wear in a busy department. A damaged cassette is likely to be impaired in function: screens may fail to maintain contact with the film or leakage of light at the edges can occur. Cassettes deserve and should have stringent care in handling. They are themselves expensive and harm to them tends to spoil other costly materials—the screens and the film. A very light cassette is pleasant to use and, while acceptable in a small

department, may prove flimsy for the hard work of a large general centre. A compromise between weight and strength must usually be accepted. (3) Ease of operation. Whatever its form of fastening the cassette should not be troublesome to open and close, particularly as this act is necessarily performed in diminished visibility in the darkroom. It should have smooth outlines and rounded corners to avoid abrasion of either patient or radiographer.

Cassettes are provided in sizes appropriate to those in which X-ray film is supplied. The latter are given in the previous chapter and, as the student radiographer will know, it is common to refer to cassettes in these terms, though their actual dimensions are necessarily a little larger. Any other nomenclature would be inconvenient. Certain specialized X-ray cassettes deserve notice for some particular features. These are described below.

Curved Cassettes

These have the front convexly curved in a shallow arc. Their object is to maintain a parallel near relationship between subject and film in anatomical regions where a plane surface may be difficult to accommodate: for example to obtain an acceptable anteroposterior view of the knee when extension of the joint is limited. They are used in the smaller sizes, for instance 8 × 10 in.

Cassettes in a Film Changer

In certain film changers designed for angiography cassettes may be stacked in a group of three to five, one behind the other. The topmost cassette in the pile is exposed and withdrawn in series. For this type of succession it is of course essential that the back of each cassette should completely absorb primary radiation, otherwise fogging of the film in each of the underlying cassettes will occur every time an X-ray exposure is made. It is possible to back each cassette with a sufficient thickness of lead. However, in preference to modifying individual cassettes, perhaps the more economical and usual practice is to place the standard cassette in a lead-lined tray for the purpose, especially as this tray can include a handle to facilitate rapid withdrawal of the cassette from the apparatus.

Cassettes and Photo-timers

The student radiographer will no doubt be familiar with the principle of controlling X-ray exposure by means of devices capable of switching the circuit when the film has received an acceptable exposure. The radiosensitive element may be a photo-electric cell or an ionization chamber.

Whichever it is, its position must be behind the X-ray film, that is behind the cassette. These cassettes then require the reverse feature of those in the angiographic film changer: not only their fronts but their backs also must be fully radioparent in order not to attenuate further the radiation transmitted by the subject.

Gridded Cassettes

Cassettes can be supplied in most of the usual sizes which have incorporated in the front a secondary radiation grid as an integral component of the cassette. They are a little deeper, slightly heavier and commensurately much more expensive than the standard cassette. However, they have marked practical advantages when radiography is undertaken with a mobile unit or when horizontal projection of the X-ray beam is mandatory. Centring is more easily determined accurately when film and grid remain aligned as a single unit; film and grid are maintained in close contact and are easy to handle; the grid is automatically protected from the kind of damage which often occurs when a cassette is placed under a grid larger than itself and a heavy patient placed on top of them both. These cassettes advisedly should carry some external indication that they contain a grid or mistakes in exposure technique are likely to occur. One manufacture obligingly colours them red but a robust labelling system would also serve.

Flexible Cassettes

Like the curved cassette, the flexible type is designed for adaptation to rounded surfaces but in this case the arc can be of surprisingly small radius. Their applications in industry, for example to girders and pipelines, are evident and numerous. In medical use they are necessary for the specialized equipment associated with pan-oral radiography. In this procedure the X-ray source actually is within the patient's mouth and the cassette placed in approximation to the external contours of the face. In the related field of rotational tomography of the jaws, the film again must be bent to a shape correspondent to the right and left halves of the maxilla considered simultaneously.

Such a curvature requires the intensifying screens to have a flexible base, for example cellulose acetate. They are mounted within a simple envelope of plastic material, folded at one end and fastened with press buttons of conventional design. Considering the highly organized needs of the apparatus for this type of dental radiography the flexible cassette appears almost fantastically uncomplicated: it is a simple and practical piece of equipment.

Multisection Cassettes

Intended for simultaneous multisection radiography these cassettes must be deep enough to hold at any one time a group of films varying in number from 3 to 7. In order to obtain a useful variety of level in the tomographic planes there should be a distance between the films of about 1 cm for most examinations, although in some cases a separation of 0·5 cm or less is requisite.

This cassette is in fact a box some 3 inches deep which contains the appropriate number of intensifying screens separated by spacers of some suitable material. The nature of the spacing substance is important since it must not be of a character to absorb or scatter X rays to an appreciable extent. At present it is usually a plastic polyfoam material, although balsa wood has been employed.

If simultaneous multisection tomography is to be a practicable and useful procedure, it is evident that every film in the group must be comparably exposed. To ensure this, special measures are necessary because of two factors.

(a) The film at the bottom of the cassette is further from the source of X rays than is the film at the top. Consequently the intensity of radiation which reaches it will be diminished in accordance with the operation of the inverse square law.

(b) Each succeeding screen absorbs some radiation, thus diminishing again the quantity reaching the last film.

Of these two effects, (a) is comparatively insignificant since the depth of the cassette is small compared with the distance between it and the X-ray source. It is (b) which is responsible for most of the attenuation of the beam during its passage from the first to the last film. To offset this a combination of intensifying screens should be employed which becomes progressively faster. For example in the simultaneous exposure of 5 layers, uniform radiographic density could be obtained by the following arrangement.

1st film (nearest to the X-ray tube)	1 high definition front screen only.
2nd film	1 standard back screen only.
3rd film	Conventional pair of high definition screens.
4th film	2 standard front screens, one in front of and the other behind the film.
5th film	Conventional pair of fast screens.

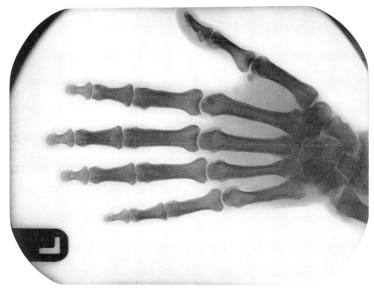

Plate 1.2. A positive radiographic image.

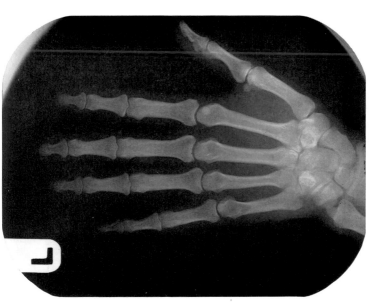

Plate 1.1. A negative radiographic image.

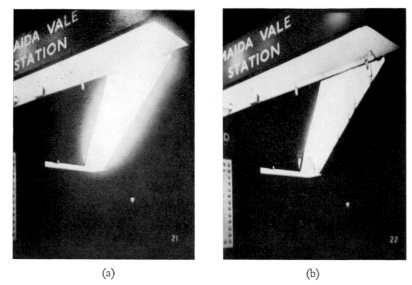

(a)   (b)

PLATE 2.1 (a) With halation. (b) Without halation. *By courtesy of Ilford Ltd.*

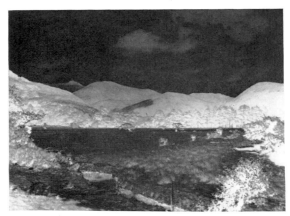

PLATE 2.2. Negative image without enlargement (original on fine grain panchromatic film).

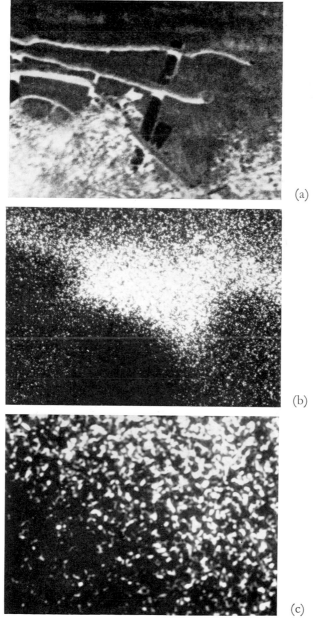

(a)

(b)

(c)

PLATE 2.3. (a) A portion of the image with × 16 direct enlargement.
    (b) × 198
    (c) × 850
The granular pattern is perceptible at × 16, and is increasingly obvious at
greater degrees of enlargement.

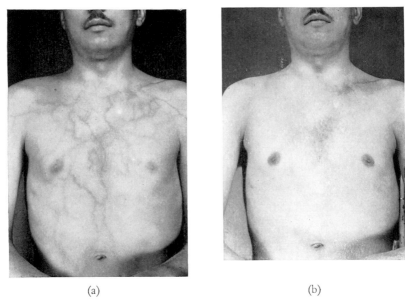

(a)   (b)

PLATE 2.4. Infra-red photography (a) reveals vessels beneath superficial tissue which are not shown by conventional photographic technique (b).

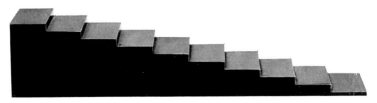

PLATE 3.1. An aluminium step-wedge.

PLATE 5.1. (Bottom right) Unsharpness curve for 200 k V X rays with high speed salt screens. (Three curves are superimposed to minimize fluctuations.) *By courtesy of The Journal of Photographic Science.*

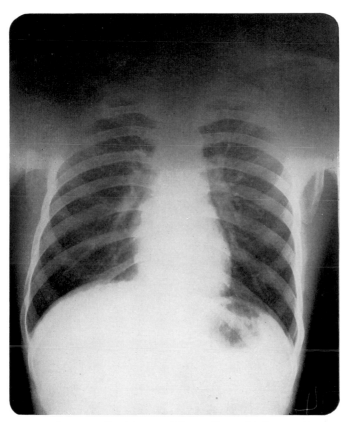

PLATE 3.2. Partial reversal in a radiographic image.

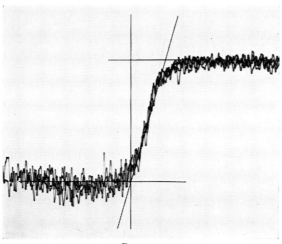

PLATE 5.1.

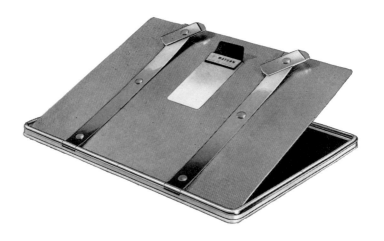

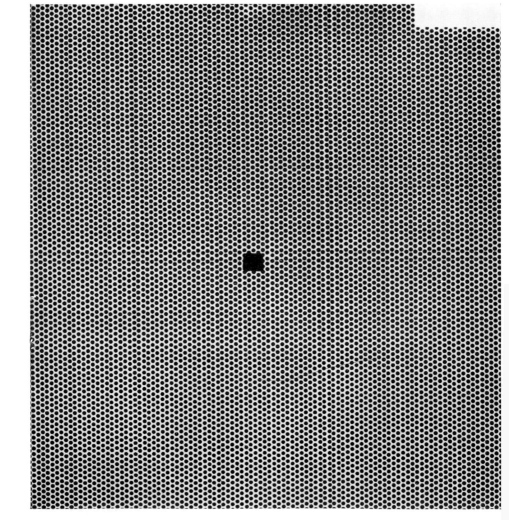

PLATE 5.2. (Top left) A typical cassette for medical radiography. The intensifying screens have not yet been fitted. *By courtesy of Watson and Sons (Electro-Medical) Ltd.*

PLATE 5.3.

(a) (Bottom left) The test radiograph of a perforated metal sheet obtained from a cassette in which screen contact is good. The central cut out area is to facilitate the measurement of density.

(b) (Below) A similar radiograph obtained from a cassette in which screen contact is poor. The sites of diminished contact correspond to the dark areas on the radiograph.

By courtesy of G.M.Ardran

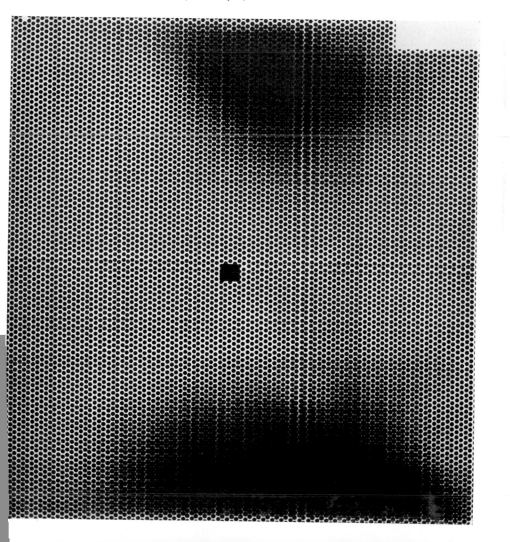

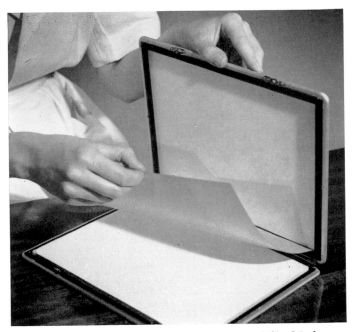

PLATE 5.4. Unloading a cassette. *By courtesy of Ilford Ltd.*

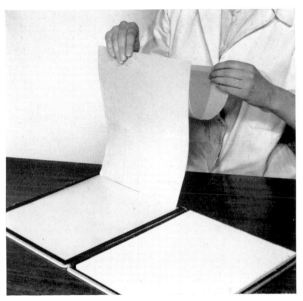

PLATE 5.5. The first stage of loading a cassette. The folder wrapping paper is drawn away from the film. *By courtesy of Ilford Ltd.*

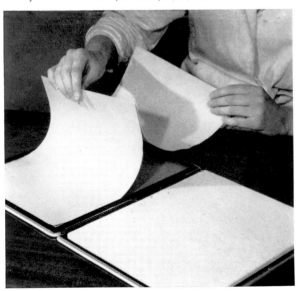

PLATE 5.6. The second stage of loading a cassette. The film has been lowered from the folder into the well of the cassette. The folder can now be discarded. The film is not touched by the operator's hand at any time. *By courtesy of Ilford Ltd.*

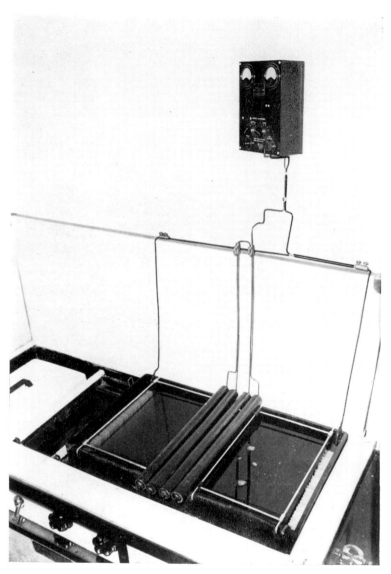

PLATE 7.1. Electrodes for electrolytic silver recovery in position in two fixer tanks. They are in full-time occupation of each tank. The control box is on the wall. *By courtesy of D. Pennellier and Co. Ltd.*

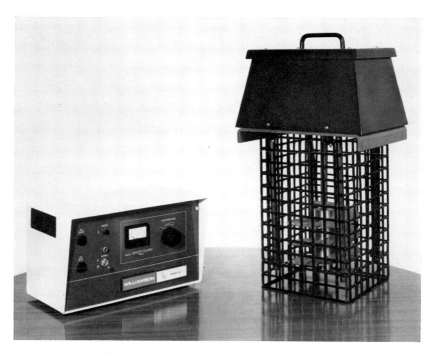

PLATE 7.2. A silver recovery unit which agitates the solution. The rotating cathode is in the form of a spiral blade and is seen in the centre of the protective wire mesh. Four carbon rod anodes are set round the cathode in a square formation. The control unit to the left is suitable for wall mounting. *By courtesy of Williamson Manufacturing Co. Ltd.*

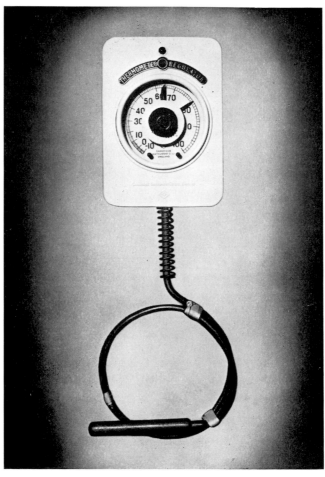

PLATE 9.1. A Cambridge thermometer regulator. *By courtesy of Ilford Ltd.*

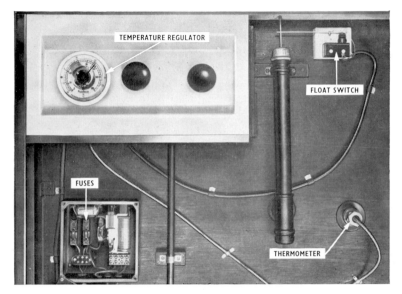

Plate 9.2. A thermometer regulator in operation in a processing unit. The front panel of the processor has been removed. The thermometer is situated in the water jacket about half-way down, and the heater (not included in the illustration) is similarly inserted at a lower level. Both are connected to the regulator. Also seen are the float chamber and the micro-switch which is operated by the float when it falls in the cylinder should the water level become too low. This safety device is shown diagrammatically in Fig. 9.4. *By courtesy of Kodak Ltd.*

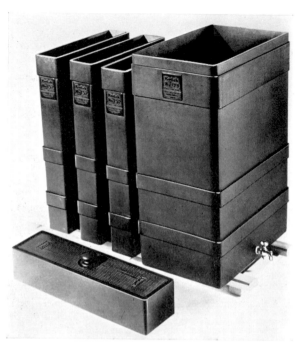

PLATE 9.3. A group of tanks suitable for processing radiographs. A lid is provided for the developer and the wash-tank has a tap for easy emptying. *By courtesy of Kodak Ltd.*

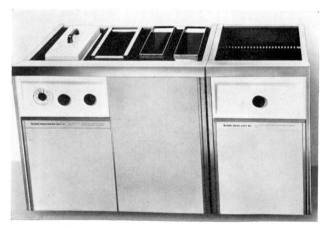

PLATE 9.4. A medium-sized unit for manual processing. It has a developer tank, a rinsing compartment and two fixer tanks within a water jacket. To suit the user, these four items can be altered in position to give a right-to-left sequence of work. The temperature of the water jacket is thermostatically controlled. The washer is of separate construction. *By courtesy of Kodak Ltd.*

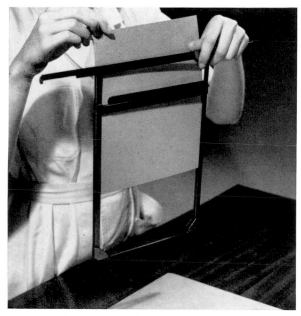

PLATE 9.5. A processing hanger of the channel type. *By courtesy of Ilford Ltd.*

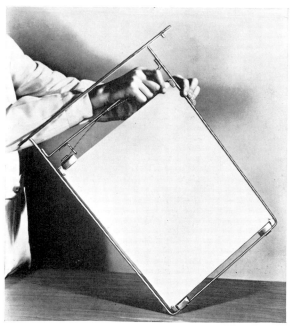

PLATE 9.6. A processing hanger of the tension or spring-clip type. *By courtesy of Kodak Ltd.*

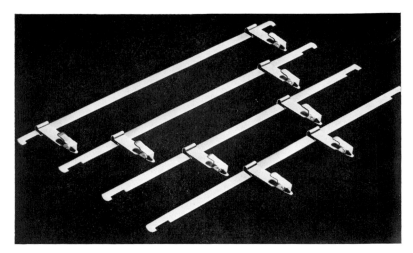

PLATE 9.7. Adjustable hanger bars to which sheet films of any size can be clipped for drying. *By courtesy of Kodak Ltd.*

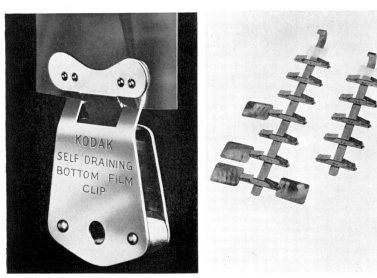

PLATE 9.8   PLATE 9.9

PLATE 9.8. A weighted clip which can be attached to the lower edge of a film to keep it flat when it is suspended and not in a hanger. *By courtesy of Kodak Ltd.*

PLATE 9.9. Hanger designed for processing dental radiographs. The patient's name or number can be written on the tablet at the end of the hanger. *By courtesy of Kodak Ltd.*

If three layers only are to be exposed at one time then the top film might have a single fast front screen, and the other two successively a pair of high definition and a pair of standard screens.

To avoid the increased hazards of damage when screens are loose and particularly the risk of placing these in incorrect sequence, it is usual to attach the screens and spacers together in the form of a book between the leaves of which the appropriate number of films can be placed. The whole arrangement is then inserted into the cassette, a little care being required to ensure that the correct aspect is uppermost.

Other multiple arrangements of screens are sometimes used in special cassettes, either to obtain radiographs in duplicate or triplicate or to record different densities (for example bone and soft tissue) during a single radiographic exposure of the subject. The principle again is the balancing of the speeds of several different screens in one cassette.

Graduated Screens

Intensifying screens are available which have a progressive intensification factor across the screen's surface. These screens are intended for the examination of regions characterized by the transmission of a long scale of radiation intensities. Examples of such regions are the leg if its full length is considered from ankle to upper thigh, and the lumbar vertebrae in the lateral projection from bodies to spinous processes.

In a pair of screens both may be graduated longitudinally; or the front screen may be longitudinal in progression and the other have a crescentic area of reduced speed at one long edge. The variation in intensifying effect is obtained by variation in either the coating weight of the screen or the density of a dye incorporated in the fluorescent layer.

CARE OF CASSETTES

Treated with kindness X-ray cassettes are good for years of hard work. Their general care is aimed at the avoidance of rough handling by all who use them. It may be helpful to mark each cassette, perhaps at a corner or along one edge, with identifying numerals which are inconspicuously apparent on each film. In a department where there are many this makes it easy to eliminate the innocent cassettes and screens, if radiographic faults are observed ascribable to damage of some kind to one or the other. Such numbering can be done with a pencil inside the cassette but it must be a small brief legend and graphite dust can sometimes be a source of artificial appearances on radiographs. If metal or

9

other opaque characters are used, room for their insertion must be made by cutting away part of one of the intensifying screens, otherwise there will be loss of contact at this and adjacent areas. Some manufacturers save the X-ray department the trouble of this exacting little task by serially numbering their screens at source.

The following further points should be noted.

Regular Inspection

Cassettes should be inspected at regular intervals to maintain them in serviceable condition. Hinges and clips are subject to stress and their proper functioning should be checked frequently to ensure that wear has not occurred.

Intensifying screens may become adrift and should be re-fixed immediately. Loose screens are an invitation to error in the darkroom for even with the best of intentions it is very easy indeed, when loading a cassette, to slip the film on top of both screens if these are unattached.

The felt pad in the back of the cassette may have become insecure or worn. This can result in failure of the intensifying screens to maintain uniform contact with the film and this in turn produces on the radiograph a localized area of unsharpness, due to the spread of fluorescent light between the screens and the emulsion. If this appearance is detected a test can be made of the suspect cassette.

Test for Screens' Contact

A radiograph can easily be taken which will show whether there is uniformly good contact between the intensifying screens and the film in a cassette. The object radiographed is a sheet of zinc—or copper—which is 0·036 in. (0·91 mm) thick and is continuously perforated; the holes should have a diameter of 3/32 in. (2·4 mm) and a pitch of 7 to the inch (approximately 3 per cm).

The density recorded on the film during the test will be more easily measured if a hole is cut at or near the centre of the zinc sheet; the diameter of this hole should be at least half an inch (13 mm). The overall area of the zinc sheet should be great enough to cover completely the cassette which is to be tested and it must lie flat and in close contact with the cassette. If wished, the zinc can be tacked for protection to a wooden frame which will keep it rigid; the advantage of a copper sheet is that it is more durable.

To carry out the test the suspect cassette is loaded with its normal film and placed on the X-ray table with the zinc sheet in front of it, so that the surfaces of the cassette and the zinc sheet are closely in touch with each other. An X-ray exposure is made at an anode-film distance of not less than 59 in. (1·5 m) using an X-ray tube with a focal spot of 1·0 mm–1·5 mm: this should be centred upon the centre of the cassette. The filtration of the X-ray tube should not be more than 2 mm Ac equivalent and the recommended kilovoltage is 50 kVp. The exposure should be sufficient to produce on the central unobstructed area of the film a density (see Chapter 11) of 2–4 on full standard development; for example perhaps an exposure of 4 or 5 milliampereseconds in the case of a film/screen combination of medium speed. The film is then processed and viewed.

Where there is a lack of contact in the cassette between the film and intensifying screens dark areas appear on the radiograph (see Plate 5.3, following p. 94). These areas will be readily visible when the radiograph is viewed in the normal way on an illuminator fitted with the usual fluorescent tubes, provided that the density of the image is high enough. The aim should be to obtain a really 'black' radiograph of the 'holes'; that is, a density in the perforated areas of 4.

At lower densities the effect is less readily apparent. It is not visible at densities of about 1·2 or less. At densities between about 2 and 3 it can be seen if the film is studied from a distance of 12 ft. (4 m) or more; or alternatively if it is viewed through a reducing lens which gives an image equivalent to looking at the film from this distance. Either of these procedures makes the test a little more complicated for radiographers than it need be and as few X-ray departments possess densitometers as standard equipment, the practical advantages of using enough exposure to obtain maximum density of the film are evident.

The results of a screen-contact test performed in this way are much easier to assess than if merely a flash exposure of a perforated metal sheet—or wire mesh—is given and the radiograph examined for evidence of unsharpness at the edges of the holes or wires. Detail unsharpness must occur whenever there is poor contact between a film and intensifying screens but blurring is likely to be less immediately apparent to the eye—especially if it is only slight in degree—than is a simple area of blackness on the radiograph. The dark patches result from scattering of the light of the screens over areas of the film which should not have been exposed as they underlie the metal of the test object. This procedure readily indicates areas where only slight loss of screen-film contact is present.

There is not much of lasting effect that can be done for a cassette which is failing to maintain contact between the intensifying screens. It is best to take a long term view of economy and discard it.

Test for Light Leakage

Following a number of fogged films physical inspection of a cassette usually makes evident the admission of extraneous light and the points at which it has entered. Broken fastenings or hinges, buckled corners or loose fronts are the likely culprits.

However if the condition is suspected rather than self-evident a test for light leakage can be made very simply by exposing a loaded cassette to an intense light. The exposure should be for 6 successive periods of 15 minutes each. Each side and each edge of the cassette in turn should face a 100 watt pearl tungsten lamp (operating at its rated voltage) which is at a distance of 4 ft. (1·22 m) from the cassette. (British Standard 4304 : 1968.) Processing the film will reveal on it patches of fog if leakage is present, the area of their situation being unequivocal evidence of where the light is entering. An edge darkening of not more than ⅛ in. (3·2 mm) is insignificant.

MOUNTING INTENSIFYING SCREENS

It was stated earlier that loose intensifying screens are a source of errors in manipulation in the darkroom. The film may not be in correct relation to the screens or the positions of the front and back screen may be accidentally reversed in the cassette. In addition to these mistakes, unattached screens are much more susceptible to damage from handling. From every point of view it is sound practice to mount the screens in permanent position within the cassette.

No attempt should be made to fasten intensifying screens into a cassette with any adhesive which may be handy in the department. Considerable attention has been given to the selection of a fixative to ensure that no chemical inter-reaction is likely to occur between this and the screens. It is not unknown for a small degree of radioactivity to be present in such an adhesive and this has resulted in bands of fog along the edges of radiographs, particularly of course if the film has lain idle for some time in the cassette.

Intensifying screens are commonly provided by their manufacturers with special adhesive tape, usually already in position on the back surface of each screen, ready for mounting. A protective layer of paper or thin plastic material must first be stripped off before the screens are positioned.

Throughout the procedure the screens should be handled gently, being held by pressure from the palms of the hands along their edges. This will avoid possible finger marks on the active surface of the screen.

The front screen is mounted first. It will be specifically named FRONT and deliberate attention should be given to its identification: it is marked clearly on the cardboard reverse aspect. The protective ribbon is removed from each strip of adhesive tape and the screen is then dropped carefully into the well of the cassette with its active surface facing the operator. No pressure from the hands or from anything else should be put upon the screen at this stage.

The back screen is then identified in the same way as its fellow and adhesive tape prepared as before. This screen is then laid carefully on top of its partner, active surface towards active surface. The back of the back screen now faces the operator. That edge of the screen which is adjacent to the hinge should not be placed too close to it or it will foul the edge and become damaged when the cassette is in use.

The last part of the procedure is simply to close the cassette, fasten it and to leave it thus for some little time, preferably overnight. This is the only pressure necessary to give the adhesive adequate hold.

CARE OF INTENSIFYING SCREENS

An intensifying screen damaged in any way is irreparably damaged. The only remedy is a new pair of screens. As they are sold in pairs, there is little to be done except replace both screens in the cassette, otherwise the odd screen must be kept in storage. Like one glove on its own, it may subsequently never have a match.

Screens are very exposed to the possibility of minor lesions. Their fluorescent emission will be affected if the active surface is even only soiled; for example by finger marks or the presence of dust or other foreign fragments such as particles of metal from the cassette itself. This makes constant attention to their cleanliness a first rule in the care of intensifying screens.

In the darkroom cassettes should not be stored or opened and re-loaded in the vicinity of chemicals. From this point of view automatic processing offers reduced hazards to intensifying screens compared with manually operated units. There is no means of removing the contamination of chemical splashes. On inspection in white light they are apparent on the screen's surface as faint brown or yellow stains and they are faithfully reproduced on every radiograph as areas of reduced density, owing to inhibition of the normal fluorescence in these areas.

Another likely source of damage to screens in the darkroom are processing hangers. If these are stored above the loading bench, as frequently they are, and the racks are insufficient for the numbers put upon them hangers may easily fall, particularly when the technician is pulling one free to use it. An open cassette lying on the bench below almost certainly will be victim to their passage, whatever may happen to the unwary technician. It is good practice always to leave cassettes closed, on a bench or anywhere else. Physical defects on the screen surface prevent fluorescence and again appear radiographically as areas of reduced density.

Heat is another agent which can diminish the efficiency of intensifying screens. Cassettes should not be left lying close to radiators or stored near hot pipes. It may be noted that film emulsions gain speed with increased temperature but screens lose it: this occurs to a greater extent and the overall effect is of loss. Furthermore when heated the screens may absorb moisture which will condense on cooling and cause the film to adhere to them. If the cassette has a plastic front this may warp and spoil the contact of the front screen.

Chemical splashes have been mentioned as a common risk to intensifying screens but there is another if technicians or radiographers are talking while putting films into cassettes. A fleck of saliva may fall on the film or on the screen during loading. It will soften the gelatine and stick the film to the supercoat of the screen. Subsequently removal of this film is likely to leave a blister on the active surface of the phosphor.

Summarizing the care of intensifying screens we can say that three good rules apply.

(1) Give regular attention to their cleanliness.

(2) Finger them as little as possible.

(3) Protect them from exposure to damaging agents such as chemicals or physical assault of any kind.

Method of Cleaning Screens

Intensifying screens should be dusted frequently with a soft brush: those sold for use on camera lenses are suitable for the purpose. During the operation the cassette should be held vertically so that loosened particles of dirt fall out of it. Dust and grit remaining in a cassette over a long period of time may become embedded in the supercoat of the screens.

Careful inspection of intensifying screens at regular intervals in a white light should be made in order to observe possible marks or defects. Screens which are old can be seen to have a fairly mottled appearance and this will be reproduced on radiographs taken with them. When this is noticed it is time to discard the screens.

In addition to dusting, the screens require washing from time to time. This should be regular darkroom practice, though on a less frequent schedule. The procedure is possible because of the protective supercoat. Items required are:

(1) An ample supply of cotton wool swabs.

(2) Good quality scentless toilet soap or a liquid detergent, such as one of the proprietary wetting agents. Never use an organic solvent, for instance ether soap.

(3) A supply of clean lukewarm water.

(4) A dry soft cloth.

Each screen is washed with a figure of eight motion, using a damp cotton wool swab which has been lightly rubbed with soap or moistened with one or two drops of wetting agent. This pad is then discarded and the screen wiped free of soap with a number of wool swabs soaked in clean water. At no stage must the screen be allowed to become excessively wet nor must water reach the back or edges of the screen. The surface is then mopped with a soft cloth, which is free of loose fibres, and left to dry by exposure to the air. The cassette should stand upright for this purpose and as far as possible the work should be done in a dust-free, draughtless atmosphere.

Grease may be removed from intensifying screens by the careful local application of carbon tetrachloride. This chemical should not be used in a confined space owing to the risk of inhaling its fumes.

Loading and Unloading a Cassette

Not least in the care of intensifying screens is the technique by which cassettes are unloaded and reloaded for further use. The following method is neat and trouble-free and if faithfully observed will assist in prolonging the life of intensifying screens. Unloading is described first as this is the sequence usually met by student radiographers working in the darkroom for the first time.

UNLOADING

The cassette is placed face downwards and opened from the back. It is then turned over and the front of the cassette tipped so that the film falls from the well of the cassette away from the front screen. This is illustrated in Plate 5.4, following p. 94. The film is removed with the free hand and the cassette closed.

If a pencilled legend has to be put on the film the cassette should *not* be used as a desk for the purpose. Repeated pressure from this source may eventually distort the cassette and spoil screen contact. Furthermore graphite dust may be thus introduced. The screens themselves may be accidentally marked by the pencil lead or indented by transmitted pressure.

LOADING

The cassette is placed face downwards on the bench and opened from the back. A film in its paper folder is removed from the box or hopper and held vertically at the folded margin. On the side nearer the operator the paper is drawn away from the film which can then be lowered gently into the well of the cassette and in smooth contact with the front screen. These two manoeuvres are illustrated in Plate 5.5, following p. 94 and Plate 5.6, following p. 94. The cassette is closed by bringing over the back and then locking the clips or bars.

For reasons of saving both money and space, many departments at present prefer to use film which is packed without interleaving paper between the sheets. In this case the above account must be modified in certain obvious respects. The guiding principle is still to avoid handling the surface of the film to any extent.

CHAPTER VI

Film Processing: Development

After an X-ray film has been exposed, it must be chemically treated or processed in order to produce a permanent radiographic image which can be viewed by transillumination. The complete processing cycle comprises development, rinse, fixing, washing, and drying; in many automatic processing units the rinse between development and fixing is omitted in favour of a squeegee action, but this is a special case and the rinse is normally an important part of efficient processing.

The object of the whole cycle is the production of a dry radiograph with an image which can be viewed, and can be kept without deterioration over a number of years if it is stored in satisfactory conditions. In this and the following chapters, the several stages of the processing cycle are considered.

THE NATURE OF DEVELOPMENT

Development is the first stage. This is the production of a visible metallic silver image from the latent one which exists in the sensitive material after exposure to light or X radiation. The fundamental change that takes place as a result of exposure and development is that the silver halide grains in the emulsion which have been exposed to light become converted to metallic silver, while those which have not received light remain largely unchanged. The conversion to black metallic silver accounts for the blackening of those parts of the film upon which light or X rays have acted.

In practice, the developer is not completely selective between those silver halide grains which have been exposed and those which have not. In time the developer will blacken *all* the silver halide grains. Anyone who forgets to take a film from the developer tank may obtain upon it an overall deposit of black silver which is convincing evidence of this eventual lack of selectivity. It is therefore more accurate to say that the function of a developer is to reduce to metallic silver the exposed grains of silver halide very much more quickly than the unexposed ones. Silver resulting from the development of unexposed grains is called *fog*. A good developer in this respect is one which shows the biggest difference in its action upon exposed and unexposed grains, and produces a radiograph with minimum fog.

A silver photographic image can be produced by the action of light alone without the aid of a developer. A piece of sensitive material left exposed without protection from light is seen to darken eventually, but the process is relatively slow. In most photographic materials the image produced by exposure to light *plus* the action of the developer is many times denser than that produced by the action of light alone. The developer may be said to amplify the action of the light and the result is that the sensitivity of the process is multiplied by a factor of about 1,000 million times; if the developer were not available the exposures required would be 1,000 million times greater than those in use. The developer is producing almost all the effect, the action of the light being one of initiation. This action is truly remarkable, for it can be produced by minute amounts of light; it is so important in beginning the formation of the image, but so slight that it produces no visible or measurable change after short periods of exposure. Photography is not possible without light or other activating radiation, but it is the use of a developer which makes it a practical proposition.

The Latent Image

The silver bromide crystals of a photographic emulsion consist of positive silver and negative bromine ions arranged in a geometric pattern known as a crystal lattice. When a silver bromide grain is exposed to light (or X radiation) the first occurrence is that some of the bromine ions in the lattice emit electrons. These electrons are able to travel through the crystal with great mobility (remaining within the boundaries of the crystal), and their extremely rapid movement carries them into what are known as electron-traps existing in the crystals.

An electron-trap is a region in the crystal of low energy called a *sensitivity speck*. These sensitivity specks are produced in the silver halide crystals during various stages of manufacture and effects on them occur particularly in the after-ripening stage of emulsion manufacture which was mentioned in Chapter 1. Electrons tend to collect at a sensitivity speck in the crystal, and they confer on the speck a negative charge; this grouping of electric charges at the sensitivity specks is a stage in the formation of the latent image.

The silver ions in the crystal have a positive charge. Not all the silver ions in the crystal are held in the lattice, some being free to move. Those that are able to travel are attracted to the negatively charged electrons in a sensitivity speck. The negative charge on the electrons neutralizes the positive charge on the silver ions, and when this happens silver atoms are formed. The silver atoms at the sensitivity specks increase in number. To recapitulate what has happened:

(i) Electrons (released by light from the bromine ions) are trapped by sensitivity specks.

(ii) Positive silver ions are trapped at the sensitivity specks by the negative charges on the electrons.

(iii) Positive charges on the silver ions are neutralized by the negative charges on the electrons and silver atoms form.

The sequence repeats itself and soon the sensitivity speck has a number of atoms of silver and is part of a photographic latent image.

This cycle of events takes place extremely quickly (one electron can travel to an electron-trap in 10^{-11} seconds), and even in a very short photographic exposure the sequence repeats itself many times. Nevertheless, unless exposure is greatly prolonged, the number of atoms of silver at each sensitivity speck is not enough for the presence of silver to be detected by ordinary tests. It is the action of the developer which most clearly reveals a difference between the exposed crystals which contain metallic silver atoms, and the unexposed crystals which do not.

The Action of the Developer

The basic action of the developer is to reduce to metallic silver the exposed silver halide grains in preference to unexposed grains. This reduction is achieved by the developer donating electrons to silver ions in the grains, thus neutralizing their positive charges and converting them to metallic silver.

As just explained an exposed silver halide crystal has sensitivity specks which contain atoms of silver. When the developer makes contact with this silver, it donates electrons to neutralize positive silver ions. This allows further silver ions to attach to the speck, and these in their turn are neutralized to metallic silver until eventually the whole crystal has become metallic silver. The negative bromine ions which formed the crystal lattice with the positive silver ions disperse into the developer solution as free bromine ions, for they have no silver ions to keep them in place.

The function of the silver atoms in the sensitivity specks seems to be to

make it possible for electrons from the developer to combine with silver
ions, and also to accelerate the process. Each silver bromide crystal in
the emulsion is surrounded by a negatively charged barrier of bromine
ions, and this of course will tend to repel electrons from the developer
and keep them out. An exposed crystal however has a gap in its complete
electron barrier where the latent image speck of silver has formed. This
allows the negative developer ions to penetrate at points where the
barrier of bromine ions is weak.

This explanation makes understandable the developer's ability to
select between exposed and unexposed grains. Only the exposed grains
have sensitivity centres which constitute weakness in the bromine ion
barrier; only the exposed grains have a combination of silver atoms and
attached silver ions. These facts increase greatly the speed with which a
developer can attack an exposed crystal and reduce the whole to metallic
silver, giving a black visible image.

This theory of the latent image and the action of the developer is
recapitulated below in general elementary terms in the hope that this
may be of help to the student.

Basic photographic action:

> Conversion of silver bromide ⟶ metallic silver.

(a) Initiated by light or X rays:

> Silver bromide = Bromine ions (negative) and silver ions (positive).

> > Bromine ions + light ⟶ electrons emitted.
> > Electrons + silver ions ⟶ silver atoms.

> These silver atoms begin to form the latent image.

(b) Continued by the action the the developer:

> > Developer ⟶ gives electrons to silver ions.
> > Electrons + silver ions ⟶ silver atoms.

Developer finds it easier to give electrons to *exposed* silver bromide
crystals; these have some silver atoms already as result of light action and
there are breaks in the negative charge round crystals containing these
silver atoms. Electrons from developer gain easier access and reduce
whole exposed crystal to metallic silver.

THE pH SCALE

This scale is used to express the degree of acidity or alkalinity of a
solution, and the student is likely to encounter it since pH values in

processing solutions are relatively critical. It will be considered before proceeding with an explanation of the constituents of developing solutions.

Probably even those of us with the scantiest chemical knowledge recognize that water is a neutral solution and that its chemical formula is H_2O. Water contains hydroxyl ions (OH) which are negative and hydrogen ions (H) which are positive. In pure water these two ions are present in equal concentrations. The concentration of each is 10^{-7} gramme ions per litre. This is the state of affairs in a neutral solution.

If the solution is made acid, the hydrogen ions are present in greater concentration than the hydroxyl ions; if the solution is made alkaline, the hydrogen ions are present in less concentration than the hydroxyl ions. A scale of acidity can be made based on the hydrogen ion concentration, and such a scale is the pH scale.

In a neutral solution, the hydrogen ion concentration is 10^{-7} gramme ions per litre, and the pH of a neutral solution is 7. So 7 is the neutral point of the scale, with the acids ranged on one side of it, and the alkalis on the other; for any given solution, the further away from 7 its pH lies on the scale, the more acid or alkaline it is. Thus:

Strongly acid	Neutral	Strongly alkaline
1	7	13

A pH 1 means that the hydrogen ion concentration is 10^{-1} gramme ions per litre; that is there are many more hydrogen ions than hydroxyl ions. A pH 13 means that the hydrogen ion concentration is 10^{-13} gramme ions per litre; that is, there are very much fewer hydrogen ions and many more hydroxyl ions. pH numbers below 7 mean greater hydrogen ion concentration, and pH numbers above 7 mean reduced hydrogen ion concentration as compared with a neutral solution.

The addition of an acid to an alkali lowers the pH towards the neutral 7; the addition of an alkali to an acid raises the pH towards the neutral 7. These therefore neutralize each other. In photographic processing, developers lie on the alkaline side of 7, and fixers are on the acid side of 7. Thus:

Acid fixing baths	Neutral	X-ray developers
5	7	10–11·5

Most radiographic developers function at a pH above 10, and require to be kept constant within 0·1 and 0·2 on the scale. Fixers are contaminated by developer carried into them, and in use their pH rises as the alkaline developer reduces their acidity.

The pH scale is logarithmic and small changes in pH mean large changes in acidity. On a logarithmic scale a change from 1 to 2 indicates an alteration which is ten-fold. In a developer this could mean a difference in activity between no development action at all, and an energy which fogged every film immersed in the solution.

THE CONSTITUTION OF DEVELOPING SOLUTIONS

Developing Agents

A developing agent is a substance able to change silver halide into metallic silver. The conversion of a salt or oxide of a metal to the metal is described as chemical reduction; the conversion of metals to their oxides or salts is described as oxidation. When reduction occurs atoms or molecules gain electrons; when oxidation occurs atoms or molecules lose electrons. From this it follows that when one substance is reduced by gaining electrons, another must be oxidized by giving electrons to it.

Photographic developing agents are thus chemical reducing agents. As explained in a foregoing section they neutralize silver ions in the silver bromide by donating electrons to them. Since the developing agents lose electrons in this transaction, they become oxidized in carrying out their function. An important characteristic in the reducing agents used in photographic developers is their ability to differentiate between exposed and unexposed grains of silver halide; lack of this ability would make a reducing agent totally unsuitable for use in a developing solution.

The activity of a reducing agent in donating electrons can be measured, and comparisons can be made between agents on this basis. They do not all donate electrons with equal freedom; those that do it readily are said to have a high reduction potential; those which do it less readily have a low reduction potential.

During the action of development bromine ions are released into the solution, and developing agents differ in their susceptibility to this increased bromide concentration. It has greater restraining action on some developers than on others; those which are readily restrained by it quickly become weaker in use as the bromide concentration becomes greater.

Numerous substances have been used as developing agents, and varieties of solution have been compounded for use in general photography. The properties of various solutions differ, though their basic components may remain much the same. It is the proportions in which these components are present which alter the results obtained. For student radiographers, however, there is no difficulty since the number of developing agents used for radiographic processing is very small.

METOL-HYDROQUINONE COMBINATIONS

For many years two particular reducing agents have been used together in one solution for the development of X-ray films (and also for general photography). These two agents (which are still in use) are Metol and hydroquinone, and solutions in which they are combined are known as MQ developers.

Metol and hydroquinone both achieve the same basic function common to all developing agents; they reduce silver halides to metallic silver. Yet they act in different ways.

Metol. This developing agent begins reduction readily, and will develop all exposed grains, including those which have received only slight exposure. Once the reduction is initiated, the process continues rather more slowly. Being susceptible to increased bromide concentration, Metol becomes weak with use relatively quickly. In the absence of any bromide to act as a restrainer, Metol tends to fog—that is it becomes unselective between exposed and unexposed silver halide grains in the emulsion.

Hydroquinone. This agent requires a strongly alkaline solution in which to act. It does not begin development so rapidly as Metol, and it has less effect on grains which have had little exposure. It functions to give high contrast. Once hydroquinone has begun to act on the exposed grains, development proceeds vigorously.

Since these two agents produce different effects it may be easily understood that when they are used in combination the solution could be expected to combine the characteristics of the two; and that alterations in the amount of each agent present could affect the result obtained. In practice there is a hidden bonus in using Metol and hydroquinone together, for the combination has photographic properties which are an improvement on the sum of those of each agent. Developers which contain Metol *and* hydroquinone produce a photographic density which is greater than the sum of two densities obtained by Metol and hydroquinone acting apart in separate solutions.

This phenomenon whereby we appear to get something for nothing —a combined effect which is better than the sum of individual effects— is known by the awkward name *superadditivity*. Not every combination of developing agents can form a superadditive system, but Metol and hydroquinone most certainly do. The phenomenon has been the subject of close investigation, and is one of the reasons why MQ developers have been so extensively used in photographic practice.

The mechanism of superadditivity is that hydroquinone regenerates the Metol in part at least, reacting with the Metol which has been oxidized in the action with silver bromide to re-form Metol and itself becoming oxidized in the process. MQ developers are still commonly used in powder form.

PHENIDONE-HYDROQUINONE COMBINATIONS

A developing agent was introduced in 1940 which in combination with hydroquinone has claimed attention and has been widely used. This new agent was first made useful by the laboratories of Ilford Ltd and has the brand name Phenidone. It shows many of the properties of Metol. It functions to give high speed and low contrast, and it tends to fog. It is not markedly affected by increased bromide concentration in the used developer particularly at pH values below 9·4.

Phenidone is frequently combined with hydroquinone in various types of developer. Such a combination is known as a PQ developer, and it shows certain advantages over the MQ type.

Phenidone and hydroquinone are superadditive together, but the bonus is even bigger and better than that given by MQ combinations, the Phenidone being from 10 to 15 times more effective. This means that smaller quantities of Phenidone can be used to achieve a given result. PQ developers are therefore usually cheaper than equivalent MQ compositions. Because only a little Phenidone in comparison with Metol is required, it is easier to prepare highly concentrated solutions. PQ combinations have therefore resulted in the use of more developers provided in concentrated liquid form.

Phenidone is regenerated by hydroquinone with greater efficiency than Metol is, and this prolongs the working life of the solution. Phenidone is much less susceptible than Metol to the restraining influence of the increased bromide concentration which inevitably occurs as the developer acts, and therefore PQ developers do not exhaust as quickly as their MQ counterparts. PQ combinations are less likely to stain clothes and hands, and carry less risk of causing dermatitis. It is not surprising that they are widely used.

Radiographic developers are compounded for high speed and contrast, long life and maintained activity. The developing solution needs more constituents than simply combinations of reducing agents if it is to act efficiently. These additional components will be considered now.

The Accelerator

In an earlier paragraph it was said that developing solutions must be alkaline. The pH of the developer has a significant effect on its activity, and variations in alkalinity alter the rate at which development takes place. Too little alkali results in the developer being sluggish in action; too much makes it over-active and uncontrolled so that it develops unexposed crystals and produces fog. A wide range of developers of varying activity can be compounded by adjustments in pH to the required level. The pH range of X-ray developers is 10 – 11·5.

Developing solutions therefore include an alkali so that they may react at the desired rate, and this alkali is called the *accelerator*. Certain developing agents need high alkalinity if they are to be active at all; hydroquinone is one of these, requiring a pH of at least 9.

The alkalis used in solutions for radiographic developers are sodium carbonate, sodium hydroxide, potassium carbonate, and potassium hydroxide. The hydroxides are strongly alkaline, and used in conjunction with the developing agent hydroquinone they result in a developer of high activity and contrast. Small amounts of the hydroxides are often added to the carbonates. The sole advantage of the potassium salts over the sodium salts is that their higher solubility allows them to be used in higher concentrations.

The Restrainer

To include a *restrainer* in the developing solution as well as an alkali to increase developer activity may sound like trying to drive a car with one foot on the accelerator, and the other just as firmly on the brake. However the manufacturers of these solutions can be expected to be more sensible than this, and there is in fact reason underlying the practice of including a restrainer.

One of the qualities of a good developing agent is its ability to act on the exposed silver halide grains very much more rapidly than it acts on the unexposed ones. The function of the restrainer is to check action on the unexposed grains, that is to prevent fog. It acts by increasing the barrier of negatively charged bromine ions which exists round the silver bromide crystals. This barrier to development (it will be recalled) exists in a complete state round unexposed crystals, and in a breached state in exposed crystals where a latent image is formed in the emulsion.

Without any restrainer the developer will be too active and will reduce the unexposed grains too readily. An excessive restrainer naturally is certain to check also the developing agent's effect on the exposed silver halide grains, and thus reduce desired developer activity. The solution must be accurately compounded so that the restrainer effectively minimizes fog during normal development, without unduly retarding the proper action of the developer which is sought. A correctly acting restrainer improves radiographic contrast by reducing or preventing fog. This is particularly important in the very low densities of the radiograph.

In Metol-hydroquinone combinations potassium bromide and sodium bromide are both used as restrainers, sodium bromide being used extensively in the U.S.A. In Phenidone-hydroquinone combinations it is essential to include in addition to the potassium bromide restrainer an organic restrainer such as benzotriazole, which is widely used. The PQ combinations are less sensitive than MQ systems to the restraining action of bromide, and a large amount of bromide would be necessary to restrain the highly active PQ developers. Organic restrainers can act efficiently at much lower concentrations than potassium bromide requires. They are also able to minimize fog effectively with less retarding action on the development of exposed silver halide grains; organic restrainers are known also as *anti-foggants*.

The Preservative

Developing agents are easily oxidized and readily absorb oxygen from the air. If nothing is done to check this, it shortens the life of the developer and discolours the solution. A chemical is therefore included which checks the rate of aerial oxidation, thus assisting to maintain the life of the bath and to prevent discolouration. This chemical is called the *preservative*. Sodium sulphite and potassium sulphite are both used as preservatives, potassium sulphite being used in liquid concentrate developers. The addition of a preservative to the developing solution does not entirely stop aerial oxidation, but it does reduce the rate at which it occurs and minimizes the more damaging effects.

As a result of being oxidized, either by air or as a natural consequence of normal developing action, developing agents produce certain oxidation products. Some of these can accelerate the process of further oxidation; the final products are insoluble and coloured, which accounts for the darkening of the solution. The action of the sulphite preservative is to form sulphonates with the early oxidation products. These are colourless and comparatively inert, so that the accelerating action is stopped and the dark final oxidation products are not formed. Radiographic developers contain a relatively high concentration of sulphite preservative, since a desired attribute is the ability to keep well over a period of time in which the solution will receive exposure to air during use.

The Solvent

The solvent used in making photographic solutions is almost always water, which has the advantages of being cheap and universally available. Unfortunately it is not universal in character as it comes out of the tap, for it then has dissolved in it various mineral salts. The nature and quantity of these depend on where the water supply originates and what treatment it is given.

However, in practice these dissolved substances are less of a photographic hazard than might be expected, and it is generally possible to use water from the tap with satisfaction. Distilled water of course is without dissolved salts, but the additional cost and effort of this process need not be contemplated when the tap water serves well, as is almost always the case.

The likely result of using water which is very hard (containing much dissolved mineral salt) is that the salts can react with photographic chemicals and produce precipitates. Such precipitates may form a chalky deposit or scum on the surface of films processed in the solutions. This will become obvious on drying and it is difficult to remove. Hard water can of course be softened before use by the addition of various agents which are available—for example the commercial product Calgon (sodium hexametaphosphate) in a concentration of ½ oz. per gallon. In practice however it is not essential to do this. Water softening agents are included in the composition of modern developers, and special treatment of tap water is necessary only in extreme cases.

It need hardly be said that water used for preparing photographic solutions must be clean and free from obvious insoluble impurities such as grit and rust or any other unexpected additions. Water which stands for long periods in copper pipes can be contaminated by copper; only a very small amount of copper present in the water used to prepare solutions leads to fog on films which are developed in them.

Other Additions

Developing solutions often contain further ingredients in addition to the basic group. These additions are for particular purposes, such as water softeners, wetting agents, and bactericidal substances. Some additions are provided in order to *buffer* the solution. A buffered solution is capable of accepting quantities of acid or alkali without much change in pH. Since pH values are so important in the activity of developing agents, adequate buffering helps to keep the activity stable; a later section (p. 123) explains the changes which occur in the developer with use and tend to alter its activity.

Buffering agents come in pairs. Examples are: sodium carbonate with sodium bicarbonate, and boric acid with sodium hydroxide.

Developing Solutions Summed-up

To sum up developing solutions, their ingredients can be listed as follows:

(i) Developing agents to convert exposed silver bromide grains to metallic silver.

(ii) An accelerator, which is an alkali, to give the developer the desired activity.

(iii) A restrainer, for example potassium bromide and/or benzotriazole, to minimize fog by checking action on the unexposed silver bromide grains.

(iv) A preservative, which is usually sodium sulphite, to maintain the bath by checking aerial oxidation and discolouration.

(v) A solvent, which is water.

(vi) Certain other additions, such as buffering agents.

Alterations in these constituents have the following effects:

(i) Changes in the amount of developing agent and in the ratio of different agents to each other in the solution alter the time needed to reach a given contrast and density—that is, they alter the development time required.

(ii) Change in the amount of alkali alters the time needed to reach a given contrast and density; increasing the alkaline content shortens the development time and decreasing the alkaline content increases the development time required.

(iii) Increasing the amount of restrainer reduces the fog level where fog exists, but results in a longer development time being required to reach a given contrast.

(iv) Alterations in the amount of preservative affect the keeping properties of the solution.

(v) Alterations in the amount of water naturally affect the dilution of the developer. The more concentrated the solution (until a certain limit is reached) the shorter the development time required. Manufacturers provide their products for use at certain specified dilutions, and these recommendations should be followed. A higher concentration may increase the fog level with little improvement in the contrast, and little shortening of the development time required. A greater dilution than that recommended lessens the activity of the developer, shortens its life, and can make it impossible to reach the required contrast however extended the development time.

THE DEVELOPMENT TIME

For some time now in manual processing the standard for developing radiographs has been immersion for 4 minutes in developer at a temperature of 68°F (20°C). (In the U.S.A. the standard is 5 minutes at this temperature.) This standard development time may not develop the film to the fullest contrast available, but keeps the fog level low.

Manufacturers recommend certain development times for specific materials in specific developers; they use sensitometric curves to derive the optimum development time. Characteristic curves of a particular material developed in a particular developer at a standard temperature for different times (Fig. 3.8 shows examples) can be used to plot more curves. These new curves show gamma, speed, and fog against time of development, and the recommended time is the one at which these quantities have optimum value.

The temperature of the solution alters the activity of the developer to a marked extent, and the developer is more active as it becomes warmer. Low temperatures imply long development times; if the developer is very sluggish at low temperatures (as some combinations are), even prolonged immersion of the film will not yield satisfactory results. High temperatures imply short development times; very high temperatures can result in fogging of the film, and in physical damage such as separation of the gelatin from its base.

The standard temperature of 68°F (20°C) is not unduly difficult to maintain in most conditions of operation in temperate climates. Automatic processing machines use temperatures around 80°F (27°C), and develop to an average of 120 seconds, but they are outside the scope of the present discussion which is principally concerned with manual processing.

Metol-hydroquinone and Phenidone-hydroquinone combinations should not be used at temperatures below 55°F (13°C). At high temperatures (above 100°F or 37.7°C) there is grave risk of physical damage to the film, even although modern emulsions are hardened in manufacture to minimize this. Within a certain range, if the developer is not at the standard temperature, adjustments can be made by developing for a longer or shorter period than the standard 4 minutes. Tables and charts have been drawn up showing the adjustments which are to be made (see Fig. 6.1).

Temperature of solution in °F	Required time of development in minutes
60	7
62	6
64	$5\frac{1}{4}$
66	$4\frac{1}{2}$
68	4
70	$3\frac{1}{2}$
72	3
74	$2\frac{3}{4}$
75	$2\frac{1}{2}$

Fig. 6.1. A typical chart showing the required adjustments in time of development at different temperatures in a correctly replenished developer.

In this connection it may be noted that different developing agents are not affected to the same extent by temperature changes. If a Metol-hydroquinone developer for use in standard conditions is used at a cooler temperature, the hydroquinone loses activity to a greater extent than the Metol, and results will be deficient in contrast. Below 55°F (13°C), hydroquinone has severe decrease in activity, but it is not true to say that below this level it does not act at all. At higher temperatures, the hydroquinone is relatively greater in activity, and the contrast in the results will be increased. This may be summed-up by saying that at the standard temperature recommended for use with a given developer, the agents in it have a balanced activity which is not maintained over a varied temperature range. The standard is chosen to give optimum speed from two different developing agents.

Modern X-ray developers which are commercially available are the results of sustained experiment and research, and are carefully compounded to meet the needs of the radiographer. They provide high contrast and speed, and give minimum fog; they keep well and have consistent activity when properly maintained; they are easy to prepare and to use. The developer should not be taken for granted. Like any other complex chemical substance, it should be treated with respect. Radiographic quality depends upon many factors, and the most careful technique in the X-ray room cannot succeed if the resultant radiographs are not developed in the optimum conditions.

TYPES OF X-RAY DEVELOPER

Concerning the various radiographic developers which are available, there are two distinct aspects which may be considered. These are (i) the form in which the developer is provided, and (ii) the work for which it is intended.

The Presentation of Developers and Preparation of Solutions

Developers are available in two forms. These are (i) dry powders from which solutions in water can be prepared; (ii) concentrated liquids which are diluted with water to form solutions of the correct working strength.

The dry chemicals are usually provided as two separate packs, one much smaller than the other. The small pack contains the developing agents, and the larger pack holds the other chemicals. The procedure is to dissolve *first* the contents of the small pack, and secondly the contents of the larger one in a certain volume of water (about $3/4$ of the total volume of solution to be obtained) at about 125°F (52°C).

The dry chemicals should be added gradually, with continuous stirring of the solution, and the contents of the small pack must be completely dissolved before adding any chemical from the second. Pouring the powder results in a certain amount of it floating about in the air;

this can be troublesome in a darkroom as the drifting chemical is a potential contaminator of films and screens and irritant to the mixer, who may inhale the powder. Any natural impatience to be finished with a tedious job must be mastered so that pouring is careful and slow. This reduces the nuisance of floating chemicals to a minimum.

The liquid concentrates are easier to prepare. The solution is simply diluted with a volume of water at working temperature 68°F (20°C) sufficient to bring it to the required working strength, and the concentrates are generally provided in volumes which make it easy to dilute to fill a certain sized tank. For example a concentrate might be supplied in a 5 gallon container for dilution with 15 gallons of water to fill a 20 gallon tank with solution of working strength; another might be supplied in a 1 gallon pack for dilution with 4 gallons of water to make 5 gallons of working strength solution.

This is certainly less time-consuming than dissolving dry chemicals, but it is important not to be led by its simplicity to evade the work of stirring. Thorough stirring is essential, and the least troublesome way of doing it is to use an efficient device such as a plunger—a broad perforated plate on the end of a metal rod. Most liquid concentrates now are packed in various plastic containers which are lighter to handle and less breakable than glass.

Available Developers

These are of different types intended: (i) for general use to develop all types of X-ray films, screen film, direct-exposure film, intra-oral films, and fluorograms; (ii) for use in rapid processing to meet the needs of operating theatre technique; (iii) for use in automatic processing machines.

DEVELOPERS FOR GENERAL USE

These are available as (i) developers of normal contrast, and (ii) developers giving high contrast. A developer of normal contrast used in the standard conditions of 4 minutes development at 68°F (20°C) gives a result of satisfactory contrast. (The expression *satisfactory contrast* may seem unsatisfactorily vague, but it is not possible to be more precise.)

A high contrast developer used in the standard conditions yields a result of perceptibly higher contrast. This is of value in medical radiography when the subject shows small differences of absorption of the X-ray beam (as in cerebral angiography for example). As well as giving high contrast in the standard time, these developers can be used to give average contrast in a shorter time—that is in 2·5–3 minutes at normal temperature. This obviously shortens processing time, and some departments with many films going through their darkrooms wish to avail themselves of this advantage.

Both these developers are designed to remain stable over long periods of time when correctly maintained, and to remain constant in activity.

DEVELOPERS FOR RAPID PROCESSING

Some applications of radiography require processing which takes very little time. The most familiar instance of this is the production of radiographs for use during surgical operations. Developers are obtainable which are specially formulated for speed; they usually have a higher pH than the general purpose developer. It might well be expected that with speed as the primary requirement, and the aim a radiograph to be viewed and used at once for a single occasion, some sacrifices could be made. Lower contrast, higher fog level, and poorer keeping properties for the solution could be tolerated, and in the earlier days of fast developers they were. Modern fast developers for theatre use, however, make minimum sacrifice of image quality, although the solutions do not keep so well in the tank as their general-purpose counterparts.

A later section (see p. 124 *et seq.*) describes the constitution of special replenisher solutions which are employed to maintain the activity of developers throughout their period of use. These replenishers can be used satisfactorily as rapid developers, and when this is done there is no need to stock a special developer for theatre processing. For example, a liquid replenisher concentrate in a 1 + 4 dilution (1 part of replenisher to 4 parts of water) used as a developer at 68°F (20°C), with 60 seconds immersion of the film, gives a result comparable with that of standard development; a 1 + 2 dilution (1 part of replenisher to 2 parts of water), used at 68°F (20°C) for 30 seconds immersion also gives an acceptable result. In Chapter ix there are some further remarks on rapid processing and a summary of available techniques.

DEVELOPERS FOR USE IN AUTOMATIC PROCESSING

Automatic processing is now in greatly increased use in X-ray departments, and the development technique applied in these machines differs from that of manual processing. Higher temperatures, shorter development times, and continuous agitation of the film are significant features in automatic processing. Some of the manufacturers market a developer specially formulated for use in their machines.

These developers may be MQ or PQ combinations. Since less

Phenidone than Metol is required to produce the same effect, it is possible to have more concentrated solutions with PQ developers, and this may help to shorten the length of time required in the processing cycle for development. What is termed a *starter* may be used. This starter solution may contain acetic acid and potassium bromide which serve to depress the very high activity of the developer solution in the first stages of its use, and thus to prevent the fogging likely to result from its energy.

The starter is added to working strength replenisher to give working strength developer which is used to fill the machine initially. During operation of the unit, replenisher is added to the developer tank by methods described in Chapter IX and Chapter X. Since the original solution is made up of replenisher plus a relatively small amount of starter, and thereafter only replenisher is required, just one developer chemical solution has to be stored in bulk. The solution stays in use up to 6 months.

The special chemicals which must be used in roller processors are further discussed in Chapter X.

FACTORS IN THE USE OF THE DEVELOPER

Certain conditions in the use of a developer alter the radiographic quality obtained. These conditions are:
(i) Temperature of the solution and length of time during which the film is immersed.
(ii) Agitation of the film during immersion.
(iii) Exhaustion of the developer.

Temperature and Time

The relationship between the temperature of developing solutions and the time of immersion of films has already been discussed. Adherence to the method of immersion for a certain length of time at a given temperature is known as the *time-temperature* technique of development. In the absence of automation it is the only way to achieve standardization, and is the most certain way of maintaining as regular practice a high quality in the image. It *should* be universal in all radiographic darkrooms.

Standardization in processing is necessary because there are so many variable factors in the radiographic image, and it is important that a given result is reproducible. Radiographs must often be compared to assess the advance or retrogression of disease, or used for comparisons between structures—for example the mastoid air cells on both sides in the same subject. If the available radiographs differ in image quality, comparisons between them cannot easily be made.

Another technique, practised but not recommended, is called *development by inspection*. In this, the radiographer takes the film out of the developer tank several times and visually judges (naturally without the benefit of white light) whether development has reached the desired level. When this point is considered to be gained, the film is taken out of the solution for the last time. No account is taken of the duration of its total immersion, and it may be that nearly as little attention is given to the exact temperature of the bath. This technique of course does *not* give a standardized result, for it is clearly subjective and variable.

T.A.Longmore once divided all radiographers into three groups; (i) a very small group which adhered undeviatingly to a time-temperature technique; (ii) a somewhat larger group which relied entirely on development by inspection, and probably did not even have an interval timer in the darkroom; (iii) the largest group of all which went into the darkroom with the *intention* of applying a time-temperature technique. Once closed up with the film they found themselves unable to resist making some inspection, and consequently took the film out of the developer if it 'came up quickly' because it had been radiographically overexposed in the X-ray room; or alternatively developed the film for somewhat longer if it had been underexposed.

The student is very likely to encounter this situation. A time-temperature technique is taught, and unfortunately in practice is frequently modified. The system has lived in use only because up to a point it seems to work (particularly where no proper replenishment technique is used) and films which would otherwise have to be repeated can be rescued from this necessity. Success in development by inspection requires considerable experience, and it is indeed regrettable that it can be achieved at all.

Fortunately with increased use of automatic processing the technique is becoming obsolescent and eventually will cease. Until that time it is perhaps true to say that the nearest approach to standardization in the darkroom with manual development is achieved by people with enough training to carry out the required manoeuvres, the temperament and inclination to do them precisely, untroubled by a sense of monotony, and absolutely no interest in the radiographic result. Or perhaps by hard-pressed single-handed radiographers who leave the darkroom carrying an interval timer to use the 4 minutes for some other job while the film is developing.

Agitation

Agitation of the film during development has two notable effects; (i) it increases within limits the rate at which development takes place, so that shorter times are required with more vigorous agitation, and (ii) it promotes uniform development.

Radiographs processed manually are suspended in stainless steel frames in a tank and usually given very little agitation. There is the disturbance of their entry to the tank and of their withdrawal, and that is usually as much agitation as they receive, apart from such movement of the solution as occurs with the entry and withdrawal of other films. The effect of agitation on development time is not a significant indication for its use in radiographic processing. Its influence on even development, however, is cause for regret that agitation is so much neglected. Even a slight agitation given 4 to 5 times during 4 minutes immersion would do much to lessen the risk of development marks which a static condition allows when films are developed in a vertical plane.

These marks can commonly take two forms. They are (i) light streaks or 'streamers' beneath heavily exposed areas of the film, and (ii) dark streaks particularly beneath areas which have been lightly exposed. The light streaks occur in this way.

In a heavily exposed area there is considerable reduction of silver bromide to metallic silver, and this is accompanied by the release of bromine ions. There is thus a local bromide concentration which has a restraining effect on development. Agitation would sweep this bromide concentration away, but a static state allows it to sink down and restrain the developer in areas vertically below regions of high exposure. These areas therefore show light streaks. PQ developers are less liable to show these effects than MQ solutions, since Phenidone is less susceptible than Metol to increased amounts of bromide.

The dark streaks occur in this way. In a static state developer from areas which are lightly exposed (this developer being largely unused) is allowed to drift downwards. Thus in regions vertically beneath these areas the developer is more active and dark streaks result. Agitation would sweep the unexhausted developer away.

Solutions which are not stirred properly also allow uneven development and the production of light and dark streaks. The object of agitation, whether of the solution or the film, is to give the developer equal access to all parts of the film at the same time, and to promote an even rate of development over the whole surface.

Exhaustion of the Developer

The activity of a developer decreases with use since the composition of the solution changes with use. Its whole function is to produce a chemical change in photographic materials, and not unnaturally the solution itself suffers chemical change in the process. It also undergoes change by aerial oxidation, and it is thus possible for a developer to exhaust with standing in an open tank.

The reactions involved are expressed below:

I Developer in use

Developing agents + silver bromide⟶
silver + bromine ions + hydrogen ions + oxidized developing agents

II Developer standing

Developing agents + oxygen⟶
oxidized developing agents + hydroxyl ions.

The following occurrences take place:

(a) Developer solution is taken out of the tank in the emulsion and on the surfaces of the film. This physically removes some amount of all the ingredients in the bath.

(b) The developing agents are changed by oxidation both in the normal developing action in which they reduce silver bromide to metallic silver and through contact with the air. There is thus constant diminution of the amount of active developing agent present in the tank. When all the developing agent is used up, the solution is completely exhausted.

(c) The oxidation products formed *may* retard the action of development. There is naturally a constant increase in the concentration of these products present in the tank. This effect, however, has little significance in reducing the activity of the bath in comparison with other factors mentioned under (b), (d), and (e).

(d) The bromine ions released with use as part of reaction I increase the bromide content of the solution. This exerts a restraining influence on developer activity.

(e) The alkaline content of the developer falls. Bromine and hydrogen ions are released in reaction I in the form of hydrobromic acid, and this is neutralized by the alkali present in the developer. This action uses up available alkali, and so the pH of the solution falls. There may be considerable reserve of alkali in the solution and it may be well buffered so that the pH is kept constant for some while, but in the end it is bound to fall. Since pH has marked effect on developer activity, the solution becomes less active.

(f) In the presence of reaction II, the sodium sulphite in the solution forms sulphonates and is used up doing so. There is thus diminution in the amount of preservative present; if the sulphite becomes completely used up, the remaining developing agents will be left without a preservative and will rapidly succumb to oxidation. As a result of the reactions taking place, there is release of sodium hydroxide in the solution and this tends to a rise in pH, which will *augment* developer activity and may increase fog level.

Aerial oxidation and oxidation through normal development action thus have opposing effects on pH. However when the solution is in use, the loss of alkalinity as described in (e) overwhelms the rise in pH that aerial oxidation causes. With this loss of alkalinity there are the other causes of reduced activity in the developer which have been shown. So used solutions are less energetic than fresh ones.

This means in practice that as the solution exhausts development times at a given temperature must be increased to reach a given contrast and density. In solutions which are nearly exhausted it may not be possible to obtain the desired density and contrast in the image, even although development time is excessively prolonged. However, for solutions only partially exhausted some compensation can be made for loss of activity by extending the time of development, or by raising the temperature.

Amateur photographers are advised to discard a solution after it has been used once, and this is reasonable practice for all occasional users of small tanks and dishes. In X-ray darkrooms a more satisfactory and economic answer is found by means of a system described in the following paragraphs.

THE REPLENISHMENT OF THE DEVELOPER

It is clear that maintenance of a developer bath in use for long periods of time requires two separate achievements. These are:

(i) That the level of solution in the bath or tank should be kept at its proper limit so that films placed in it are totally submerged.

(ii) That the activity of the bath should be kept constant. It is insignificant to the user if there are alterations in the chemical composition, provided that the activity and the results obtained do not change.

Distinction has been made between these two essentials. The physical maintenance of the level of solution has been called *replenishment*; the chemical manoeuvres required to maintain constant activity have been called *regeneration*. In radiographic darkrooms the common practice has been to use only the term *replenishment*; this means that a replenisher solution is put into the developer both to maintain its level and at the same time to regenerate it.

Factors Affecting Fall in Solution Level

Barring any accidents with plug-holes or similar disasters, the level is reduced mainly by solution being carried out of the tank when films are removed. The volume of solution removed for a given area of film put through the tank is known as the *carry-over rate*, which can be expressed with more convenience and fewer syllables as C.O.R. Radiographic darkrooms in general hospitals using manual processing seem to show a C.O.R. which varies from about 1 to about 2 ounces of solution per square foot of film put through. (In automatic processing the rates are very much lower, being about 0·5–1·0 oz./sq. ft. and at a minimum for roller-type machines; but these are not under consideration here.)

Some of the factors affecting the loss of solution are:

(i) Size of film and type of hanger.

(ii) Technique used.

(iii) Drainage time given.

SIZE OF FILM AND TYPE OF HANGER

Developer is removed from the tank (a) in the gelatin and on the surfaces of the film, and (b) in the hanger which supports it during development. Obviously larger films can be expected to remove more solution than small ones. In expressing the C.O.R. in oz./sq. ft. it is assumed that the carry-over rate is proportional to the size of the film, and in practice in most hospital departments this assumption is close enough to the truth to serve. In departments where the films used either are mainly small or are mainly large in size, this assumption holds a more significant degree of error.

The two types of hanger encountered are (a) the channel type which holds the film in grooves, and (b) the tension type which holds the film by means of a clip in each corner. Most radiographers answering from a general impression of experience would say that the channel type of hanger removes more solution than the clip type. In fact this is true, though the difference between them as found experimentally is not so great as might be anticipated, and oddly enough in practice the type of hanger used does not markedly affect the carry-over rate. The two remaining conditions are greatly more significant.

TECHNIQUE USED

The important points are these: Is the film put into the developer and taken out once only at the end of the development time? Or is it taken out several times during development to inspect progress? When it is taken out, does the solution carried on the film drain back into the tank, or is its destination disregarded and developer scattered impartially over any adjacent parts of the processing unit? Obviously the technique of development by inspection must lead to an increase in the carry-over rate, and combined with failure to let the drainings return to the tank it can result in a very high C.O.R. in some cases.

DRAINAGE TIME GIVEN

When films are transferred from the developing tank to the next stage of the processing cycle, they may be moved directly over or they may be allowed to drain before being carried over. There have been many opinions on the length of drainage time that should be allowed, and to review these discussions is not our purpose now. Perhaps all that need be said here is that a very short drainage time results in a high C.O.R.; careful drainage of moderate duration (say 5–10 seconds) results in a low C.O.R.; prolonged drainage may be tiresome to do, and consumes time; furthermore it can lead to excessive accumulation of bromide in the tank.

Individual radiographers adopt their own techniques. Doubtless in some cases they consider and rationalize their choice of drainage time, and in some cases they adopt short periods because they are always busy and are not prepared to spend time patiently holding each film over the tank of developer. Which technique they choose is less important than that it should be standardized as far as possible so that the C.O.R. in a particular darkroom does not show wide variations.

Since the factors which most affect C.O.R. are those relating to an individual's technique, they are susceptible to much variation and in theory are impossible to standardize. However in a given darkroom surprisingly it is possible to achieve what amounts to practical standardization. Perhaps for most of the time one person is undertaking the development, or perhaps a group of people are successfully adhering to a precisely stated technique.

Maintaining the Activity of the Developer

In order to maintain the activity of a developing bath, the solution added to it should counteract the effects of exhaustion. It should be added so that counteraction is at a rate that matches the rate of exhaustion and allows equilibrium to be achieved. If these conditions can be met, it is possible to maintain a developing bath in use without altered activity for an indefinite period of time.

It was once the practice to discard a developer and fill the tank with fresh solution when the volume of replenisher which had been added over a period of time was equal to that of the original developer. Thus the contents of a 5 gallon tank would be discarded when 5 gallons of replenisher had been added. This was known as 100 per cent replenishment.

In recent years replenishers have been studied and formulated on a more scientific basis than before. If they are used with care and added at the correct rate, it is possible to maintain a developer in use with replenishment to 500–1,000 per cent, the activity being unchanged. Experiments have been described in which given developers were kept in use for 1–3 years with a carefully adjusted replenishment technique. In practice most X-ray departments discard their developers after much shorter periods of time, and probably below 500 per cent replenishment. This is not for loss of activity of the bath, but because of other factors such as the advisability of cleaning out the tank. Prolonged replenishment saves the chore of frequently cleaning tanks but it is doubtless a malpractice to leave them uncleaned for long periods of time.

THE CONSTITUTION OF THE REPLENISHER
Given an understanding of the processes which occur in the developer during use, it is easy to see in general outline the requirements of the replenishing solution which is to restore its activity.

(i) Since the developing agents are used up, the replenisher should contain them in somewhat higher concentration than did the original solution. As it is mainly the hydroquinone that is used up, the replenisher contains more extra hydroquinone than extra Metol or Phenidone.

(ii) Since with use there is increased concentration of bromide which restrains the developer, bromide is not included in the replenisher. This does not really solve the problem of the formation of bromine ions, but at least it does nothing to aggravate it. Since Phenidone is less susceptible than Metol to the bromide build-up, PQ combinations are more easily maintained than MQ developers.

(iii) Since the pH of the developer falls in use, the replenisher contains a high concentration of alkali (usually sodium hydroxide) to offset this.

(iv) Since the preservative in the developer is used up, some extra sulphite must be included in the replenisher. Its presence prevents aerial oxidation of the replenisher as it stands.

(v) There may be other additions to maintain adequate buffering of the solution.

A replenisher is designed to be used with a particular developer, and modern replenishers are formulated with care and scientific understanding. They are available like the developers in powder form to be made up into solution, or as liquid concentrates, and they are used in the form appropriate to the developer to which they relate.

The liquid concentrates are now widely employed as they are so convenient; like the developers they need only dilution with water to the manufacturer's specification. A modern result of research into the developer and its appropriate replenishment is the formulation of a single solution which acts as a developer at one dilution and as replenisher at another; this is known as a self-replenishing developer.

USING THE REPLENISHER

A few paragraphs earlier it was stated that to maintain the activity of a bath of developer the rate of regeneration must match the rate of exhaustion. This is a crucial point. There are several factors which affect the loss of activity, and these factors are so variable that in theory a replenisher can be formulated only for a particular group of conditions. However, the manufacturer would find it impossible to sell a single replenisher formulation for his developer if this theoretical consideration were stringent in practice. Fortunately for those who manufacture and those who use the products, developer/replenisher combinations can be formulated on the basis of certain average conditions, and the prevalence of the average in practice enables the system to work very well indeed. Factors which affect the efficiency of replenishment are as follows:

The carry-over rate. This obviously determines the rate at which the level of the solution falls, and therefore determines the volume of fluid that must be put in to restore the level. The loss of activity of the developer however, is determined not by this physical condition, but by the amount of chemical work it has been required to do; this is the important factor in determining the amount of *regeneration* the developer requires.

Now clearly if the system is to function efficiently over a period of time these two factors must be in the correct relationship to each other. The volume of solution required to restore the working level must bring sufficient regeneration to match the loss of activity. If the operator in the darkroom removes films very carefully and drains them patiently, allowing the drainings to fall back into the tank and never inspecting the image during development, the fall in solution level will not be great. Not very much replenisher will be added, and if at the same time the developer is processing many films the result will be under-replenishment, and loss of activity in the bath. If on the other hand the operator is so energetically active in the darkroom as to spray developer liberally about with every removal of films, employs no drainage technique, and inspects frequently, then the fall in solution level will be great and much more replenisher will be added. This could lead to over-replenishment; though on the whole it seems the less likely situation of the two.

Knowledge of the C.O.R. is thus very important in the formulation of developer/replenisher combinations, and clearly the C.O.R. in any particular darkroom cannot be known by the manufacturer. Average rates, however, are known, and in hospitals an average rate of 1·5 oz./sq. ft. is assumed. It is possible to work to the manufacturer's directions satisfactorily with replenishers formulated on the basis of this average. It is clear, however, that a department with a C.O.R. very different from this average, or with a darkroom practice allowing of wide variations in C.O.R., could find itself in difficulty in the use of replenisher solutions.

The remaining factors affecting the efficiency of replenishment are concerned with the chemical work which the developer is required to do.

The radiographic subject and the film used. Since the developer's work is to reduce silver halide to metallic silver and it is required to perform this on *exposed* regions of the film, the amount of work it has to do varies with the radiographic subject. A posteroanterior view of the chest on a 12 × 15 in. film, two views of a metatarsus on a 6 × 8 in. film, a lateral view of the skull on a 10 × 12 in. film all contain less silver from the conversion of silver bromide than, say, an anteroposterior view of the elbow on a 6 × 8 in. film, or a study of the barium filled stomach on a 10 × 12 in. film.

Thus the amount of work done by the developer per unit area of film put through it depends on the radiographic subject. It depends also on the size of film used for that subject, and other such esoteric factors as the amounts of silver in the sensitive materials and the proportions of silver bromide and silver iodide in the emulsion. In a general X-ray department the proportion of silver developed varies over a considerable range with the different subjects examined. However, general departments are alike in handling more or less the same mixture of subjects, and any one department over a period of time uses only one or two types of film. For any particular busy department the average quantity of silver halide developed per unit area of film will be more or less standardized. An average figure of 30 per cent of the total available silver (taking into account the size of film generally used for particular examinations) can thus be assumed as a basis for formulating the developer/replenisher combination. Special departments such as chest clinics or obstetric units may find themselves too far from this average, and it will be necessary for them to keep this consideration in mind in devising their replenishment technique.

Technique of Adding the Replenisher

There are several possibilities here as considered below. One requirement is certainly common to them all; after replenisher is added the contents of the tank must be well stirred before films are processed.

(i) Perhaps the most common practice is to use the replenisher simply to restore the developer solution to the correct working level. This is done as necessary at the beginning and during the course of each working day, and the amount added is simply that required to allow the bath to cover totally the films put in it.

For such a system to be successful it is necessary, as has been seen, for the loss of solution from the bath to be matched to the loss of activity by the developer. Many departments act on the assumption that this is so, and find such a technique of replenishment satisfactory, the bath being maintained without noticeable alteration in its activity during the period of use.

(ii) Another method takes more account of the work done by the developer, and replenisher is added in relation to the area of film which has passed through the tank. After a certain area of film has been processed a certain volume of replenisher is added. If this is not enough to raise sufficiently the solution level, fresh developer is added; if it looks as if it will be too much, some of the used developer is taken from the tank and discarded. This naturally involves keeping records of the area of film processed, but it is not necessary to do this by recording the separate areas of all the film sizes used. The assumption on the basis of averages that 1 film = 1 sq. ft. gives sufficient accuracy.

(iii) If the replenisher is one of the liquid concentrates, the above method can be modified by adding to the tank a certain quantity of replenisher *concentrate* and bringing up the level by the addition of water. If the replenisher is designed to be normally diluted (1 + 4), then 30 oz. (1 ½ pints) of concentrate can be added for every 100 films processed.

(iv) It is possible by keeping records to calculate the carry-over rate in a given department. The area of film developed in a given period (say 1 week) divided by the volume of fluid added in the same period to maintain the level in the tank gives the C.O.R. in oz./sq. ft. If this is significantly different from the average, practical compensation can be achieved by using the replenisher at different dilution from the normal recommendation. A C.O.R. of 1 oz./sq. ft. would require a (1 + 3) dilution in place of the normal (1 + 4); a C.O.R. as high as 2 oz./sq. ft. would require a (1 + 5) dilution.

The foregoing paragraphs apply to manual processing. Automatic processing units have their own systems which are described later.

Sensitometric Control of Replenishment

The most satisfactory and positive way of checking the performance of a developer bath and assessing replenishment is by regular sensitometric tests. These are performed by means of radiographs of step-wedges of the type described and illustrated in Chapter III. Such testing can be done in the following way:

In addition to the step-wedge for the purpose of the radiographic exposure, a densitometer is required in order to be able to measure density in the result; the step-wedge should be a wide one. A radiographic exposure is made with such a wedge placed over the film. It should be positioned so that the longer dimension of the wedge corresponds with the longer dimension of the film. If a strip of completely radio-opaque metal is placed at one end of the wedge *across* the film (i.e. parallel to a short edge), it is posible to test for fog.

When it has been exposed, the film is cut into strips *along its longer dimension* (i.e. cutting parallel to its long edges), so that the result is a series of narrow strips containing all the steps of the wedge, plus a portion which has received no exposure because it was screened by the radio-opaque metal at the foot of the wedge. These step-wedge strips are developed one by one at intervals regularly during the period of use and replenishment of the developer bath, the first one when the bath is fresh.

On each strip, by means of a densitometer, the following are measured:

(i) The maximum density attained.

(ii) The contrast, this being calculated from the density differences between two steps of the wedge—two which represent mid-tones in the radiograph.

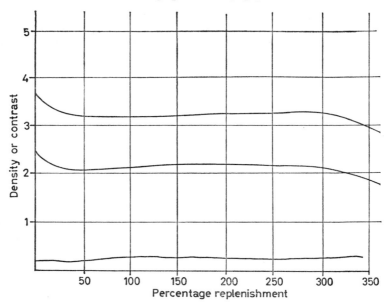

Fig. 6.2. Typical curves showing (upper curves) maximum density, contrast, and (bottom curve) fog plotted against percentage replenishment of a developer. It is shown that after an initial fall, contrast and density remain virtually constant until at 300 per cent replenishment there is a marked fall in both quantities. (These curves are hypothetical, and do not record the results of actual tests.)

(iii) The fog density, measured in the part of the film screened from exposure.

These quantities are then plotted on a graph against the extent of replenishment; Fig. 6.2 shows the type of result that might be obtained. If these values remain constant, the activity of the bath is being consistently maintained and replenishment is satisfactory. Inadequate replenishment is revealed by a slow drop in the contrast and maximum density obtained; over-replenishment leads to a rise in all three values.

X-ray departments in practice seldom perform these tests as routine checks on the performance of replenished developer baths where manual processing is used. With some automatic processing installations they are regularly done through the recommendation and co-operation of the manufacturer. The service provides a supply of previously exposed step-wedge films which are processed at certain intervals (say once a week) and sent to the manufacturer for sensitometric evaluation.

CHAPTER VII

Film Processing: Fixing

When a film is taken from the developer, the exposed and developed crystals of the silver halide emulsion have become black metallic silver and a complete image has been formed. The unexposed silver halide is not developed. It is practically insoluble in water, and at this stage remains in the emulsion as a light-sensitive material. If left there, it will darken and spoil the image when any prolonged exposure to light takes place.

The fixing process is therefore required to fix or make permanent the image by removing the silver halide, leaving the metallic silver image unaltered against a translucent background. The silver halide is removed by being changed to a complex silver substance. The compound formed is soluble in water, and it therefore dissolves in the water content of the fixing solution and is further washed away in a later stage of the processing cycle.

Secondary purposes of the fixing bath may be to stop further action by the developer absorbed in the swollen gelatin of the film, and to harden the film to prevent physical damage. Some hardening, as already mentioned, is done by the manufacturer who makes the emulsion, but it is helpful if the film can be further hardened while it is being processed; it is convenient to do this during immersion in the fixing solution. These secondary purposes will later be discussed in more detail.

INTERMEDIATE RINSE

In manual processing it is customary to use between development and fixing an intermediate stage known as a *rinse*. This is discussed in detail in Chapter VIII, and for the moment it will be left alone.

CONSTITUTION OF THE FIXING SOLUTION
The Fixing Agent

This is the constituent which converts the silver halide. To be suitable for the job the fixing agent is required to:

(i) react with silver halide to form a soluble compound;
(ii) leave the gelatin undamaged;
(iii) have no appreciable effect on the silver image;

Sodium Thiosulphate

The most commonly used agent for this purpose is sodium thiosulphate, known to succeeding generations of photographers as 'hypo'. In an earlier nomenclature it was given the chemical name hyposulphite of soda, but today this is considered incorrect. Although the formal name is now sodium thiosulphate, the old abbreviation is firmly fixed, one might say, in common usage. It may be wrong to the pedants, but every photographer knows exactly what substance you mean when you say 'hypo'.

The chemical action of the hypo with silver bromide is to form a somewhat polysyllabic compound. The reaction can be expressed simply thus:

Silver bromide + sodium thiosulphate⟶
    sodium salt of monoargento-dithiosulphuric acid + sodium bromide

Probably only a chemist can call this complex acid by name with familiarity. To remember the name is less important to a student radiographer than to realize the nature of this argentothiosulphate which forms: a soluble compound resulting when the fixer acts on silver halide. The solubility allows it to be removed by water.

Sodium thiosulphate can be obtained in two forms—crystalline and anhydrous. The crystalline form in smallish fairly clear crystals is cheaper, and is likely to be used by those making up their own fixing baths from separate chemicals. This is indeed a most uncommon practice in hospital X-ray departments today. Radiographers, however, may want small amounts of a plain hypo solution for after treatment of a film (see page 435 and following pages in Chapter xix). For this purpose crystalline hypo is likely to be obtained from the hospital pharmacy.

The anhydrous form is a fine white powder and is very suitable for the ready-packed chemicals for fixing baths which are commercially available. It has more hypo in less bulk than the crystalline form, and it mixes readily with the other constituents provided to complete the fixing bath. As fine powder to be dissolved in water, it has the disadvantage of floating about in the air which was mentioned in connection with the developer; when inhaled it produces an acrid taste at the back of the mouth which makes a tedious job actively unpleasant. Slow and gentle pouring with thorough stirring is well advised. Furthermore large amounts of hypo falling into the solution result in a cake of chemical most difficult to dissolve.

AMMONIUM THIOSULPHATE

In recent years there has been increased use in radiographic darkrooms of another fixing agent—ammonium thiosulphate. This is used in proprietary products supplied as liquid concentrates. To make a working solution these concentrates are diluted with a suitable volume of water according to the manufacturer's recommendations. The liquid concentrates are obviously more conveniently prepared for use than is the powdered form.

The reaction between ammonium thiosulphate and silver bromide can be expressed thus:

Silver bromide + ammonium thiosulphate—→
ammonium salt of monoargento-dithiosulphuric acid
+ ammonium bromide

It is thus similar to the action of sodium thiosulphate in that the result is an argentothiosulphate and a bromide which are soluble in water.

The ammonium complexes which form are less stable than the sodium complexes produced when hypo is the fixing agent. This is significant in practice from two points of view: (i) if the films are not completely washed, subsequent staining and deterioration in the image will be quicker in onset than if a hypo fixing bath is followed by inefficient washing; (ii) if ammonium thiosulphate fixers in use are splashed on to organic materials such as radiographers' coats, stains develop which are not removed by ordinary laundering. Their appearance is accelerated by the heat of the processes applied.

Ammonium thiosulphate solutions fix more rapidly than their sodium thiosulphate counterparts in equivalent concentration. Some rapid fixing solutions are therefore based on ammonium thiosulphate.

Other fixing agents are known in photography but they do not appear in radiographic darkrooms; here sodium thiosulphate and ammonium thiosulphate are the only ones used.

In addition to the fixing agents, other constituents are present in X-ray fixers. These are considered below.

The Acid, The Stabilizer, The Buffer

Development must not be allowed to continue in the presence of fixing agents. The function of an intermediate bath between the developer and fixer is to stop the action of the developer before the film reaches the fixing stage. Developer carried into the fixing bath in or on the film and continuing its action can have certain possible effects.

(i) Development continuing in the presence of the fixing agent can cause *dichroic fog*. This is an unmistakable stain which appears greenish-blue when examined by reflected light, and pinkish when viewed by transmitted light; hence its name which means showing two colours. The stain is really a deposit of silver finely divided, and it is produced by the action of the developer reducing silver salts which the fixer has put into solution. It can thus occur both when the fixing bath (which is usually acid) is contaminated by developer (which is alkaline), and when the developing bath is contaminated by the fixer. So it is sound practice never to let these two meet.

(ii) Developer transferred to the fixing bath can produce another type of stain—that of the brown final oxidation products of oxidized developer. This becomes particularly obvious under the influence of electrolysis which may be applied to the bath for the purpose of silver recovery. (Electrolytic silver recovery is discussed in detail later in this chapter.)

(iii) Prolongation of development after the film leaves the developer can produce streaks on the radiograph.

In order to preserve the film from these ills, it is usual to include in the fixing solution a suitable acid. Since the developer needs an alkaline environment before it can act, acidification of the fixing bath halts the further action of any developer which may be left in the film; some developer is *bound* to be carried into the fixing bath. The acidity of the fixer is important also in its effect on the efficiency of hardening agents as discussed in the next section.

Strong acids spoil hypo and precipitate sulphur with an accelerating deterioration of the bath. So a weak acid is used, and acetic acid is frequently chosen. There is still some tendency by the thiosulphate solution to decompose and precipitate sulphur, even although the acid is not strong. To prevent this, it is usual to include in the solution a preservative or stabilizer. This can be a sulphite, a bisulphite, or a metabisulphite; with acetic acid as the acidifier the preservative is often sodium sulphite.

An alternative method of providing for acidification and stabilization is to use one compound to do the work of two. Such a compound would be an acid sulphite such as sodium metabisulphite or potassium metabisulphite; these are commonly used.

There is another function to be considered—that is buffering the solution. The bath is acidified to a pH of about 4·5 to 5·0, but in use this figure tends to rise owing to the carry-over of some alkaline developer in the films. It is therefore general practice to buffer acid fixing baths so that the pH will be maintained. Pairs of agents used for this purpose are sodium acetate and acetic acid; and sodium sulphite and sodium bisulphite.

To sum up: (i) It is required to include in the fixing solution (a) an acid, (b) a stabilizer, and (c) a buffer. Some of the compounds used are able to serve in more than one capacity. (ii) A typical combination is: acid—acetic acid, stabilizer—sodium sulphite, buffer—acetic acid and sodium acetate. (iii) Sodium metabisulphite and potassium metabisulphite each can be used for the double function of providing both an acid and a stabilizer, and they have some buffering action as well.

The Hardener

The emulsion layer of a film absorbs moisture and swells during processing. As Fig. 7.1 shows, it can become several times thicker than it was in the dry state. This swelling is most marked during the water-

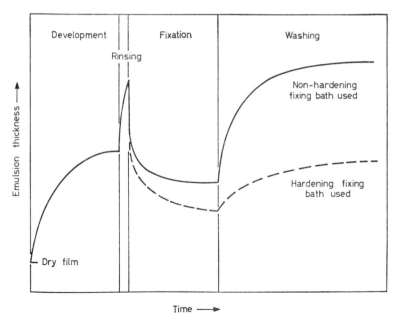

Fig. 7.1. Changes in emulsion thickness during processing. *By courtesy of Ilford Ltd.*

rinse and washing stages because where solutions have a high salt concentration (as in the developer and fixer) only a limited amount of swelling takes place. For the same reason, swelling is greater in soft water than in hard.

Hardening of the emulsion during fixing, as the graph shows, results in its being less swollen at the end of the wet processing cycle. Efficient hardening has certain beneficial effects.

(i) The temperature at which the gelatin softens is raised. This means that much higher temperatures can safely be used for drying films.

(ii) The gelatin absorbs less water, and therefore can be dried more quickly.

(iii) The film is much less susceptible to physical damage such as scratches, abrasions, and other marks on the surface.

(iv) The radiographs can be put safely through rapid driers at high temperatures.

All these are points of considerable practical importance. Shorter drying times are advantageous to busy X-ray departments, where almost anything is welcome that reduces the time-lag on the dry-to-dry film journey. Radiographs manually processed in large numbers, often at the same time and frequently sent wet to the hazards of clinics and out-patient departments, do not lead sheltered lives. Any process that armours them against damage is helpful.

X-ray films are hardened by manufacturers by means of hardening agents incorporated in the emulsion, but it is necessary to do some further hardening during processing if the desired results are to be obtained. Hardening *can* be a separate stage of the processing cycle, and it *can* be initiated during development as is done in automatic processing by roller processors. However, it is conveniently, commonly and in radiographic darkrooms universally done during the stage of fixation.

Hardening agents are incorporated as constituents in fixing baths; it is doubtless now clear to the student why a radiographic fixing solution is described as 'acid hardening fixer'. A solution containing hypo alone is called a plain fixing bath. As will be seen, the hardening agents used are effective only in acid solution, and this is a further reason for acidifying the fixer.

Three hardening agents have been used for fixing baths in X-ray darkrooms. These are (i) chrome potassium alum, (ii) potassium alum, and (iii) aluminium chloride. It is because the pH of the bath is important to these agents that the solution must be well buffered, so that it can accept without much rise in pH the alkaline developer which is carried into it. If the pH of the hardening fixing bath is too low, there is danger of yellow sulphur being deposited in the solution; if it is too high, hardening efficiency is lost.

The buffering of fixers used in automatic roller processors must be particularly good as the films pass straight from developer to fixer.

CHROME ALUM AS HARDENER

This for a time was commonly used and a fresh solution of it is a very efficient hardening agent, said to be more efficient than a solution of potassium alum. For radiographic darkrooms in which the fixing bath is expected to be maintained in use for a long period of time without renewal, chrome alum as a hardener has a great disadvantage; it does not keep its efficiency for more than a few days. Once the solution has been made up, this loss of hardening action will occur whether it is being used or is simply standing in a tank and the hardening action will fall to zero in a few days; it is a fact that very prolonged keeping will restore the hardening action, but perhaps this is not very useful in view of what happens first!

Chrome alum is therefore suitable for a hardening fixing solution which is to be used soon after preparation and not used for long. At the present time it is met in the fixing tanks of X-ray darkrooms less often than in fixing solutions for use in processing for operating theatre techniques.

Chrome alum is critical in its demands concerning the pH at which it works effectively and the range is 3.5 to 4.7. Above 4.7 there is little hardening action, and chrome alum hardens most efficiently at the lower pH; but where it forms part of a hardening fixing bath there is the risk of sulphurization at that level of acidity.

POTASSIUM ALUM AS HARDENER

At the present time this is the most widely used hardener in radiographic fixing solutions. It retains its hardening properties well with time, almost indefinitely, and has its greatest efficiency at a higher pH —from 4.5 to 4.9. At raised pH, hardening continues up to the region of 5.5 but it does not survive a pH above 6.

In acid hardening fixing baths there is danger at pH values beyond 5.5 that a white 'bloom' (a precipitate of aluminium hydroxide with potassium alum hardener) may appear on the film.

ALUMINIUM CHLORIDE AS HARDENER

This aluminium compound can be used in a concentrated hardener solution. It is normally associated with the rapid ammonium thiosulphate fixers and allows hardening to be completed in the very short time that the film remains in such a bath.

In the composition of any acid hardening fixing bath sufficient hardener is allowed for the bath to keep its hardening properties as long as it is in use, and for it to harden films efficiently during the length of time allowed for their immersion.

The Solvent

The solvent and diluent for fixing solutions is always water, and the reader is referred to page 113 where water as a solvent for photographic chemicals is discussed.

Other Additions

Boric acid is introduced into the solution to function as an anti-sludging agent. The sludge in question is the white precipitate which appears in fixing baths when the pH rises too high, particularly with potassium alum and aluminium chloride hardeners. Boric acid delays the precipitation of this sludge.

FACTORS AFFECTING THE USE OF THE FIXER

The first stage in fixing a film material is diffusion of the fixing agent into the gelatin of the emulsion. This is followed by a chemical action involving fixing agent and silver bromide and oxygen from the air to form soluble complexes and soluble halides in accordance with the relationships given on pages 134 and 135. These substances go into solution, and in the last stages of fixation are diffused to some extent out of the emulsion.

The process is accompanied by an observable effect—the disappearance of visible traces of the unexposed and undeveloped silver halide on which the fixer is acting. The milky-yellow regions of the image as it comes out of the developer vanish in the fixing bath, and the deposits of black metallic silver are seen, not against an opaque yellow ground, but on a clear transparent base.

When this observable effect is complete the film is said to be *cleared*, and the time which is taken by this is called suitably enough the *clearing-time*. The time taken for the whole process in its three stages is known as the *fixing-time*. In certain circumstances the clearing-time and the fixing-time can be considered to be the same. In practice radiographers, recognizing that it is difficult to say with accuracy when a film is wholly cleared, have followed the custom of leaving films in the fixing bath for longer than the clearing-time. The fixing-time is usually taken to be twice the clearing-time. A longer period of immersion not only allows certainty that the film is fully cleared, but permits effective hardening to take place; it has been said that 10 minutes' immersion should be allowed for maximum hardening; in potassium alum acid fixers 5 minutes is more than adequate.

It may perhaps be worth noting now what happens at the other extreme when films are given long immersion in a fixing bath—for example they are left for an hour or more or even are forgetfully abandoned overnight. Sodium thiosulphate given time exercises a weak solvent action on the silver image itself, particularly in an acid solution; ammonium thiosulphate can do this too, somewhat more quickly. The result can be a film which emerges from the fixing bath as a pale shadow of what it was when it went in.

Several factors affect the rate of clearing and the fixing rate. These are listed below.

(i) The type of fixing agent used.
(ii) The concentration of the fixing agent.
(iii) The temperature of the solution.
(iv) The presence of aluminium salts such as potassium alum or aluminium chloride used as hardeners.
(v) The film material—screen-type or direct-exposure film.
(vi) Agitation of the film during fixing.
(vii) Exhaustion of the fixing bath.

The Fixing Agent Used

We need be concerned here only with the two fixing agents which have been previously discussed—sodium thiosulphate and ammonium thiosulphate. As mentioned in the previous discussion, ammonium thiosulphate is more rapid in action than sodium thiosulphate when they are compared in equivalent concentrations.

The Concentration of the Fixing Agent

For wet films it is true to say that higher concentrations of fixing agent result in shorter clearing times. In normal conditions, however, there is not much difference between the fixing rates of a 40 per cent solution of crystalline hypo and a 60 per cent solution. In practice, sodium thiosulphate is used at concentrations of about 40 per cent of crystalline hypo, and ammonium thiosulphate at concentrations of about 15 per cent.

The Temperature of the Solution

Temperature affects the clearing-time, which decreases as the temperature of the solution is raised. Generally at higher temperatures diffusion processes take place more quickly and the gelatin is more readily permeable. It is, however, unnecessary to control the temperature of fixing baths in radiographic darkrooms as strictly as that of developing solutions. There should not be too marked a difference between the two, and obviously if the fixer is at too high a temperature the gelatin will swell too much, may soften unduly, and can give rise to many difficulties.

In practice, the optimum temperature for the fixing bath lies between 60°–70°F (15°–21°C). At 60°F the fixing-time allowed should be increased by about 50 per cent of the time allotted at 68°F (20°C).

The Presence of Hardeners

Potassium alum and aluminium chloride lengthen the clearing-time of solutions in which they are present. Where speed in fixation is a primary consideration—for example in radiographic processing for the requirements of an operating theatre—the rapid fixing agents which have been mentioned are often used. These proprietary products supplied as liquid concentrates may have the hardener solution provided separately so that it can be eliminated from the fixing bath; the fixing rate is increased as a result.

When a non-hardening fixer is used, the films must be hardened *after* they have been fixed. This is achieved by immersing them in the separate hardening solution or in a normal acid hardening fixing bath before washing, after they have been viewed in the theatre.

The physical hardness of an emulsion does not have much effect on the rate of fixation. An unhardened emulsion offers less hindrance to diffusion, but at the same time it is more swollen and diffusion paths are consequently longer.

The Type of Film Material

Various features of a photographic emulsion alter the rate at which the material clears. These are: (i) The silver halide used: silver bromide fixes more quickly than silver iodide. (ii) The grain size: small grains not unexpectedly dissolve in less time than larger grains. (iii) The thickness of the emulsion layer: since most of the fixing time is taken up by diffusion of soluble salts out of the emulsion layer and not by chemical action, and since diffusion can take place more rapidly in thin layers, thinly coated materials clear more quickly.

The operation of these facts is doubtless appreciated by radiographers who see them in practice. We soon realize as a matter of experience that screen-type film clears more quickly than direct-exposure film, and that the fine-grain materials which may be used for fluorography clear more rapidly than either of the others. Different proprietary brands of film can differ greatly in clearing-time.

Agitation of the Film

Since the fixing process mostly depends on diffusion, agitating the film increases the rate at which it clears. Agitation prevents the collection of a layer of exhausted fixer near the film surface; fresh fixer can then swirl against the film and will significantly decrease the time required for clearing.

Most radiographers at one point or another have stood in darkrooms and vigorously agitated in the fixing bath a film which they wished to clear and view quickly. Apart from this, many radiographs manually processed receive little agitation in the fixer. Lack of agitation in the early stages is regrettable. If the film is agitated in the first few seconds of its arrival in the fixer bath, any developer carried with it is soon neutralized.

Exhaustion of the Fixing Bath

Practical experience again soon teaches us that a used fixing bath takes longer to clear films than a fresh one does. Indeed this longer time is taken as an indication of the state of exhaustion of the bath. With use the following changes occur in the composition of the solution and slow its action:

(i) There is increasing dilution of the bath as water from the rinse is carried in and fixer is carried out with the passage of films. There is thus reduction in the concentration of hypo; another cause of reduced concentration is that the fixing agent is used up. From either cause this decreased concentration materially affects the clearing rate.

(ii) There is steady accumulation of soluble silver complexes—the argentothiosulphates resulting from the reactions on pages 134 and 135. When these compounds are in solution silver ions are liberated, and the presence of these ions retards the chemical action.

(iii) There is steady accumulation of soluble halides in accordance with the previously mentioned reactions. In fixing solutions used for processing radiographs, these halides will be bromides and iodides. Both slow down the fixing action, particularly the soluble iodide even although it may be present in a very small amount.

REGENERATION OF THE FIXING BATH

The Effects of Exhaustion of the Fixing Bath

The points in the previous paragraph relate to the fact that as the fixing bath is used it becomes much weaker in its action. From what has been said previously it will be realized that this is not the complete picture of what is happening. To sum up, the effects of using a fixing bath which is nearly exhausted are:

(i) Slow clearing-time and eventually inadequate fixing. There is a tendency for the film to retain unfixed silver halide and unstable silver complexes which may not be eliminated by washing. The end result possibly is a stained film.

(ii) The film may be inadequately hardened.

(iii) The film may have developer stains.

(iv) The film may be marked with deposited scum.

Estimation of Exhaustion of the Fixer

The duration of useful life for a fixing bath depends upon the following factors:

(i) Number of films passing through the solution.

(ii) The silver halide content of the emulsions which are processed. This refers to such matters as the amounts of silver, and silver bromide/iodide ratios in the materials used.

(iii) The area of silver halide which is left for removal in the fixing bath. It will be recalled from the previous chapter that different radiographic subjects result in different amounts of silver halide being made developable; the rest must be removed in the fixing bath. It is said that in 'the average radiograph' in a general X-ray department about 2/3 of the silver halide is not developable and is removed in the fixing solution.

(iv) The operator's technique. Dilution of the bath by the transfer of rinse water into it and of fixer out of it with the passage of films will vary. An operator who drains the film carefully over the rinse and over the fixing bath in turn, so that the drainings return to their source, will minimize (but not prevent) this dilution.

One way of estimating the exhaustion of the fixing solution is to record the number of films which pass through it, and then discard the bath when it has dealt with a certain number; for example 400 films of 10 × 12 in. size, or their equivalent, through a 10 gallon tank. Because the number of films fixed is only *one* factor in its exhaustion, and the others as previously listed are variable, this method of determining exhaustion may be misleading.

A modification of it dispenses with the record-keeping, and the fixing bath is simply renewed at a regular *time*—for example every Monday morning the X-ray department begins its week's work with a fresh fixing solution. One week's work has very much the pattern of all the others, the number of different emulsions used in any one department at a given time is not great, and the number of films processed does not vary very much from week to week. All these considerations make it possible to relate the probable exhaustion of the fixer simply to the length of time it has been in use in a radiographic darkroom. This method is a reasonable one, giving satisfactory results, but it is not economical.

Increase in clearing-time is commonly used as indication that the fixer is exhausted. A bath is said to be exhausted when it takes twice as long to clear a film as when it was fresh. In practice a fixing solution can be used satisfactorily when its clearing-time is longer than this, and to discard the bath when its clearing-time has doubled certainly gives a generous margin of safety.

Regenerating the Fixer

Something is being done to prolong the life of a fixing bath if it is replenished with a solution containing:
(i) the fixing agent to make good the effects of dilution;
(ii) an acid to counteract the decreasing acidity;
(iii) a hardener to offset the loss of hardening power;
(iv) a sulphite to maintain the quantity of preservative since this is falling with oxidation.

Despite this regeneration, the used solution continues to accumulate soluble silver complexes. Unless a means of removing the silver content is employed, it is of little value to attempt to maintain the bath in efficient activity simply by adding to it fresh acid hardening fixer. Its fixing-time will become inconveniently prolonged, and the presence of a high concentration of soluble silver complexes can result in stained films. Test papers can be bought which will indicate the silver content of a used fixer.

Methods *are* available for removing silver during use of the bath, and these will be considered in more detail shortly. For the present it can be said that in radiographic darkrooms using manual processing, the practical answer found to the problem of fixer exhaustion depends on whether silver recovery during use of the bath is practised. The situation is summarized below.

WITHOUT SILVER RECOVERY DURING USE

The bath is discarded when it is considered to be exhausted on the basis of one of the following: (i) after a given period of time; (ii) when it has fixed a given number of films; (iii) when its clearing rate has become greater than that of the fresh solution by a given number of times —perhaps twice, which gives a good margin of safety. Method (i) is the least sound economically.

The two-bath technique. This is a procedure frequently used to ensure that fixing will be complete; it may incidentally extend the effective life of the bath. *Two* fixing tanks are used; the system is first begun by preparing and filling *both* with fresh solution. When radiographs are removed from the developer, they are put in tank A after the rinsing stage, and they are left in tank A until they have cleared. They are then transferred to tank B for an equal period.

Tank A is doing most of the work, while the contents of tank B remain relatively fresh since it is doing little but remove soluble silver compounds which are still in the gelatin. When tank A is considered exhausted it is discarded and a new bath is prepared. Tank B now is used for first immersion of films coming from the developer, while tank A with its fresh solution assumes the secondary role. In its turn tank B is discarded, and is refilled with fresh solution; tank A is brought back to first place in use, and the cycle begins to repeat itself. This technique ensures both efficient fixing and economy in the use of chemicals.

It is common practice to subject *discarded* solutions to one of the methods of silver recovery, since not to do so is in effect to throw money with the solution down the drain. The high value of silver and the large volumes of used fixer from radiographic darkrooms have made the recovery of silver economically a worthy procedure.

As the bath is not for further photographic use, silver can be recovered from it by what is known as sludging; in this method chemicals are added to the exhausted solution, and silver is precipitated. For example, the addition of sodium sulphide to a used fixing bath which has been made alkaline precipitates silver sulphide; sodium hydrosulphite added to an alkaline fixer precipitates finely divided metallic silver. The fixing solution is made alkaline first in order to avoid the production of hydrogen sulphide, an evil-smelling gas to which photographic materials are sensitive. Another method involves precipitation by metals; iron and zinc, added to the solution as iron filings or zinc dust, deposit silver as they dissolve. The precipitates which result from these reactions can be removed from the vessels in which the action takes place and can be sold to a silver refiner.

X-ray departments do not undertake their own sludging. The process is as unattractive as it sounds, and in hospital there is usually lack of time and space in which to do it. Instead discarded fixer is often kept in a container to be collected regularly by silver refiners, who pay the hospital an appropriate sum of money for the transaction.

WITH SILVER RECOVERY DURING USE

If an electrolytic method is used to recover silver from the fixing solution during use, the bath can be successfully regenerated. This allows the bath to be used for extended periods without fixing-times which are inconveniently long and with much less risk of staining. A regenerated bath in these circumstances shows clearing-times which are somewhat longer than those of a fresh solution; but it is a stabilized clearing-time which shows no further increase while the bath is used.

The bath is replenished by adding the normal acid fixing salts with hardener which are commercially available, and from which the bath was originally prepared. The use of these ensures that the fixing salts are added in concentrated form, either as dry powder or as liquid concentrate. Furthermore, other components—the acid, and the hardening and preservative agents—are included with the fixing salts. Where the commercial preparation is accompanied by the hardener as a separate pack, this is added with the replenishing fixer in the same proportion as in the bath originally prepared.

With this system of regeneration, careful checks on the acidity of the bath are required. Further details of regeneration technique connected with silver recovery are explained in the next section.

SILVER RECOVERY

There are various methods by which silver can be recovered from used fixing solutions. Radiographers need concern themselves simply with those likely to appear in X-ray departments, and there are two general methods to be considered. These are:

(i) Electrolytic recovery. This can be carried out while the fixing bath is in use.

(ii) A metal exchange method which is used to recover silver from the overspill of fixing solutions issuing from automatic processing units in operation. This method causes chemical change which spoils the fixer for further use.

Electrolytic Silver Recovery

Electrolytic silver recovery sounds a simple process indeed, for it entails putting two electrodes into a silver-salt solution and establishing a voltage between them. Silver then plates out upon the cathode.

The process is a straightforward one when the solution for electrolysis contains a simple silver salt in which the silver is present in the form of positively charged silver ions. The silver ions are naturally attracted to the cathode, their charge is there neutralized, and silver is deposited. It requires only a small potential difference to be maintained between the electrodes, and the greater the electrolytic current flowing the more rapidly is silver deposited.

The first problem in electrolysis of a used fixing bath is that the silver which loads it is not a docile positive ion. It will be remembered that we are dealing here with complex argentothiosulphates in solution. The ions involved are negatively charged, and will migrate not towards the cathode but away from it (Fig. 7.2).

These complex ions do make some concessions in so far as they undergo dissociation, and give rise to a very small proportion of positive silver ions. These few positive ions move to the cathode, and silver is deposited. As these few silver ions are reduced, there is further dissociation to a limited extent to make up their number, and thus a slow continuous deposition of silver can theoretically take place.

It can be seen, however, that the reluctance of the complex argentothiosulphate ions to approach the negative electrode results in a deficiency of them in the region of the cathode, and a deficiency also of the positive silver ions which they produce on dissociation. The cathode therefore will quickly be at a loss for silver ions. Since it is a determined acceptor of positive ions, in the absence of silver the cathode attempts to plate out some of the thiosulphate ions of the fixing salt itself. This has a disastrous result, for the thiosulphate ions break up. One of the products formed is silver sulphide, and this has the power to react with

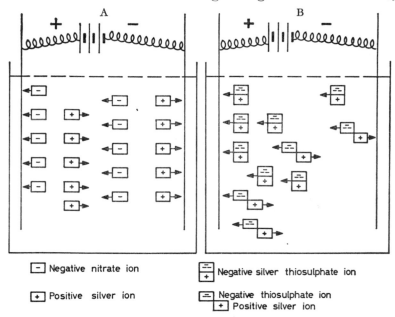

Negative nitrate ion

Positive silver ion

Negative silver thiosulphate ion

Negative thiosulphate ion
Positive silver ion

FIG. 7.2. A: electrolysis of a simple silver salt solution (silver nitrate). B: electrolysis of a used fixer.

In the used fixer the complex silver thiosulphate ions are negative and are attracted to the anode. They can dissociate to give a small proportion of positive silver ions.

unexposed silver halide. Films put into a fixing bath where silver sulphide has formed become the victims of sulphide fog. The fixing solution is soon unusable and must be discarded, an expensive, wasteful, and exceedingly trying necessity.

These disasters are avoided in a solution which is violently agitated all the time that silver recovery is in progress. Agitation forces the argentothiosulphate ions to go where they are wanted—towards the cathode—and this reduces the risk of sulphiding which is promoted by lack of silver ions near the negative electrode.

It is difficult in practice to arrange to fix films and at the same time to agitate the solution, and for many years electrolytic silver recovery did not appear in hospital darkrooms. Only large photographic concerns, for example those of the motion-picture industry, would embark on the costly equipment and the multiplicity of tanks required so that films could be fixed in one tank, and silver recovered in another.

However, in 1937 it was discovered that sulphiding can be avoided in a static bath provided that the potential difference between the electrodes is kept sufficiently low, there being critical levels of voltage at which sulphiding begins. Following this, the development of equipment suitable for use in the radiographic darkrooms of hospitals made forms of electrolytic silver recovery commonplace in X-ray departments.

A silver recovery unit consists of an electrode assembly inserted in the fixing solution, and a control box which operates from the alternating current mains. Equipment within this box supplies unidirectional current at the required voltage for the electrodes, and a means is provided for controlling current and/or voltage. Current (and in some cases voltage also) is recorded on a suitable meter on the control box. The complete control assembly can be fitted conveniently to the darkroom wall.

Low Current Silver Recovery

As has been shown, it is important that the potential difference between the electrodes is kept low when the solution is static. The electrodes may take the forms of a separate anode and cathode placed at opposite ends of the tank, or sometimes they are put together in a single assembly, the cathode being placed round the anode. The metal cathode is large in area—it may be a stainless steel plate or a sheet of silver gauze—and the anode is usually a carbon plate or rod. Large cathode area allows higher current to be used, and increases efficiency in the process (Plate 7.1, following p. 94.)

These electrodes are in full-time occupation of the fixing tank, and it is therefore important that they should take up as little space as possible. This is an obvious limit on cathode size. Details of design show marked variation, and some units demand more space than others. Two electrodes in a single assembly may take up less space than separate ones on the opposite sides of the tank, but they present problems for their cleaning and servicing. Separate electrodes may result in more efficient recovery of silver since the electrolytic action involves the whole tank, instead of a small volume between the anode and the cathode.

These units work at potentials of up to 500 millivolts. It is not possible to give a certain voltage as a fixed figure above which sulphiding occurs, for the value depends on several variables. These include factors which vary with the amount of work the fixer is required to do.

With features of a unit's design and circumstances of its use, the current varies greatly. A wide range of currents seems to be employed, and figures from 0·04 to as high as 0·8 amps have been mentioned; the meter is scaled usually in milliamperes. In relation to the area of the cathode, the current-density should be one or two milliamperes per square decimetre of cathode. Larger cathodes clearly allow the use of higher currents without rise in current-density above this figure. The student may see these units described as low current-density units.

If the current is too low, the results are what we might expect. Silver is not being recovered at a sufficiently high rate and builds up in the bath, retarding the chemical action and leading to markedly increasing clearing-times. Too high a current can lead to sulphiding of the bath. The symptoms in this condition are that the silver deposited on the cathode looks grey-black and loose, the fixer looks dark brownish-black, and there is an unpleasant smell. Firm white or cream silver on the cathode is a healthy sign, and indicates that the current is at a correct value for the conditions of use. (Brown colouration of the fixer is not of itself a cause for alarm, since the solution can receive this tone from the coloured oxidation products of developer carried into it.)

For any electrolytic silver recovery to be really efficient, silver should be recovered at a rate matched to that at which it forms. Any slower rate than this is wasteful; some of the fixing solution is always carried over to the wash tank with passage of films, and the higher the concentration of silver carried with it the more wasteful the process is in terms of hard cash. It does not seem possible to make low current-density units highly efficient, owing to the lack of agitation to keep plenty of silver ions near the cathode.

In certain cases some degree of agitation has been provided. One method is to put the fixer into motion by bubbling nitrogen through it, but in one trial this was not found to improve efficiency to a great extent. This may have been because the level of agitation cannot be very high in a tank in which films are being processed simultaneously with the agitation.

In Chapter XI darkroom design is discussed, and it is mentioned that a pass-through tank can be used to pass films from the darkroom into an adjacent viewing room. This pass-through tank can be a fixing-bath or a washing–bath. If a fixing-bath, then it cannot be used to contain electrodes for silver recovery. The problem has been met by inserting the electrodes in a small tank adjacent to the pass-through tank, the fixer being circulated between the two by means of a pump. The function of the pump is not to agitate the fixer in order to improve silver recovery, but simply to circulate the solution between the tanks and it is not highly active motion. It probably does little to improve efficiency in recovering silver.

HIGH CURRENT SILVER RECOVERY

Some years ago a unit was introduced which was designed to apply violent agitation, and to use a high current-density so that silver could be recovered at a more rapid rate. The agitation is achieved by a cathode in the form of a screw which is rotated at high speed when immersed in the fixer. This cathode is a strong construction in stainless steel. Four carbon rods for anodes are set vertically round it at the four angles of a square formation. The whole assembly is surrounded by a protective cage (Plate 7.2, following p. 94).

The rotation of the screw forces a stream of solution vertically downwards, and the liquid in the whole bath is kept in brisk motion. This unit is an efficient one. Running at a current up to 3 amps, it gives a good recovery rate, but time and care must be devoted to it if it is to operate at maximum efficiency.

It is not possible to use the tank for fixing films while this unit is in action. It has therefore been employed to recover silver during the night and at week-ends when no films were being processed. This has been a satisfactory routine, for the high recovery rate allows the silver concentration in the bath to be kept to a low level even with an intermittent recovery. To meet the common problem of a darkroom which never stops work through the demands of an emergency service, a two-tank system can be applied. One tank is in use for films and the other is subjected to silver recovery, with alternation of their roles. Care should be taken not to recover too much silver by these methods.

To sum up these electrolytic methods of silver recovery:

(i) Low current-density units can be used, with little or no agitation, and may be operated while the bath is in use.

(ii) High current-density units can be used, with brisk agitation and with greater efficiency, but without use of the bath during recovery.

(iii) Several makes of unit are available. They have differences in design and their own advantages and disadvantages. Actual techniques of use show considerable variation; so also do the proportions of silver recovered per unit area of film, different techniques giving very different results.

FACTORS WHICH AFFECT SULPHIDING DURING SILVER RECOVERY

The first of these is electrical and the remainder are chemical in nature.

(i) The current-density. This has already been discussed, and the salient facts are repeated now. In the absence of brisk agitation, any attempt to recover silver too rapidly by an increase in current can lead to sulphiding and deterioration of the bath. Where violent agitation is applied, a higher current-density can be used with safety.

(ii) The silver content of the bath. When there is little silver anywhere in the bath, sulphiding is very likely to occur. There is a certain minimum concentration of silver below which this disaster is a certainty at even the lowest current-density, or with the greatest agitation. This is why it is important not to attempt to recover silver from a fresh fixing bath. Only use can load it with silver; it is general practice therefore for a fresh fixing solution to be in service for a day or two before the silver recovery unit is switched on. Similarly it is important during periods when the tank is not in use and not accumulating silver, either that the recovery unit should be switched off, or that the current should be reduced to half its normal value. If these procedures are not followed, the silver concentration in the bath may fall to a dangerously low level. The safe minimum concentration has been given as 2 g/litre; in practice silver recovery units are often operated so that concentrations do not fall below 5 g/litre, and they are frequently much higher than this. As said earlier, test papers are available for estimating the silver content of the fixer. They can be used to determine (a) whether the silver content has reached a level that makes silver recovery desirable, and (b) whether the silver recovery unit has operated to bring the silver content down to the required low value.

(iii) The sulphite concentration. If this is high there is less tendency for the sulphiding reaction to take place. In use of the bath, the concentration of the preservative falls with oxidation, but it is not likely to fall to a critical level in view of the fact that the technique of regeneration adds sulphite with other constituents of the fixing solution.

(iv) The pH of the bath. The optimum value seems to be one not greater than 5, so pH values which ensure adequate hardening are also helpful in not promoting the sulphiding reaction.

REGENERATION TECHNIQUE

When an electrolytic silver recovery unit is working satisfactorily, re-generation of the bath can be accomplished with relative simplicity. It may be useful to enumerate again the important changes which occur during use.

(i) Increasing dilution of the bath, and thus a fall in concentration of the fixing agent.

(ii) Steady accumulation of silver complexes.

(iii) Steady accumulation of soluble halides.

(iv) Loss of acidity by transfer of alkaline developer.

It is now clear that the argentothiosulphate build-up under (ii) is dealt with by the silver recovery unit. Soluble halides increasing under (iii) cannot be treated, as it is not practical to attempt to remove them from solution. The clearing-time gradually increases to something greater than it was when the solution was fresh, and with regeneration the bath reaches a stage of equilibrium in which the concentration of soluble halides does not rise, and clearing-times do not increase.

In carrying out regeneration with electrolytic silver recovery, the practical procedures necessary are to deal with (i) and (iv) by maintaining (a) the concentration of fixing agent, and (b) the correct acidity.

Maintaining concentration of the fixing agent. When the fixing agent is present in less concentration, there is alteration in the specific gravity of the solution. Test of the specific gravity is a simple and satisfactorily exact method of determining when additional fixer must be put into the tank. If the fixing agent is added in the form of a packed proprietary agent, then other required ingredients for the fixing solution (whether they are all in one pack, or provided in 2 or 3 separate packs) are added at the same time. We need not worry then about decreased concentration in respect of the hardener and preservative.

The method is to test the specific gravity when the fixing solution is fresh and has not been used; it is then checked regularly during the week. The exact intervals will be determined by working conditions and the number of films processed in the fixer; it might, for example be every third day. When the specific gravity has fallen by a certain amount, a given quantity of fixer is added. As an instance, a certain commercially available acid fixing salt with hardener (prepared as a single powder) has specific gravity 1·170 when it is freshly made. The manufacturers recommend that when this has fallen to 1·155, the contents of a gallon tin of the powder should be added to a 10 gallon fixing bath. This will restore the specific gravity to 1·170. This method eliminates guesswork from the procedure.

The commercial preparations will be added either as powders or as liquid concentrates. Powders must be added with great care, especially if the work is being done in the darkroom. Here particles dispersed in the air contaminate sensitive materials, as well as embarrass the operators. The addition of liquid concentrates is less messy, but a possible source of discomfiture to those doing it is that the added volume of fluid may be too much for the tank. If the level of the solution looks too high for what is to be put in, some must be taken from the tank before any addition is made; this is always regrettable since it wastes silver-containing fixer.

Maintaining correct acidity. When the fixer salt has been added, the acidity of the bath should be checked, some of the solution being removed in a test-tube for this purpose. The acidity of fixing baths can be tested with indicator papers which have a narrow pH range. Alternatively, if the solution is a colourless one such as sodium thiosulphate fixer with potassium alum hardener, bromo-cresol green indicator solution can be used. When a few drops of this are added to the fixer a bottle-green colour is the reaction sought; bluish-green indicates that the solution is lacking in acid, yellow-green that it is over-acidified.

Fixers employing chrome alum as hardener are green anyway, and bromo-cresol purple can be used. However, since the hardening power of chrome alum falls off in a few days whether the bath is being used or not, there is really little point in putting it into a tank which it is expected to retain in service for a long period of time with the aid of these regenerating techniques. In practice there would seem to be little need to use the bromo-cresol purple test.

If tests reveal that the bath is under-acidified, acetic acid is added—for example 15 ml of a 50 per cent solution of acetic acid per gallon of liquid in the tank.

By means of these techniques a bath can be kept in use for very long periods of time—perhaps indefinitely. However, regeneration interminably extended is not good practice, though it may seem attractive because it saves emptying the tanks, cleaning them out, and preparing new solutions. It is suggested that the fixing bath should be changed not less often than once every 6 months. Over a long period of time the bottom of the tank accumulates gelatin if nothing else (other items such as missing dental films and even their hangers, plastic pegs or rings used to identify individual radiographs, and other oddities have been found). The presence of gelatin at first helps deposition of silver on the cathode, but it may eventually lead to a poor colour in the silver, and an excessive amount of gelatin can encourage sulphiding of the bath.

Silver Recovery by Metal Exchange

If base metals such as iron filings, zinc dust, steel wool, or tinplate scrap are put into a solution containing silver salts, the base metal dissolves and the silver is deposited out of solution in exchange. This reaction can be used to recover silver from photographic fixing solutions which it is not proposed to use again. As a result of the exchange, metal salts are put into the fixer which prohibit its further use for photographic processing. This method therefore cannot be used in X-ray departments for fixing baths which are being kept in use. It can be employed very satisfactorily to treat fixing solution issuing as overflow from automatic processing units. The process is cheap and extremely efficient.

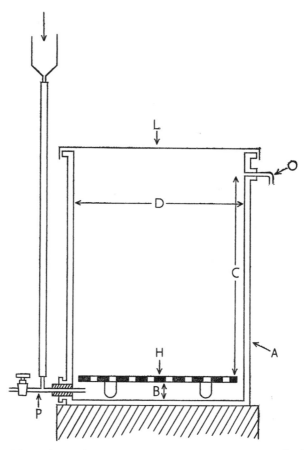

FIG. 7.3. Fixer solution from the processing machines is fed into the funnel at the left and enters the recovery vessel at P. H is a perforated platform supported about 1½ in. above the bottom of the vessel. C is the space in which steel wool is packed. Desilvered fixer overflows at O. *By courtesy of* RADIOGRAPHY, *The Journal of the Society of Radiographers.*

A metal exchange unit has been devised (Fig. 7.3) using a vessel which contains steel wool. This steel wool is in the form of disc pads of a type used in some floor-cleaning machines, and this is a very convenient form in which to use it. The pads are available in various sizes, and they can be selected so that they fit into a cylindrical vessel—perhaps 30 of them arranged like a pile of waffles just lightly touching the sides of the container. The lowermost one does not lie on the floor of the container, but rests on a perforated disc standing on little legs which keep it clear of the bottom of the vessel by about 1½ inches; this allows the solution which enters at the bottom free and uniform access to the steel wool. The vessel must be of acid-resisting material, for example glass, well glazed earthenware or plastic, and the perforated disc which supports the steel wool pancakes must be chemically inactive and of a strength to bear several pounds weight of silver.

The fixer from the automatic processing unit served by the silver recovery system is fed in at the bottom of the vessel and rises up through the steel wool, desilvered fixer being discharged at the top. The steel wool pads are converted to silver in the exchange process, and when all the pads are spent the appearance of the top one can be seen to have become black from light grey.

So long as the effluent fixer from the top of the unit contains no silver, the steel wool is not fully exhausted, but as soon as there is silver in the discharge the pile of steel (now silver) wool must be changed, and the vessel must be charged with new discs. The frequency with which this needs to be done depends on many factors; each charge of steel wool is likely to last for a period of some weeks. Silver in the effluent fixer can be detected by holding a bright copper strip or coin in the flow; if silver is present it will plate out on the copper.

Given the right conditions this recovery process is remarkably complete, and there should be hardly any silver leaving the unit with the effluent fixer bound for the drain. For fuller details of the operation of such a recovery unit, the reader is referred to publications by Levenson and Frank listed in the bibliography at the end of this book.

The Value of Silver Recovery

Silver recovery in hospital X-ray departments now seems firmly established, and doubtless is likely to remain so on economic grounds. It has been estimated, for example, that a darkroom processing 200 films per day throws £600 per annum down the drain with its discarded fixing solutions; and that 12,000–30,000 average radiographs processed in a year result in 100–400 troy ounces of silver going into the fixing solution during that time. Where electrolytic recovery is used and the fixing bath is regenerated, there is said to be a saving in chemicals of up to 75 per cent; the efficient recovery achieved by the steel wool method has been able in one case to pay for all the chemicals used in two automatic processing units.

These statements may bring a gleam into the eye of any officer concerned with hospital finances, but perhaps they leave radiographers less elated. While regeneration of the fixing bath saves a recurrent task in renewing solutions frequently, silver recovery has a certain nuisance value in the X-ray department. If the discarded solution is to be sold to a refiner, putting large volumes into a suitable container is an unattractive task. If electrolytic methods are used, space in the fixing tank is lost, and running the unit and regenerating the bath require a certain amount of time and attention. The steel wool method looks trouble-free to run, but again involves some time spent on an unpleasant task in renewing the charge of steel wool. It is unlikely, however, that these considerations will bring the practice of silver recovery into disuse.

As a final comment it can be said that the electrolytic method in practice shows remarkably wide variation of efficiency; this arises through differences in the technique used. It has been stated that the variation was found to be between 4·3–29·6 troy ounces of silver recovered per 1,000 sq. ft. of film processed. This is a considerable range, and it seems certain that units are often run at a low level of efficiency accompanied by unnecessary loss of silver. Perhaps the existence of *some* silver recovery system which seems to work reasonably well keeps everybody happy, and it is doubtless true to say that in many X-ray departments the senior staff are quite unable to spare for a silver recovery unit the time and attention required to run it at *maximum* efficiency.

CHAPTER VIII

Rinsing, Washing, Drying

THE INTERMEDIATE RINSE OR STOPBATH

This refers to the stage in the processing cycle which is between development and fixation. Its object is to prevent film materials from carrying active developer with them into the fixer. It has already been seen that the presence of developing agents in the fixing bath can result (i) in dichroic fog; (ii) in staining from the brown final oxidation products of oxidized developer; (iii) in increased alkalinity of the fixing bath as the developer solution contaminates it.

Correct use of the intermediate rinse minimizes or prevents these troubles. This part of the processing cycle is somewhat disregarded, not in the sense that it is left undone, but in the sense that it may be done without much care. Inefficiently carried out, it can fail entirely in its object.

In automatic processing units the rinse may be omitted. Its omission saves time in the processing cycle, and its inclusion has proved unnecessary. Risk of staining is reduced by agitation of the film during its period of travel through the wet parts of the processing cycle, and the quantity of developer carried by the film into the fixing bath can be brought to a minimum by the squeegee action of rollers; furthermore the fixing solution is well buffered.

In manual processing there are two possibilities for this intermediate stage.

(i) To *slow* the action of the developer and to remove it from the surfaces of the film by simply diluting it with water. This is done by a *plain rinse bath*.

(ii) To *stop* the action of the developer by neutralizing it in the emulsion layer and also to remove it from the surfaces of the film. This is achieved by putting the film in an acid solution known as an *acid stopbath*.

Of these two, in X-ray departments the acid stopbath is much less commonly used than a plain rinse. In radiographic darkrooms, fixing baths are almost always acid so that the action of the developer is stopped at that stage, and the previous acid bath is unnecessary. It may be appreciated that a plain rinse *must* be followed by the use of acid fixing solutions.

Plain Rinse

This can be (i) a static bath, or (ii) a bath of water continually renewed because it is in the form of a spray (a spray rinse) or because there is running water continually entering and leaving the bath (a running rinse).

The static bath is extremely simple—it is just a tank full of water—but it must be warily regarded as a potential source of damage by being kept in use too long. As films pass through it, the liquid contents become loaded with developer, and what began as plain water becomes an alkaline solution. It will cease to be effective in slowing the action of the developer. The most important thing to remember about a static rinse is that it must be renewed frequently. This is the dip-rinse to which reference is made in Chapter ix.

A spray-rinse is described in Chapter ix. It looks an advantageous system since the water is always fresh, being provided as a number of jets directed on the film, and it is economical since the water flows only when films are passing through the rinse. It is, however, liable to certain inefficiencies as explained in Chapter ix. A critical factor is the available water pressure. Errors can arise through careless use of the rinse, poor positioning of the jets, and lack of maintenance of the sprays.

The running rinse, also described in Chapter ix, is a system whereby there is a flow of water through the tank, the water entering at low level and leaving at the top. It is a commendable and efficient system; the principal disadvantage is lack of economy in the use of water.

Acid Stopbath

An acid stopbath clearly must be a static system since the provision of acid solutions on tap is not practicable. The need for frequent renewal is thus present as in the case of a plain water rinse; since the acid bath is a chemical preparation, its renewal has not the complete simplicity of filling a tank full of water. As an approximate guide, it may be renewed after processing films equivalent to 120 sq. ft. per gallon. Some acid stopbaths have an indicator in solution which changes colour when a certain degree of alkalinity has been reached. This change in appearance shows at once when the bath is contaminated by alkaline developer to a point where it is no longer sufficiently acid to perform its function.

A solution of 3 per cent acetic acid is commonly used; greater concentrations may liberate bubbles of carbon dioxide in the gelatin of the material. Stronger acids, such as sulphuric acid, can wreck the fixing bath when they are carried into it with the passage of films.

The period of immersion required in rinse or stopbath varies with factors such as the carry-over rate of the developer, and the agitation achieved either by movements of the film or by movements of the water in a spray or continuous flow. Agitation clearly improves the efficiency of the process, aiding removal of the surface developer and permeation of the gelatin. The suggested times are a minimum of 5 seconds immersion under jets, and 10 seconds immersion in static baths.

WASHING

This stage in the processing cycle follows fixation. When the film comes out of the fixing bath, it carries in its emulsion layer (i) the argentothiosulphates which have been formed in the chemical action of the fixer; (ii) residual sodium thiosulphate, or alternative fixing agent; (iii) remaining salts which are the other constituents of the bath. If no effort is made to remove these, more than one form of disaster awaits the film.

The results are (a) the colourless argentothiosulphates decompose after a while to form silver sulphide, which produces a yellow-brown stain; (b) the residual sodium thiosulphate decomposes, and substances are produced which attack the silver image and form silver sulphide, resulting similarly in a yellow-brown stain and loss of the image; (c) all the residual salts crystallize on the film surface and make the radiograph difficult or impossible to view. Since all these substances are water soluble, they can be removed by water, the process being one of diffusion.

The object of washing thus is to remove from the emulsion substances which it has acquired during fixation, and which will deteriorate the image if they are allowed to remain. It can be done by subjecting the film to a flow of water, or by putting it into a series of baths of clean water, the water being changed for each bath.

Student radiographers may recall with horror their meeting with an exponential relationship in the absorption of X-ray beams, but one thing about it is easily remembered: that exponential absorption results in the radiation never being totally absorbed. Some fraction tantalizingly remains. Diffusion of residual salts into the washing water results in their exponential removal; this is never complete and some fraction always remains. The aim of washing is to reduce the residual salts not to zero but to a level so low that they can do no harm.

The question then arises as to what this level is. All the substances to be removed wash out at more or less the same rate, and it is usual to express the level of what remains in terms of one salt only; the chosen one is hypo. Tests can be done to determine the amount of hypo remaining in an emulsion, and the results are expressed in micrograms of hypo per square inch of film. The lowest level measurable by usual tests is 5 microgm/sq. in. The level above this which in fact is safe depends upon several considerations, which include conditions of storage; perhaps the most important is the length of time for which it is expected to keep the films. A distinction has been made between what is termed normal commercial storage (which would be a few years only), and what is termed archival storage (which is an unspecified period considered to be permanent or 'for ever'). In the latter case, for many photographic records the hypo content may be required to be so small as to be undetectable. For radiographs it has been suggested that a maximum level for permanent records is 40 microgms/sq. in. (This is 20 microgms/sq. in. per each emulsion.) In practice it is probably unnecessary to achieve so low a level of hypo content, since most hospitals have not the filing space to keep their films permanently, and are doing well if they can keep them 10 years.

The Washing Rate

This term is a convenient expression for the rate of removal of hypo in the water bath, and it is affected by various factors which will be reviewed in due course. Before doing this, the diffusion process itself is now considered more closely.

At the time when the film is put into the water there is high hypo concentration in the emulsion, and (we hope) none in the water; there is thus a big difference between the hypo concentration in the two. In these circumstances, the hypo diffuses out of the emulsion into the water, and eventually the relative concentrations are evened, the level becoming the same in the emulsion and in the water (a weak hypo solution by now). If matters are left like this, no further diffusion of hypo from the emulsion is likely to take place.

If the film is now put into a fresh bath of water instead of being left in the previous one, there is again difference in hypo concentration between the emulsion and the water. The process of diffusion begins again and continues until equilibrium is reached. Passing the film through several changes of water thus results in the removal of certain fractions of the hypo content, until eventually what remains is so slight as to be disregarded or as to be unmeasurable. For each change of water the washing rate begins at a maximum and falls to nothing when the state of equilibrium is reached.

It can be appreciated that a sufficient number of changes of water is more important to adequate washing than the volume used; a certain volume used as a static bath gives a very much less efficient result than a smaller volume used to provide several changes. Water is most economically and efficiently used when it is employed to give as many changes as possible of as small a volume as possible, and when time is allowed for each change of wash to reach the point of equilibrium just described. It may be difficult to achieve this in practice and keep the processing cycle within a realistic time-limit.

Factors Affecting the Washing Rate

Hypo Concentrations in Emulsion and Wash-Bath

The importance of the difference in hypo concentration between emulsion and wash-bath has been explained already. The concentration difference can be maintained at a maximum if a constant supply of completely fresh water impinges on the emulsion, as by the use of a spray, the water running at once to an outlet. This gives very rapid washing, and saves time but not water. It would in any case be difficult to adapt for washing large numbers of radiographs. In X-ray darkrooms the method used is immersion of the films in a large tank through which water is kept flowing.

The Temperature of the Wash-Bath

The washing rate increases if the temperature of the water is raised, but there is an obvious limit here. If the water is warmer than 77°F (25°C), the gelatin may be removed from the film base, particularly if it has not been adequately hardened at an earlier stage. At temperatures below 60°F (16°C) the washing rate is very slow.

The Nature of the Fixing Bath

The hardening agents used in the fixing bath affect the rate at which hypo elimination takes place in the wash. It was found that where potassium alum is the hardening agent and the pH of the fixing bath is at a level to give efficient hardening, the washing rate is slow.

Increase in the pH of the fixer improves the washing rate, so that washing can be done in a shorter time. It will be remembered, however, that increased pH results in loss of hardening action. It follows then that with potassium alum hardeners it is not possible to achieve efficient hardening in the fixer and rapid removal of the hypo in the subsequent wash. The same is true of aluminium chloride hardeners.

Chrome alum hardener in the fixing bath seems to have no effect on the subsequent washing rate. Since chrome alum has the disadvantage of losing its hardening power in a few days (as discussed in the previous chapter), the fixer may soon be a non-hardening one.

A neutral or alkaline fixer promotes rapid washing, but, as well as its failure to harden, its inability to halt quickly the action of the developer encourages the formation of stains. The situation can be summarized by saying that the use of acid hardening fixer solutions is incompatible with a rapid washing rate, but that for the sake of other advantages which accrue from the use of these fixers some sacrifice in regard to the washing rate is necessarily accepted.

AGITATION

If agitation is applied, fresh water is brought continually against the films and the washing rate is improved. In radiographic darkrooms some agitation is provided by the flow of water through the tank in which washing is done.

THE USE OF HYPO CLEARING SOLUTIONS

It has been found that when films are put into the wash-bath after previous soaking in solutions of certain sodium salts (such as sodium sulphite), the washing rate is considerably increased. Manufacturers now provide various solutions of this nature, by the use of which washing times are shortened by a factor of 5 or 6 or even more, water is saved, and an efficient process of washing is more certainly achieved. These are real advantages in any X-ray department.

These solutions for reducing washing time are sometimes described as hypo eliminators; the same term is used also for solutions which have an action somewhat different to the one mentioned above. When residual hypo is brought into contact with hydrogen peroxide in an ammoniacal solution, the hypo is converted to inert sulphates soluble in water and resistant to atmospheric oxidation and subsequent change. This therefore is elimination of the hypo by its conversion to something else, whereas the process mentioned earlier is one which simply hastens removal of the hypo in a water wash. The use of hydrogen peroxide and other substances for chemical change of the hypo has been regarded by photographers with some doubt. The present-day hypo clearing solutions to improve the washing rate are enjoying greater popularity and wider use, certainly in radiographic darkrooms where manual processing is still employed.

Some Practical Points

In radiographic darkrooms with manual processing, the method used for washing is to immerse the films in a large tank, or in a series of tanks, through which water is kept flowing. This method is not particularly economical of water, but it is adapted to the washing of a large amount of material, and it makes minimum demand on the attention of the operator, an important consideration since the psychologists tell us that we cannot do two things at once.

In such tanks, the water in practice often enters at the bottom and leaves near the top. This is not the ideal arrangement since the hypo content tends to sink to the bottom of the bath; it is better for the outlet to be at the bottom, the tank draining by a syphonic arrangement. When films are put into the tank, the point to be remembered is that the films should enter near where the water leaves, and should leave near where the water enters. The reason here is that this allows films to have their last washing with water which comes fresh to the tank, and has not been heavily loaded with hypo by films newly arrived from the fixing bath. An arrangement of the inlet and outlet for achieving this is siting the inlet at the bottom of one side of the tank, and the outlet at the top of an opposite side, the flow of water being in the direction counter to the travel of films through the tank.

If only one tank is used, it must be recognized that if a batch of films is placed in the tank and is adequately washed, placing another batch of films alongside the first introduces more hypo which is diffused into the bath. This can contaminate the first group of films. The risk is minimized by careful observation of the correct progression for films through the tank. It is better still if two separate tanks are available through which films are progressed; equally well the tanks can be used completely to wash one batch at a time, each tank being employed alternately to take the films as they first come from the fixing bath.

The question that remains to be answered is how long washing actually takes. There is no single answer to this since many variables influence it, and several conditions would need to be specified in giving such an answer. However, it has been said that if the rate of flow of water through a washing tank is such as completely to change the water once every 15 minutes, adequate washing will be achieved in 10 minutes (this assumes the use of no hypo clearing agent). In practice this time is often extended to 20–30 minutes for the sake of certainty and convenience. The length of time taken to change the water in the bath can be assessed by discolouring the water in the tank, and timing the period required to remove all discolouration.

The main risk in extended washing, particularly with unhardened emulsions, is undue swelling and softening of the gelatin; these effects will be worse if the water is above 70°F (21°C). Unnecessarily prolonged washing is of course uneconomical of water. If the film becomes unduly softened by washing it for too long and/or at too high a temperature, difficulties will be encountered if it is afterwards put into a rapid drier. The softened gelatin will stick to the rollers in the drier and successful transport of the film will be impossible.

DRYING

So far all the stages of the processing cycle have had at least one common factor—they all have made it necessary for the film to become wet. In fact it becomes very wet indeed, and by the end of the washing stage an emulsion contains several times its own weight in water. It is clearly necessary to dry films before they can be used conveniently and the object of this last part of the processing cycle is to remove most of the water in the gelatin. The final product must be an undamaged emulsion free from dust particles, crystalline deposits, stains and marks. It is described as being a dry film, but the term is a relative one; it is very much *drier* than it was. A fully dehydrated emulsion is brittle and will crack, so this extreme state is to be avoided. At the end of the drying process, the film looks and feels dry, but it should contain about 10–15 per cent of its own weight of water.

Drying is a procedure which often takes longer than the rest of the processing cycle, even when it is going well and a satisfactory level of efficiency is achieved. Breakdown in drying arrangements produces in the X-ray department a severe 'bottleneck' almost at once, while to see good radiographs marked through faulty drying is an exasperating experience.

It is important that this last stage in the cycle should not be lightly regarded because it is the last stage, generally involves no chemical complexities, and usually can proceed with little attention from the operator.

Factors affecting Drying Times

The length of time required to make a film look and feel dry is determined by the quantity of water to be evaporated. In automatic processing units drying is rapid, and the most important factor in achieving this is physical removal of excess water, usually by means of the squeegee action of rollers. (This squeegee action also reduces the washing time required; it takes from the film water which is loaded with residual fixing salts that otherwise must be removed in washing.)

An unhardened emulsion (as shown in Chapter vii) swells more in washing than a hardened one, and it therefore holds more water when the film comes out of the wash-bath. Unhardened emulsions thus take longer to dry than hardened ones do. Where rapid drying is to be done, the correct hardening of the emulsions is significant from two aspects; (i) because less water will be present in the emulsion to remove, and (ii) because a hardened film is better able to withstand the raised temperatures which may be used. Rapid drying devices which transport films by rollers require strict adherence to the manufacturer's recommendations on hardening since (as said before) emulsions which are too soft in the heat stick to the rollers.

The most usual method of drying photographic materials is by air, and in the drying rooms of X-ray departments hot air methods are most widely used. The films are put in drying cabinets which keep a current of warm air on them. Any photographic materials which are dried in this way should previously be hardened, and the air which circulates on them must be free from dust.

There are three features which are important. These are (i) the temperature of the air; (ii) the humidity of the air; (iii) the flow of air past the emulsion.

Raising the temperature of the air increases the rate at which moisture evaporates from the gelatin and thus shortens drying time. There seems to be no 'right' temperature, and opinions move up and down the thermometer scale in debate on the optimum level. Figures varying from 100°F (38°C) to even as high as 160°F (70°C) have been quoted; most people would regard this upper level as very high, and certainly emulsions would need to be well hardened before they were subjected to it. Conventional driers on the market use temperatures of 110°F–

118°F (43·3°C–47·7°C), and one of the rapid driers uses a temperature of 120°F (48·8°C).

The humidity of the air is significant in this way. The difference in percentages of water in the gelatin and in the air surrounding it determines the rate at which water is removed from the emulsion. The lower the humidity of the air, the more rapid is the loss of moisture from the emulsion to it.

Flow of air past the emulsion is very important, more important than temperature. Adequate flow of air, even if it is relatively cool, can dry films much more quickly than hot air which is static. The air in a drying cabinet is moved by a fan, and saturated air in the immediate neighbourhood of the film surfaces is swept away, and is replaced by fresh air of lower humidity. This accelerates the drying process. When drying devices break down, the loss of the service of a fan is a greater trial than the absence of a heater.

The Use of a Wetting Agent

Wetting agents are compounds of which small amounts in solution enable liquids to spread more easily. They are useful in photography both when dry surfaces are to be made wet, and when wet surfaces are to be made dry. If the film, on its removal from the wash-bath, is immersed briefly in a solution of a wetting agent, the surface tension of the water on the faces of the film is reduced. On coming from the wetting agent, the film is at once hung to drain and is afterwards put in the drier. The water runs freely and uniformly from the vertical surfaces of the emulsion, and is thus removed without more ado.

This prevents the collection of droplets of surplus water on the surfaces of the film. These spots can take a period of time to dry which is surprisingly long to an impatient radiographer and even to a patient one. The use of wetting agents spares us this delay of waiting for a last refractory spot to dry. More importantly they spare us drying marks which the droplets of water can produce; the uneven drying results in an area of uneven density on the film, a mark which can be permanent.

Chemical Methods of Drying

Since the delay in waiting for photographic materials to dry is significant if the result is to be used without loss of time, various methods for speeding up this part of the processing cycle have been sought. The most promising approach seems to be to use hot air as already known, and to shorten drying times by providing plenty of air at raised temperature.

One drier on the market provides in this way (combined with the squeegee action of rollers on the film) a dry radiograph in 80 seconds.

There are chemical methods available by which to accelerate drying, and these can be used in the lack of special equipment. Some of them are for use only on certain materials by resolute and skilful operators— for example, soaking paper prints in spirit and then flaming it off by igniting the spirit at a bottom edge. Such a method could not be applied with success to radiographs, or to any materials by nervous practioners.

In the X-ray department, chemical methods of drying are not used as routine practice. They may be applied to the occasional special case when a dry radiograph is wanted very quickly. Today automation is present in an increasing number of departments, and shorter processing times and equipment for rapid drying are widely available. It seems that radiographers need hardly concern themselves with a chemical method. For the sake of completeness and providing an extra ace up the sleeve, one is mentioned now.

If the washed radiograph is bathed in an alcohol solution, its water content is replaced by alcohol. This is much more volatile than water, and when the film is hung to dry it dries more rapidly. There are risks in the procedure. One is that strong alcohol can distort film base. Films coated on both sides are less liable to this damage, and can safely be treated with aqueous solutions not more concentrated than 70 per cent of spirit by volume. Another risk is that moisture will be removed from the upper emulsion layers very rapidly, while leaving the water content of the lower layers unable to get away. The 'dry' radiograph then has a cloudy appearance.

Industrial or surgical spirit can be used (not domestic mauve methylated spirit, for this becomes milky when diluted with water). The washed radiograph is bathed for 2–3 minutes in 70 per cent spirit and is then hung to dry. This technique should not be applied to radiographs which will be used to obtain accurate measurements of the dimensions of the image—for example in foreign body localizations—when distortion of the base might cause error.

CHAPTER IX

Film Processing: Equipment

In this chapter will be given some closer account of the practical methods which are used to obtain development and permanence of the latent radiographic image, discussed so far mainly from the viewpoint of chemical and physical theory. In particular some of the equipment designed for this work will be described and its salient features explained.

In terms of essential needs, a group of three dishes, a means of warming the solutions and a sink with a cold-water tap will serve the purpose of processing a radiograph. In the past it has been done like this on a small scale, for instance in a darkened theatre dressing room to obtain films which assist in controlling orthopaedic surgery: and emergency may require processing to be so performed from time to time.

However, dish development of radiographs clearly has nothing in its favour except that it can be made to work. Its disadvantages may be listed briefly.

(1) Control of temperature is difficult.

(2) Exposed solutions oxidize rapidly.

(3) Only one film can be processed at a time.

(4) Films necessarily receive more handling and this is likely to be harmful since the emulsion is swollen and softened by processing liquids.

(5) Processing is difficult to standardize and dependent for success upon a practised technician. Failure to cover the whole film rapidly or to keep it covered in a shallow depth of solution; adherence of the film to the bottom of the dish, either momentarily or throughout most of the procedure; variable agitation or total lack of it; each of these is a potential hazard and at one time or another has spoiled radiographs.

(6) It is a fatiguing and exacting form of work.

Because of these disadvantages the routine processing of radiographs is undertaken in various systems of tanks. They have in their favour features which are the converse of the points just noted.

(1) Temperature control is easier when the volume of solution is large and surface exposure relatively small.

(2) Oxidation is decreased in a tall tank because the surface area is reduced. Often a lid can be used and this will further lessen the exposure to air. The solution therefore keeps better.

(3) Several films may be processed simultaneously and if the developer tank is fitted with a lid the darkroom need not be continuously under safe-light illumination.

(4) There is no direct handling of vulnerable emulsions.

(5) Processing can be more nearly standardized. Both plane surfaces of the film are equally exposed to the action of solutions—unless a tank is improperly crowded. Agitation may be performed mechanically or manually at certain defined intervals.

The principles of tank processing are embodied in several practical forms. This may be:

(a) a set of separate tanks;

(b) a group of tanks built into a larger one to make a processing unit which is either completely or very nearly self-contained;

(c) machinery for automatic processing.

The first two represent manual operation; (b) is no more than an elaboration of (a). They have certain common features which scarcely require separate discussion. The equipment under (c) must be considered on its own.

However, before either type of apparatus is described recognition must be given to the importance in any processing equipment of (1) correct temperature control, and (2) the nature of the material of which the equipment is made. Solution temperatures, as we have seen, profoundly influence development. Substances used for the manufacture of processing instruments are of significance since they must meet certain requirements and possess certain characteristics whether the item concerned is a complete processing unit, which if it is automatic will have moving parts; a plumbing system to serve such a unit; or a minor accessory such as a stirring rod or mixing bucket. Both these factors are considered in the next sections.

TEMPERATURE CONTROL

In this context of processing equipment, control of temperature can be obtained in a number of ways. If we consider the United Kingdom and indeed many other countries, the implications are that this control involves *raising* the temperature of processing solutions to some appropriate level above that of the ambient temperature. In a tropical environment the reverse is likely to be true and means must be found of keeping solutions sufficiently cool for satisfactory operation. However, methods of heating, being numerically more important, will be considered first. They are as follows.

(1) A simple immersion heater. This is the system which will operate if the processing equipment comprises a number of tanks not collectively linked by a heating system.

(2) A thermostatically controlled heating element. This system is the one found in many self-contained processing units.

(3) A water-mixer. This device can be used to fill a sink with tap water at some desired temperature so that the contents of tanks standing in it can be heated to a similar degree. In general X-ray departments, which usually do not depend on sinks and tanks for processing, a water-mixer may be found now in association with certain automatic units.

Immersion Heaters

These simple devices are manually operated. An immersion heater of this type is an electrically heated poker of a length and design suitable for suspension from the rim of a processing tank. The shaft or element is made of a non-corrodible metal, such as stainless steel coated with lead. The metal parts should be earthed and the handle well insulated. The poker is put into the developing solution, being supported in the tank by shoulder plates, and is allowed to remain until the desired temperature is reached: processing of course cannot be undertaken while this is being done. Occasional stirring of the solution with the poker will help the diffusion of heat throughout the tank.

Some practical precautions in using the immersion heater should be observed.

(1) The heater should be inserted into the developer *before* the plug is fitted into the wall socket and the heater switched on.

(2) The plug should be of the three-pin variety.

(3) The current should be switched off *before* any attempt is made to withdraw the heater.

(4) On removal from the developer the heater should be transferred at once to the rinse bath. This procedure (a) prevents overheating of the element; (b) washes it and removes oxidized products which might contaminate the developer on the occasion of the next use of the heater.

(5) The developing solution should be well stirred following removal of the heater and the temperature taken again to check that it is satisfactory.

Immersion heaters suitable for use in X-ray processing tanks usually have a power consumption of 500 to 750 watts. Some of them will raise 3 gallons (13·5 litres) of solution from average room temperatures to 68°F (20°C) quite rapidly, that is within 3 or 4 minutes. They should not be left without frequent attention or they may overheat the solution. Some heaters are supplied with a bracket so that they may be conveniently suspended on a wall when not in use. If this is not provided some care should be exercised in disposing of the poker. Darkroom benches have been seared before now in this way.

TANK THERMOMETERS

A thermometer is necessary to register the temperature of tank solutions. Even if the darkroom has a processing unit where these temperatures are controlled by a thermo-regulator and indicated on the same instrument, a simple thermometer is an important accessory. It may be helpful on occasion in order to check the accuracy and efficiency of thermostatic apparatus or to use in association with specialized processing equipment on a minor scale, such as that for cinefluorograms, which may not be thermostatically maintained.

Thermometers designed for X-ray tanks are usually 9–10 inches in length. The tube of mercury is mounted on a flat back-plate of white plastic material which sometimes may be strengthened with stainless steel. This has a clip to fit over the edge of the tank, a guard to protect the mercury reservoir, and a hole or ring at the top to allow the thermometer to be suspended at a deeper level if required or from a wall hook when not in use. It has a temperature range usually from about 50°F (10°C) to 80° or 90°F (27° or 32°C) and it is customary to mark the standard processing temperature, 68°F (20°C), with a particularly bold calibration. When not required the thermometer should be kept vertical in order not to break the mercury column and it is good practice to wash the instrument in *cold* water after every use.

Thermometer Regulators

A heating element which is under automatic thermostatic control is included in nearly all processing units. The function of this combination is to regulate the temperature of a volume of water in which the processing tanks normally stand. This volume of water constitutes a *water jacket* the temperature of which will affect the temperature in the tanks which it surrounds, owing to heat exchange between them.

A water jacket is not a particularly rapid method of altering the temperature of processing solutions. Some hours are likely to be required for the stabilization of individual tank temperatures. In order to be convenient the heating system of the jacket should be in continuous operation, even during periods, for example at the weekend, when processing is not expected to be undertaken. While this may appear to be an extravagant use of electricity, it is not really so. The power consumed in maintaining solutions at a given temperature is probably no greater than that required intermittently to heat them to the same temperature once they have become cold.

Electrical heating apparatus which is to remain like this in potential operation must have automatic control to ensure that the current is cut as soon as the desired temperature is reached. A thermostatic device for this purpose in processing equipment is a *thermometer regulator*, the one best known to radiographers being the Cambridge pattern which appears in many X-ray darkrooms on different units. However, it is not materially different from other thermometer regulators.

The Cambridge model is illustrated in Plate 9.1, following p. 94. Its main features are:

(1) a large dial with calibrations between o and 100°F;

(2) two pointers on this dial, a red one which can be manually adjusted with a key to lie opposite the chosen value of temperature, and a black one which records the temperature actually obtaining in the water jacket;

(3) a lead-covered capillary tube terminating in an expanded portion or bulb which in practice will be situated about half way down the depth of water concerned, in order to record its mean temperature. This bulb is the sensitive element in the thermometer.

It may be noticed that the Cambridge thermometer regulator does not depend on the familiar response to heat of a column of mercury but upon the expansion and contraction of a volume of gas. This is a more accurate method of measuring temperature.

In most cases the water jacket is warmed by a lead-covered, coil-type immersion heater situated near its base. Sometimes the element is within a stainless steel tube. Depending on the size of the volume of water to be heated the power of this heater is likely to vary from 300 to 1,000 watts. In Plate 9.2, following p. 94, which illustrates the practical arrangement in a typical processing unit, the thermometer and the regulator can be seen in circuit. The thermometer bulb is connected by means of its capillary tube to the regulator, and the heater also through a connection box with fuses. As the temperature of the water jacket rises, the black pointer on the regulator dial will move round the scale until its position coincides with that of the previously set red pointer. When this occurs, a micro-switch in the regulator operates a control switch in the heater circuit and the current supply is terminated. When the temperature falls sufficiently, the two pointers on the dial are again separated and a similar sequence of events results in the restoration of the heating current. The processes alternate continuously.

It will be appreciated that a thermometer regulator of this kind is simultaneously a measuring and a regulating instrument. Its practical application in a processing unit usually includes a safety device to prevent overheating of the elements if the level of the water jacket for any reason falls below the site of the thermometer; in this event the regulator itself would no longer be in charge of the situation and could not terminate the current supply. The operation of this safety switch is discussed in a later section of this chapter in which the water jackets of processing units will be generally described.

Water Mixers

A water-mixing valve is illustrated diagrammatically in Fig. 9.1. It operates by combining hot and cold water from the tap supply to produce a mixture at the desired temperature. Possible applications of such a blend are:

(1) as a water jacket for processing tanks;
(2) in automatic processing systems for washing purposes or for heating chemical solutions.

This method of controlling water temperature is both compact and relatively inexpensive: it is properly described as a thermostatically-controlled, manually-adjusted mixing valve. Reference to Fig. 9.1 demonstrates its main features. These are described below.

(1) Separate inlet ports for the hot and the cold supply.
(2) An outlet port for the tempered water.
(3) A handle for selection of the desired temperature, which is manually adjusted by the user. Such a valve might be capable of supplying water at any chosen value between 60° and 100°F (15°C and 38°C), irrespective of fluctuations in the temperature or pressure of the supply. In some valves the handle may be removable after adjustment in order to avoid accidental tampering with this control.

14

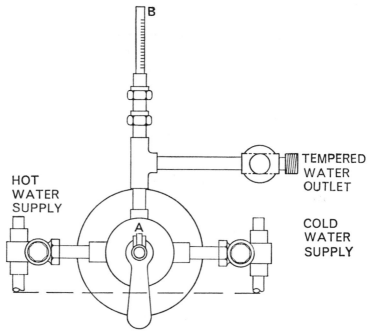

Fig. 9.1. Water mixing valve. *By courtesy of Kodak Ltd.*
    A   Handle which is manually adjusted by the user to select the temperature of the tempered water.
    B   Column thermometer inserted in the outlet pipe.

(4) A thermometer, of which the bulb is inserted in the outlet pipe. The one in the diagram is of a column type but a dial thermometer is equally suitable.

(5) A thermostatic motor the function of which is to maintain the selected water temperature.

Fig. 9.2 shows the thermostatic motor in section. It is not suggested that student radiographers should know in detail the operation of this but some may feel a little curiosity about the motor's method of work. Without our considering the finer points of the diagram, it can be seen that the hot and cold water enters the motor chamber at two slightly different levels; and that a movement of the valve assembly and shut-off disc forwards through the chamber in a direction tending to cover the hot water inlet must at the same time tend to uncover the cold water inlet.

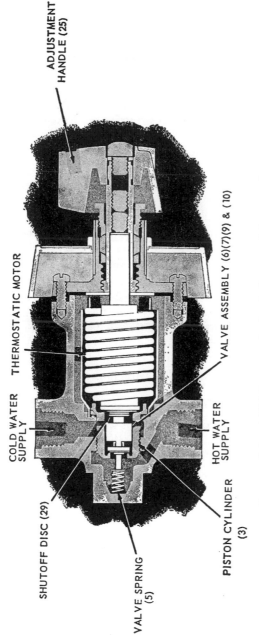

ADJUSTMENT HANDLE (25)

THERMOSTATIC MOTOR

COLD WATER SUPPLY

SHUTOFF DISC (29)

VALVE SPRING (5)

VALVE ASSEMBLY (6)(7)(9) & (10)

HOT WATER SUPPLY

PISTON CYLINDER (3)

FIG. 9.2. Pakorol XM Processor. Sectional diagram of thermostatic motor which maintains the selected temperature in a water mixing valve. By courtesy of Pako Corporation.

The motor chamber is liquid-filled and this liquid expands if the temperature of the blended water is higher than that set by the adjustment handle. The expansion results in a movement of the valve assembly towards the hot water seat, thus decreasing the flow of the hot and increasing the flow of the cold supply. If the temperature of the mixed water is lower than it should be, contraction of the liquid in the motor chamber reverses the movement of the valve assembly and with it the effects on the hot and cold supplies. Furthermore, change in the temperature or pressure of either of the latter similarly causes the motor to reposition the valve assembly in order to maintain the required delivery temperature.

An efficient mixing valve of this type will hold the temperature steady to ± 0·5°F (0·3°C) under normal conditions; and to ± 1°F (0·6°C) under conditions of difficulty, for example a pronounced fall in inlet pressure or excessive fluctuation in the temperature of the hot water supply. It may be noted that for effective operation of the valve, the minimum temperature of the hot water should not be less than 30°F (18°C) above the value selected for the tempered water. Equally the maximum temperature of the cold water should be at least 10°F (6°C) below that of the blend; if it is higher than this it should be cooled by refrigeration before being supplied to the regulator. In areas where the water is very hard, the mixing valve is likely to require cleaning from time to time to remove salt deposits. It should also be examined for rust along spring parts as this can readily cause faulty operation.

Methods of Cooling Solutions

We have considered so far only equipment which *raises* the temperature of solutions from their standing value to the level required for correct processing procedure. In climates where the ambient temperature normally exceeds 75°F (24°C), it becomes necessary to *cool* solutions before they can be employed in accordance with standardized techniques.

We can recognize that if cooling equipment either is unavailable or proves inadequate in producing working temperatures of a more normal value, then some modification of the recognized procedure is required. This modification can be summarized under the following headings:

(1) minimizing the increased amount of softening of the film emulsion which will occur in warm solutions;

(2) reducing the time spent by the film in each stage of processing, particularly those of development and washing, in order to prevent undue swelling of the gelatin.

In practice this entails the use of anti-swelling agents in the developer and of hardening baths, both between development and fixation and even prior to development if the temperature range is from 90°–105°F (32°–41°C).

It is not proposed to give here in any further detail the chemicals usually employed for this purpose. Unless the work is being undertaken in an extremely precarious and unfavourable situation it seems likely that radiological units will have the command of cooling apparatus of some kind, even if it is only as simple a device as a covering of wet rags or perhaps ice packed round the tanks or immersed in an impervious bag in the solutions. Our present purpose is to consider briefly some aspects of equipment for cooling.

The working temperatures of processing solutions can be reduced either if the ambient temperature of the darkroom is held sufficiently low or by the use of a refrigerator unit which will cool the water jacket, in a manner comparable with its heating in more temperate climates. If seasonal variations are such that cooling is required during some months of the year and heating at others, the supply circuit should have a switch of the throw-over type, in order to avoid the possible accident of attempting to conduct both processes simultaneously. In some circumstances sufficient reduction of the darkroom's ambient temperature can be obtained if a system of air-conditioning is in use. In this case no modification of the processing equipment is necessary.

However, in many cases cooling of the water jacket becomes essential and usually this is effected by a separate refrigerating unit which—unlike the heating element described in the previous section—is not an integral part of the processing unit itself. If room temperatures are *not* appreciably above 90°F (32°C), a small refrigerator may simply be attached by a bracket to one end of the processor: from it, stainless steel pipes carrying the coolant pass into the water jacket, one going to the front of the processing tanks and the other to their rear. An adjustable thermostat provides control of the water jacket's temperature. In the use of a cooling pipe running through the water jacket we have a close analogy with the principle of heating by means of immersion devices, such as those earlier described.

It should be noticed, however, that in the design of many processing units the water jacket normally embraces developer and fixing tanks but does not include the washing tank, since in temperate conditions no special treatment of the washing water is required. In these circumstances the wash water will be at the temperature of the mains supply.

If the difference between this and the other tanks is very great then local strains in the gelatin as a result of contraction and expansion may produce a creased or cracked appearance of the emulsion known as *reticulation*. In a unit in which the developer, dip rinse and fixing bath are cooled to the standard 68°F (20°C), and the mains water is above 80°F (26°C), then the thermal disparity of the solutions must be considered as too great.

In this event a refrigerating unit is likely to be used which will cool the water *supply* and deliver a sufficient quantity of cooled water for the normal operation of the processor. This type of refrigerator should be situated outside the darkroom, since its condenser radiates a certain amount of heat. The unit is in continuous operation under thermostatic control and typically might provide 20–25 gallons (90–122·5 litres) per hour at a final temperature of 68°F (20°C) from an initial maximum of 90°–95°F (32°C–35°C), the ambient air temperature being up to 110°F (43°C).

In some cases a *flow control* is included in the water circuit. This device will limit the flow of water through the cooler in the event of temperatures rising above the pre-set value: restriction in the amount of water will result in greater efficacy of cooling and thus ultimately a reduction to the required temperature.

MATERIALS FOR PROCESSING EQUIPMENT

A considerable amount of study has been given to the correct selection of substances suitable for the manufacture of items of photographic equipment. The following factors are relevant to the problem.

(1) The material should have no effect on the photographic properties of the solution concerned. For example galvanized iron might be fairly suitable for a washing tank, but when it is used for developing or fixing solutions the zinc in it is liable to react with sodium bisulphite and give rise to chemical fog, as a result of the formation of sodium hydrosulphite.

(2) The material should be capable of resisting the most corrosive fluid with which it is likely to be in contact. Again galvanized iron can be taken as an example: it is readily attacked by fixing solutions and carry-over from the fixing bath could be a danger to washing tanks made of this substance.

(3) The period of time during which a material is likely to be exposed to chemical action and the probable dilution of the solutions concerned.

These considerations might make some substances suitable for a washing tank or a plumbing system but not for storage of chemicals or for use as developing or fixing tanks.

(4) The cost of the material. Tantalum for instance appears to be inert to all photographic solutions but is too expensive for any but small items of equipment.

(5) The mechanical adaptability of the material for constructional purposes. Glass for example is highly resistant to chemical actions but is too fragile in many situations, especially of course if the equipment is large.

In selecting a material for photographic use the first criterion is obviously its chemical suitability. If this is satisfactory then the other factors mentioned can be considered. Costs and mechanical adaptability *are* important but become irrelevant if the substance concerned has chemical characteristics which are inappropriate.

As distinct from the possible production of photographic disasters of the kind described under (1) above, the most likely chemical hazard is that of corrosion of metals as a result of the action of solutions. Several forms of corrosion are recognized.

(a) General corrosion or uniform dissolution of the substance.

(b) Pitting or localized corrosion which will eventually lead to perforation of the material.

(c) Intergranular corrosion which results from attack near the boundaries of grain structure within the substance.

(d) Stress corrosion cracking: this is a specialized form of attack which appears to result from a combination of stress and unfavourable environment. Usually the material simply cracks without apparent cause and with very little evidence of corrosive destruction. In the case of exposure to photographic solutions this effect occurs more often with thermoplastics than with metals.

However, to the user in general, corrosion is simply corrosion. Its exact nature is of less significance than knowledge of the conditions which tend to give rise to it, since if we know these we may delay its occurrence, if only by such a simple measure as careful cleaning of certain parts of containers. Conditions favourable to corrosion are found in the following situations.

(1) Where there is electrolytic action between two metals in contact in a solution.

(2) At the surface of a solution where both solution and container are in

association with air, particularly in a closed container as a result of vapours condensing on areas above the surface of a solution.

(3) At points where a solution is trapped and becomes static.

(4) Where dissimilar solutions are in contact with each other.

(5) At localized points where metal is in contact with a non-metallic material, for example wooden duck boards, or other supports for a tank in a sink or processing unit.

(6) Where there is continuous mechanical stress, for example bending of the material or even the movement of solutions at high velocity.

Consideration has to be given not only to the material of which any article is constructed but also to those substances which may be used with it to make joints or watertight connections. For instance any solder containing tin will cause fog, as also will cheap rubber if sulphur and metallic sulphides are present as impurities.

It is to be remembered, too, that any coated material, for example steel lined with rubber, is only as good as the thickness and durability of the coating substance. If the coating is worn, scratched or cracked, or if it contains blemishes or pores, the exposure of the base metal which is likely to result can contaminate solutions or cause corrosion. Coating materials should be neither brittle nor thin. To prevent the formation of pinhole defects they should be used in at least three applications to a total minimum thickness of 0·005 inches.

The association of different materials has a further danger if the article concerned is manufactured from one metal plated by another. If the plating wears off or becomes damaged the effect of two metals in solution is to form an electrolytic cell: the resultant process of electrolysis leads to the destruction of one of the metals. Whenever possible metal equipment should be made from a single metal or alloy and electro-welded from the outside. If two dissimilar metals must be used electrolysis between them can be decreased if they are separated from each other by a layer of some insulating material.

Among metals, stainless steel is very suitable both chemically and mechanically for all types of processing apparatus. The best steel for the purpose, because it is most resistant, is of the kind described as having an 18/8 analysis (18 per cent chromium, 8 per cent nickel) and containing 2–4 per cent molybdenum: it should have a carbon content no higher than 0·2 per cent and preferably less than 0·08 per cent. A high proportion of carbon in the alloy results in the segregation of carbides at welds, with resultant corrosion. It is to be remembered that the ability of these steels to resist corrosion is found largely in their highly polished surfaces. If they become dirty or scratched, chemicals are likely to affect them.

Modern processes have made available a wide range of synthetic thermoplastic materials which are easy to manufacture and resistant to most photographic solutions. While chemically suitable, however, some grades have a mechanical disadvantage as they tend to be brittle.

Wood is a naturally occurring material which has certain good qualities. It is cheap and very simple to construct. The best woods are those which are hard and relatively impervious. A number come into this category but suitable examples are cypress, spruce, beech and teak. All woods, however, absorb fluids to some degree and are prone to warp, to accumulate slime from the action of bacteria, and to crack when penetrated by crystalline deposits, for instance at the rim of a chemical solution. These disadvantages can be lessened if the chosen wood is impregnated with paraffin wax or lined with some other material—a facing of metal for instance—or painted with a resistant lacquer. Distortion may be prevented by bracing deep tanks or sinks with steel rods, rather than merely screwing their components together. However, woods are less often used than they were, owing to the greater suitability of modern materials for most applications.

Darkroom plumbing no doubt is a matter which student radiographers may well feel to lie beyond their scope and control. However, it is to be observed that the previous discussion of materials appropriate or inappropriate for the manufacture of processing equipment is relevant equally to agents for the disposal of discarded processing solutions.

Provided they are well diluted, exhausted developers and fixers can be passed without special treatment into the normal drainage system. Brass or copper pipings, however, should not be used, owing to their readiness to corrode. Whenever possible a material should be chosen which is resistant even to full strength processing solutions. The following substances are applicable: for large drains—earthenware pipes with joints set in acid-proof cement; for smaller connections—18/8 molybdenum stainless steel, steam-quality screwed iron piping, or synthetic substances such as polythene or polyvinyl chloride (P.V.C.).

All outlets should have detachable strainers of stainless steel. The fitting of plugs to give easy access to pipes which turn through an angle is often a useful measure. Some water in association with processing products tends to form a gelatinous deposit which can obstruct a drain over a period of time. The possibility of reaching likely sites of obstruction easily should be available.

Material	Chemical suitability for X-ray developers and fixers	Mechanical suitability			Comments
		Tanks	Racks Sprockets rollers etc.	Pipes	
Metals:					
Iron				√	
Lead				√	Only other use is for sink linings.
Stainless steel 18/8 Molybdenum	√	√	√	√	Note that the term stainless steel itself means very little. It should be of specified quality.
Metals coated with:					
hard rubber	√	√		√	
P.V.C.	√	√			
Thermoplastics:					
Rigid P.V.C.	√	√	√	√	Heat distortion occurs at temperatures above 158°F (70°C). Some grades are slightly brittle.
Polythene (Polyethylene)	√	√		√	Some types are susceptible to stress-corrosion cracking.
Polystyrene	√	√		√	Some grades are brittle.
Wood					Now usually encountered in the form of plywood which is bonded with waterproof phenolic resin and finished with a protective coating, e.g. a facing of P.V.C.; it is used for the main structure of processing units or for sinks to contain photographic dishes.

FIG. 9.3. Table showing chemical and mechanical suitability of certain materials for different photographic purposes.

Pipes for the water *supply* are in a less hazardous position than drainage systems. Brass or copper piping is very satisfactory. Rigid P.V.C. can also be used, though it may be brittle. Lead is relatively expensive and owing to its soft nature must be well supported.

It should be observed that developer is not immune to the presence of copper; indeed one part in 1,000,000 of this metal is capable of contaminating a solution. It is good practice when preparing such solutions first to run off the static contents of any supply pipes before using the water. Condensation on copper pipes above a developing tank may result in droplets falling into the solution and this has been known to fog films during development.

By way of summary of the subject, the table in Fig. 9.3 lists certain materials which are commonly employed for the manufacture of photographic equipment at the present time and likely to be found in X-ray departments. It shows their chemical and mechanical suitability for certain applications.

MANUAL PROCESSING

Processing Tanks

At the present time the routine manual processing of radiographs is most likely to be undertaken in an inclusive unit. Tanks which are not linked together in this form are usually for a specialized purpose. Examples of this specialization are those available for processing fluorographic roll film. However, whether a tank is supplied by itself or is an insertion in a larger container, neither consideration affects its general requirements of structure and design.

Materials generally suitable for the construction of processing tanks have been described in the previous section. At the present time those most likely to be found in use for the purpose are:

(1) hard rubber;

(2) perspex;

(3) stainless steel.

The first of these is the least and the third the most expensive. Hard, vulcanized rubber is a light, reasonably strong substance but is liable to bulge if repeatedly filled with hot water, particularly of course if it is not thick enough. The plastic materials have replaced porcelain and enamel, both of which were prone to chip and thus lead to chemical contamination and erosion; porcelain tanks also had the grave disadvantage of being very heavy. Tanks made of stainless steel with welded seams are no doubt the best. They are not brittle, or prone to distortion, nor do they otherwise deteriorate. However, they are about three times the price of vulcanized rubber.

It is usual to supply a lid to fit the developing tank. One for the fixer may also be recommended as a protection against any accumulation of dust on the surface of the solution and to prevent crystallization at the rim. However, it is doubtful if this practice in fact is often followed. Indeed the vapour from an acid fixing bath which is covered can readily attack a stainless steel tank, particularly if the steel does not contain molybdenum.

A minimum of four tanks is necessary for processing, one each for the separate stages of development, rinsing, fixing and washing. These may all have the same capacity, but perhaps better is to make the wash tank larger than the others as a rule and to have a fixing tank of twice the volume of the developer. Such a group of tanks is illustrated in Plate 9.3, following p. 94.

In this outfit the wash tank has a capacity of 10 gallons (45 litres) and is equipped with a tap below for easy emptying. The other three tanks each contain 2 gallons (9 litres). A base board is provided and the complete assembly can readily be arranged in a sink to form a composite unit.

The tanks shown are 21 ½ in. (54 cms) in height and this is representative of many. The sink intended to house them should not have its base more than 12 in. (30 cms) above the floor or the working level may be too high for convenience. Both hot and cold water should be provided for general purposes, though only cold is essential to the functions of rinsing and washing. It can be fed to the tanks in question by means of flexible rubber or plastic tubing which should be weighted and long enough to reach to the bottom of each in order to obtain a complete volume exchange; otherwise water trickling in at the top of the tank may quickly overflow and the major contents remain stagnant.

Tanks of this kind are provided in a number of standard sizes. 2-, 3-, 5-, 10-, and 15-gallon (9, 13.5, 22.5, 45, and 67.5 litres) are a typical, although not the only available range. If films for processing include those of dimensions 14 × 17 in. a 3-gallon tank (13.5 litres) is probably the minimum capacity which should be considered.

A processing system on these lines is efficient enough up to a certain point. Its main disadvantage is the difficulty of maintaining solutions at a constant temperature over a number of working hours. If processing is necessary at some isolated time, for example during an emergency call at night, the unit is not ready for use. In these circumstances a frequent practice is to put an immersion heater into the developing tank and leave it while the patient is received and the X-ray examination made. It is a matter of chance and probably rather an unusual occurrence if the radiographer finds on returning to the darkroom that the temperature of the developing solution is precisely the desired one. If it is not, the tendency to 'make it do' is naturally pronounced.

A 5-gallon tank (22.5 litres) cannot safely contain more than 6 films at once without a risk of their touching each other at some time. This is rather a limited capacity. Larger volumes have the disadvantage that an immersion heater requires longer periods to bring them to the correct working temperature. Because of these features the use of a self-contained unit with thermostatic control of temperature is much to be preferred.

Processing Units

Self-contained processing units are available in a number of designs and sizes. A typical one is shown in Plate 9.4, following p. 94. Essentially each such unit consists of a set of tanks inside a larger one. The outer tank in reference to its function as a container for the water jacket is designated generally by that name.

GENERAL CONSTRUCTION

It can be seen that the unit illustrated has a developing tank with a lid, a compartment for rinsing, a fixing tank and a final, larger section for washing purposes which is independent of the water jacket. The developing tank shown has a capacity of 5 gallons (22·5 litres) but in a larger unit it would be 10 gallons (45 litres). These figures, and similar ones quoted elsewhere in the section, will have greater meaning for the student if they are related to the practical observation that in a 10-gallon (45 litre) tank it is possible to put 12 to 15 hangers at one time without undue risk of films being in contact with each other.

The processing unit has a fixing tank which holds 10 gallons (45 litres) of solution. This is considered the minimum size suitable for most forms of silver recovery equipment. If such apparatus is not to be used, the single tank could be replaced by a pair having a capacity of 5 gallons (22·5 litres) each: students no doubt will see this arrangement in many smaller X-ray departments. Processing units designed to handle a larger flow of work might have one or two 18-gallon (80-litre) tanks for fixing purposes.

Tanks are likely to be made of perspex, polyvinyl chloride (P.V.C.) or stainless steel. They are usually arranged for a left-to-right sequence of work but as a rule the reverse progression can be obtained on request to the manufacturer. The photograph in Plate 9.4, following p. 94, illustrates a unit in which the rinse section is flexibly connected to its water supply: this means that its position in the water jacket can be moved at will and the other tanks arranged in suitable order on either side of it. The washing section is completely separate and can stand equally well on the left of the water jacket. This adaptability of design makes either sequence of work readily available; indeed the user can alter it at any time to his own convenience.

The basic structure of this processing unit is a shell of 1-inch resin-bonded plywood reinforced with steel tie rods. Externally the unit is panelled with melamine sheeting: this is a laminated material presented under a number of trade names of which perhaps the one best known is 'Formica'. Internally the unit is clad with a facing of P.V.C. All the exposed edges are capped with stainless steel.

These are all typical modern materials. They provide a hard-wearing structure which is chemically suitable, trim and pleasant in appearance and easy to keep clean.

The Water Jacket

The water jacket usually has inlet and outlet valves operated by control knobs on the front panel. However, in a small processing unit the jacket may be fed by the less sophisticated device of a hose connected to some external supply tap: it is emptied by removal of a rubber bung from the outlet pipe. A chain and lever considerately attached to the plug make its withdrawal feasible without immersion of the hand and arm in the full depth of water: the proximal end of the chain is hooked over the edge of the unit in a convenient situation when the bung is in position.

As we have seen, the temperature of the water jacket is usually under automatic control by means of a heated element at its base and a thermometer regulator. Included in the system is a device which will prevent overheating of this element should the level of the water fall below a critical level. It operates by means of a float switch which breaks the current supply to the heater.

The float switch. In Plate 9.2, the external appearance of the float switch can be seen. The device consists of a float in a small chamber which is attached to the front of the water jacket and is in communication with it. The level of water in the two is necessarily the same: if it falls in the main compartment it is bound to do so equally in the chamber of the float switch.

In Fig. 9.4 we have a schematic diagram which shows how the movement of such a float in response to alteration in the water level can be used to operate a micro-switch, depicted in the diagram above it. Closure of these contacts, made when the float switch falls a critical distance, operates others in the thermometer regulator which break the circuit supplying the heater.

When the level of water rises again, the float opens the first pair of contacts and the current supply to the heater is then restored by the reverse sequence of events.

A float switch of this type is a simple device. However, it requires regular maintenance no less than more elaborate pieces of electrical apparatus. Particularly in areas where the water is hard, salt deposits may collect round the sides of the chamber at the surface, or round the edges of the float, and this accumulation can readily prevent free movement of the float. If it becomes completely or virtually immobile, of course it will fail to operate the micro-switch. The manufacturers recommend that at

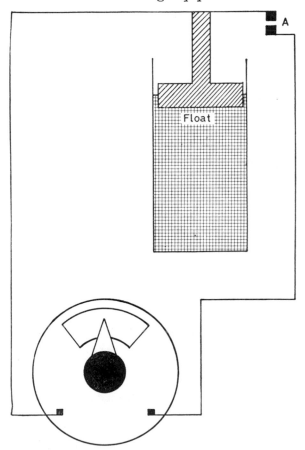

Fig. 9.4. Diagram to illustrate the operation of a float switch in a processing unit. The level of water in the float chamber is the same as that in the water jacket. If this level falls, the float will move downwards, thus activating the micro-switch at A. Closure of the contacts at A operates others in the circuit of the thermometer regulator which break the supply to the heater. The external appearance of the float chamber and switch can be seen in Plate 9.2.

least once a year a competent electrician should check the electrical equipment of the processing unit: this survey will include an examination of the float switch.

When it is necessary to empty the water jacket radiographers and technicians sometimes rely on the operation of the heater's safety devices and do not switch off the regulator at the mains before allowing the water to drain. This is a careless practice which has led to trouble on occasions when the float had in fact become stuck. The possibility of fires in processing units has led to a government recommendation in the United Kingdom that a relay which is thermally operated should be included in the heater circuit in addition to the float switch. This may appear perhaps as a 'braces-and-belt' approach to the risk, when adequate safeguard no doubt is provided by the simpler measures of regular maintenance and the consistent habit of switching off immersion heaters at the point of mains supply whenever it becomes necessary to empty the water jacket. In any event these practices are wise and should have routine application in any X-ray department.

THE RINSE

The rinsing section of the unit shown in Plate 9.4, is movable but in others of different design it is probably not a discrete tank but a built-in compartment of the water jacket. In either case it provides one or other of two forms of rinse: these are (a) a spray rinse, (b) a dip or running rinse.

Spray rinse. In this system two rigid tubes are fitted at the top of the compartment. They run the full extent, one on each side, and are parallel to the plane surfaces of a film suspended within the compartment. One end of each tube is connected to a water inlet valve: the distal ends are closed. A series of perforations along each tube is directed towards each other so as to throw a fine spray of water on the opposing surfaces of the suspended film. The water supply is turned on and off as needed by a control lever at the front. A drain at the bottom of the compartment is permanently open to allow for the water's escape as it is used.

This system can be efficient but it has potential faults which may easily be present for a time without the operator's noticing. These are of the following kind.

(1) If the position of the tubes is not carefully adjusted the angle of the jets in relation to the film may be such that they impinge on it at too low a level. They should be directed of course at its upper extreme border and if they are not then a portion of the radiograph is unrinsed.

(2) The perforations are very fine and a number of them may readily become blocked. The strip of film opposite these again will not be rinsed. Their condition needs constant attention with a stylet or pin, especially in areas where the water is hard.

(3) If the water is not turned on fully enough, or if for any reason the pressure is low, then the trickle from the jets may not even reach the

film. In diminished illumination and in haste this occurrence is not always recognized.

Dip or running rinse. Because of the inherent weaknesses of the spray rinse, a dip or running rinse is to be preferred. To use these it is necessary to close the drain at the bottom of the compartment, generally by means of a bung which can be removed at need by pulling on an attached chain. A single tube positioned vertically at the near end of the compartment feeds water into this section at a low level and it escapes by overflow at the top through a cavity which is in communication with the drain at the base. Two methods of work are possible.

(a) The compartment may be filled with water and used to rinse a number of films. When it becomes cloudy the whole volume is discarded and renewed.

(b) Water is allowed to trickle continuously into the section so that its renewal is a gradual process. These are known respectively as a dip rinse and a running rinse. The second is no doubt the more efficient of the two, since the first may be allowed to continue in use rather too long if the operator is busy and feels that there is not time to renew it.

Either system has the advantage over a spray rinse that a number of films may be placed in the tank simultaneously without loss of the rinse's efficacy. This means that a small group can be transferred from the developer to the rinse in immediate sequence and then taken in the same way from the rinsing to the fixing bath. Consequently there is closer control of the development period of the later films in the series, as they do not have to wait for their removal from the developer until rinsing of their predecessors is complete: equally the rinsing of the earlier ones is more likely to be effectively performed over a sufficient interval.

THE WASHING SECTION
The washing section has usually a greater capacity than the other tanks. It may be simply a compartment in the body of the unit which is independent of the water jacket, or it may be a separate structure as it is in Plate 9.4 and many larger installations. A self-contained washer is more flexible in arrangement and has the further advantage that it can readily be duplicated. Two or more may be placed in tandem with a processor which has developing, rinsing and fixing sections, and where the disposal of a large number of radiographs is involved this can prevent overcrowding at the washing stage. A washer or washers of this kind may be put equally well alongside a pass-through unit in a viewing room where wet radiographs

are checked for quality: this system of work is described in Chapter XI.

The washing section of the unit illustrated in Plate 9.4 can accept a total of 24 hangers at any one time and the unit is designed to process 50–60 radiographs per hour. In larger washers this capacity is doubled. Whether the washing section is a discrete entity or an integral division of a self-contained processing unit, its general features are likely to be similar.

Water enters through a spray- or rose-feed at the bottom of the tank and its flow is controlled by an inlet valve situated at the front of the unit and operated by a screw knob. When fully open this is capable of filling the tank quite rapidly and also of flooding the darkroom if it is left like this too long. Once the washer is full, the supply of water should be diminished until a smooth flow is obtained which can be kept running continuously without harm for whatever period the darkroom is required to operate. The rate should be sufficient to change the water in the tank at least four times in every hour. In the case of a tank containing 50 gallons, a flow of 3½ gallons per minute is necessary.

Water can leave the tank at either of two points.

(1) An overflow pipe at the top. This is its normal outlet during processing procedure.

(2) A drain in the base of the unit which is ordinarily closed by a gate-valve or bung and opened when it is desired to empty the unit for cleaning or other purpose.

The significance in effective washing of arranging the flow of water from a low to a high level through the tank, or in the reverse direction, has already been noted.

Hangers are supported in the washer at a height below the water level by stainless steel racks, usually slotted to separate each film from its neighbour and allow a free current of water between them. These may be fitted either at right angles to the front of the unit or parallel with it. Other considerations being equal, the latter arrangement is perhaps the more convenient in operation since it maintains the hangers in the same plane as they have occupied in the other tanks: otherwise the technician must turn them through 90° as they are moved into the washing section.

In some processors there is free space available within the washing compartment for the insertion of a 3-gallon tank (13 litres) of wetting agent if it is desired to use this.

Specialized Processing Equipment

The processing units described in the previous pages are of a kind likely to be found in a general X-ray darkroom and are designed to handle a continuous flow of all sizes of film. For certain types of specialized work, processing equipment planned for the purpose may often be used. Examples are found in that designed for the processing of roll film or again in the small tanks suitable only for dental radiographs.

Much of what has been said in this chapter is applicable in the context of any specialized processing equipment and students should not have difficulty in relating to these general observations practical features of some particular apparatus which they may handle in the course of experience. In Chapter xviii the processing of fluorograms will be more fully considered in view of the special problems involved.

PROCESSING IN THE OPERATING THEATRE

The student will be aware that radiographs are often taken in the operating theatre to control the course of certain surgical procedures. Special methods are likely to be employed for the processing of these, in order that films may be viewed and operative technique planned by the surgeon without lapse of time; any undue delay may add considerably over the course of the operation to the period for which the patient is under anaesthesia and thus to the risks of the procedure.

A number of means are available for obtaining rapid processing in the operating theatre.

(1) A standard X-ray replenisher used in a dilution of 1 + 2 or 1 + 4 which will give complete development within 30 or 60 seconds respectively.

(2) A standard X-ray developer used at elevated temperatures.

(3) A specially formulated developer designed to give complete development within 15 to 30 seconds.

(4) An image transfer system employing the Polaroid radiographic cassette and processor.

The last of these requires the use of other, quite different equipment and the principle is described in Chapter 1. Though it is relatively expensive in material costs, it is very fast and provides a dry processed print in about 10 seconds.

Methods (1) to (3) imply a conventional form of processing apparatus, though it is often of specialized design. For instance, the tanks and thermostatically controlled water jacket may be mounted on a trolley:

this is likely to have an extensible section to serve as a loading bench and may include its own safelight and cupboards to store chemicals. The whole assembly is quite mobile and can be plugged into a mains socket in any handy room which is capable of being totally darkened.

Perhaps more important than the equipment used is the actual processing technique. When development occurs very rapidly it becomes more difficult to control and radiographs taken in the operating theatre are often seriously flawed by processing marks. These are likely to be due to:

(a) uneven dispersal of the developer solution over the whole surface of the film;

(b) dichroic fog formed because the film is inadequately rinsed and active development continues in the fixing solution.

To avoid contamination scrupulous care and cleanliness of method are essential, particularly when a very small rinse tank is used. The following further points are also worth notice.

(1) There should be constant agitation of the film during processing.

(2) The addition of a few drops of wetting agent to the developer or preliminary immersion of the film in plain water will break down surface tension and facilitate contact of the developer with all points of the emulsion simultaneously.

(3) The use of an acid stopbath between development and fixation should make certain that the developer is fully neutralized before the film enters the fixing solution.

(4) The correct selection of radiographic exposure factors may be significant. When working in the operating theatre, radiographers have a natural tendency to overexpose films so that time spent on processing them may be reduced. However, it is well to remember that many chemical actions cannot be hurried and at the same time successfully controlled. Exposure factors which result in an image of sufficient density after 10 seconds' development or less are better reconsidered if films are seen to be streaked and fogged. For example, when using a standard replenishing solution in a dilution of $1 + 4$, factors should be selected which allow the film to go for the *full* development period of 45 to 60 seconds. It is no help to provide the surgeon with a radiograph which has been rapidly processed if the detail of the image is unreadable; better far, to spend an extra half a minute in the darkroom and obtain a clean film, free from processing faults.

Processing Hangers

Films are suspended for processing in tanks in metal frames known as hangers. These are designed:

(a) to support the film and allow it to be manipulated without handling of the emulsion;

(b) to permit a number of films to be processed simultaneously and to keep them separate from each other during the procedure.

There are two general varieties of hanger: these are the channel type and the tension type.

CHANNEL HANGERS

In this design of hanger the frame is a double structure on either side of the film and forms a groove which holds each of its edges. At the top of the frame a hinged lip can be raised to allow the film to be inserted and this is then closed. A hanger of this type is illustrated in Plate 9.5, following p. 94.

The good features of the channel hanger are:

(1) it is quick to load;

(2) the film is securely held and in normal conditions is unlikely to suffer accidental release during processing.

Less convenient features are as follows.

(1) Since the sides of the frame overlap the edges of the film this area is protected during drying and radiographs dried in these hangers remain wet at the edges long after the rest of their surface is ready. In practice this makes it necessary to remove films from channel hangers and suspend them by another means for drying.

(2) Channel hangers are difficult to clean. If inadequate attention is given to them, chemical deposits and other residues are prone to accumulate in the grooves. If a film is not removed from its hanger for drying, the heat may raise the temperature of the metal sufficiently to melt the emulsion in contact with it. This mishap not only damages the immediate radiograph but has the capacity to inflict similar harm on its successors, since the sticky emulsion remaining in the hanger may adhere to another film when the hanger is again heated in the drier.

(3) While the film cannot readily become detached, it is not a close fit in the channels. The play available creates some tendency for the larger sizes of film to bow away from the vertical plane under the pressure of attempted immersion in a deep solution. This may bring one surface of a film into contact with its neighbour or—if the hanger is worn and the

top of the frame either broken or missing—may in fact pull the film from the hanger. Any hanger, whatever its pattern, which is in a state of even slight disrepair, should be discarded until it can be serviced or replaced.

TENSION HANGERS

Tension hangers have a steel-rod framework which normally does not touch either plane surface of the film. Each of four small clips perforates one corner of the radiograph and maintains it within the hanger; the lower two clips are attached directly to the frame and the upper two by means of a spring bar, the purpose of which is to hold the film under slight tension and keep it flat. A typical tension hanger is illustrated in Plate 9.6, following p. 94.

In loading this hanger it should be inverted and the film attached first to the two lower clips. The upper clips in turn can then be brought to meet the parallel edge because of the mobility given them by the spring bow. If the film is not flat in the hanger it is usually because it is incorrectly placed in the lower clips and adjustment to these should be made if required.

Tension hangers have the convenience that they can be used to suspend films in a drier and are easier to keep clean than those of the channel type. However, they require rather more care in loading and sometimes during processing a film will pull free from one of the clips; both these features are accentuated if the film used has the rounded corners now presented by manufacturers.

HANGER BARS AND CLIPS

Hanger bars are virtually essential accessories to the use of the channel type of hanger, since they are designed mainly to support the film during drying. Their appearance is illustrated in Plate 9.7, following p. 94 and is largely self-explanatory. The position of the clips along the bar is adjustable so that each is appropriate for any size of radiograph. A film can be attached to a bar either before being put into a channel hanger or after removal from it before entry into the drying cabinet. Some care must be exercised in positioning the clips to avoid bowing of the film and the use of a weighted clip on the lower edge is helpful in keeping it vertically taut in the drier. A clip of this type is illustrated in Plate 9.8, following p. 94.

These accessories could be used together to replace a processing hanger if required but they are not very convenient as a normal practice. Other smaller varieties of single film clips are available and can be seen in manu-

facturers' catalogues but on the whole they have few applications in
general X-ray departments.

DENTAL HANGERS

A special type of hanger is used for the processing of dental radiographs.
This is illustrated in Plate 9.9, following p. 94 and again is self-explanatory in appearance. The hanger usually includes an ivorine tablet for
record purposes. In attaching dental radiographs to these hangers the
technician should avoid impaling the film at the point where its surface
is embossed to identify the tube aspect. This can lead only to doubt and
confusion.

Care of Tanks and Processing Units

If nowhere else, in the darkroom at least cleanliness is next to godliness.
A little attention regularly given is worth far more than a large-scale
attack sporadically conducted. The technician who has for the darkroom's equipment the pride of a ship's engineer for his engines and can
be discovered habitually going round with a cloth in his hand is of in-
estimable value in the production of good radiographs.

Modern materials are easy to maintain in smart condition simply by
being regularly and often wiped over with a clean damp cloth; the operative words are 'regular' and 'often'. In the case of many plastic materials,
stains usually penetrate beyond the surface. If they are not removed
within a few hours of formation their subsequent removal may be very
difficult indeed. Warm water and a little soap solution are effective in the
first instance.

The steel capping on some processing units may be polished after
washing by the use of impregnated wadding, such as 'Dura-Glit'.
Deposits on the surface may be removed with fine pumice, and troublesome rust deposits usually respond to a 5–10 per cent warm solution of
citric acid followed by simple washing. Abrasives and wire wool never
should be employed for this purpose.

When chemicals are changed the opportunity should be taken to scrub
tanks thoroughly with clean warm water and a long-handled brush.
Very hot water is detrimental in action to hard rubber and will distort
tanks of this kind. At no time should it be used indiscriminately on tanks
of plastic material. Narrow tanks require a double-sided brush and one
designed for the purpose is easily obtainable.

A hard scale sometimes forms on the sides of developing tanks and
can be difficult to remove by scrubbing, particularly if it is of long

standing. A 10 per cent solution of acetic acid put into the tank for a while may help to loosen the deposit and it can then be dislodged with a scrubbing brush. After this treatment, thorough rinsing of the tank with clean water is essential.

The presence of bacteria in the processing water is a potential hazard to radiographs. As a result of their action sulphites may be converted to sulphides which affect photographic emulsions and produce chemical fog. Because of this risk it may be thought advisable to sterilize processing tanks from time to time. This can be done by filling them with a bacteriostatic solution. For this purpose a suitable substance is dichlorophen, obtainable as the proprietary preparation 'Embatex'. Four ounces (115 ml) of 'Embatex' to 10 gallons (45·5 litres) of water is an appropriate strength. Alternatively a domestic bleaching preparation such as 'Parazone' or 'Domestos' may be used in a dilution of 1 + 5. Such a solution should not be left for any length of time in stainless steel tanks, as a reaction between the metal and the bleach will occur. After sterilization, tanks should be thoroughly washed before further use.

The tendency of static volumes of water to accumulate slime is well known to us all. The water jackets of processing units are prone to gather bacterial growth because such micro-organisms flourish in conditions of warmth and where light intensity is low. Their presence not only is unpleasant to sight, touch and sometimes to our sense of smell, but is likely to promote corrosion of the unit's structure and can effectively insulate processing tanks: this will retard the transfer of heat from the water jacket to the developing solution.

The growth of algae can be prevented in a water jacket by the introduction of chemical agents. The water jacket of the unit illustrated in Plate 9.4 holds about 20 gallons (90 litres) of water. One ounce (28·5 g.) of sodium pentachlorophenate added to this makes an appropriate bactericidal solution. Alternatively, 'Embatex' in the proportion of 1 oz. (28·5 g.) to 10 gallons (45·5 litres) may be used.

Care of Hangers

Processing hangers are made of stainless steel of a specified quality such as was described in a previous section. They repay regular attention. A hanger which is dirty or damaged, or one which is not the correct size for the film but employed because of shortage, almost certainly will originate a number of artefacts during processing. Indeed it is not an unknown occurrence for a film even to be torn if it is forced past the edge of a neighbouring film which is partly adrift from its hanger in a processing tank.

As well as being periodically inspected for serviceable condition, hangers should be cleaned on a regular rota. Abrasives must not be employed for this purpose. Dry scrubbing with a stiff brush, if undertaken at frequent intervals, is simple and effective. It should be combined with a regular wash in clean hot water to dissolve any obstinate chemical residues.

Hangers which have been allowed to become very dirty may need more powerful treatment. A suitable cleanser for this purpose is 5 oz. (64 ml) of glacial acetic acid with the addition of water to make 80 oz. (1000 ml) of fluid altogether. Glacial acetic acid can be obtained from the pharmacy. Hangers should be steeped in this solution for an hour and then scrubbed in three changes of hot water.

AUTOMATIC PROCESSING ON THE IMMERSION PRINCIPLE

The subject of automatic processing will be examined fully in the next chapter. At this stage it is proposed to consider only those processors which operate on the immersion or dunking principle. These depend upon mechanized methods of dipping a film into a tank, withdrawing it after a specified interval and moving it into another tank. They require the use of a hanger, usually only a bar to which the film is clipped by semi-automatic means, and it is both convenient and appropriate to consider these processors as a logical extension of a manual procedure. They usually employ conventional chemicals at a higher concentration than is used for tank processing and developing temperatures are higher (70°F–80°F) (21°C–26.5°C).

Processors of the dunking type are less commonly in use than the more sophisticated units which have roller transport. Their processing cycle is generally slower—though it is often more flexible—and they need more space. Their good points are:

(a) they put very little restriction on either the size of film or type of emulsion processed;

(b) in the event of a breakdown it is possible—though by no means convenient—to continue to process a film by hand;

(c) they are much less expensive than roller units.

A number of processors which work on the immersion principle are available and students may meet one or another of them in use in their departments. The account which follows is of a typical unit of this kind. Details are bound to vary between different processors.

Loading the Film

Processors of the immersion or dunking type cannot handle a film unsupported and consequently it must first be loaded into a suitable hanger. In an automatic system it is particularly important that the hangers should be efficient; a film adrift in the developer may be seriously overdeveloped in a matter of seconds. The hangers, therefore, are of special design and are likely to be in fact only a single bar to which is fitted a row of clips or pins at short intervals. The bar and the film to be loaded are put together in a clamp incorporated in a loading bench or table. This is operated by a handle or treadle. Its action is to open the clips or pins sufficiently to permit insertion of the film, which is then firmly held or impaled when the clamp permits them to close again. This procedure takes longer to describe than to perform and is in fact both rapid and simple even in darkness.

The Processing Scheme

Fig. 9.5 is a cycle diagram of a typical processor employing clip bars and operating on the immersion principle. It will be seen that there are seven compartments in the unit: one of these is for developer and two each for the remaining stages of fixing, washing and drying. At each of two stages the film is taken between a pair of squeegee rollers which remove surface moisture from it (a) after development and (b) after the second washing. The first is an important factor in the omission of the rinse from the processing cycle and the second shortens the drying time of the film.

The following account of the processor's operating sequence should be studied with the aid of the diagram in Fig. 9.5 and the photograph in Plate 9.10, following p. 206. On the right of the drawing can be seen the loading ramp where a number of clip bars, with a film in position on each, have been stacked. Up to six clip bars can be put on to the ramp at one time and the unit will automatically feed itself with these during the ensuing 7 minutes.

Plate 9.10 shows the processor from its loading aspect in the darkroom. Looking into the unit one sees at the top of the picture empty clip bars which are on a storage rack ready for use. In the lower half of the photograph we see the seven processing compartments; above each there is a

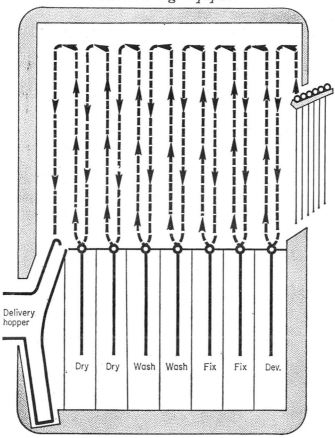

Fig. 9.5. Cycle diagram of an automatic processing machine operating on the immersion or dunking principle. *By courtesy of Ilford Ltd.*

linear arrangement of guides which are designed to prevent a film from curling as it is lowered into its appropriate processing section. The empty loading ramp is above these guides.

Higher up, towards the top of the photograph, can be seen the front edge of a metal carriage to the sides of which are fixed a number of hooks or claws. During operation, this carriage moves in an upward and down-ward direction and also backwards and forwards to a more limited extent owing to the eccentric revolution of an endless chain arranged vertically at the side. This—and other chains in the processor—are driven by an electric motor of fractional horsepower.

As the carriage moves during operation of the unit, any pair of hooks attached to it can pass beneath and then lift a clip bar placed either on the loading ramp or in the processing compartments.

We may appropriately begin our description of events in the processor at a moment when we may assume that the carriage is passing the loading ramp on an upward journey. The following sequence then occurs.

(1) A clip bar on the loading ramp will be collected by the hooks.

(2) The carriage completes its upward trajectory and descends, lowering the clip bar and its passenger into the developing tank.

(3) The motor stops for a predetermined interval selected on a clock or interval timer (the uppermost dial in Plate 9.10).

(4) When the interval timer reaches zero the motor restarts and the carriage begins an upward movement, lifting the film from the developer.

(5) As the film leaves the developing tank it is passed between a pair of squeegee rollers which were previously open but now close on either side of it.

(6) The revolution of the chain suspends this first film over the fixing tank while other hooks on the carriage collect a second film from the loading ramp.

(7) The carriage is again lowered, putting the developed film into the first fixer and the second film into the developer.

(8) The motor again stops, halting the carriage for the predetermined processing interval during which the developed film is partially fixed and the second film developed.

This cycle of events is repeated indefinitely as films are taken through each of the seven processing compartments, there being only one film at a time in any one section. Squeegee rollers, similar to those above the developing tank, operate in the same way as the film leaves the second wash, removing surface moisture from it.

The drying sections of this processor operate on the principle of employing large volumes of air at moderate rather than high temperatures. The word *large* here should be considered in relation to the film, for the actual capacity of each drying compartment in cubic feet is very small compared with a conventional drying cabinet; the real point is that each section of the unit deals with only one film at a time. The temperature of the air is under thermostatic control and the air constantly recirculated by a fan. A duct in the roof of the unit allows continuous escape of an adjustable portion of the circulating air. This avoids excessive

humidity; it also alters—and thus is a means of controlling—the temperature of the drying compartments.

After the second drying section, transport is by a single pair of hooks
each mounted on another endless chain on either side. By these means
the clip bar and its freight are lifted from a ramp and passed along a
guide plate which holds down the leading edge of the film while the clip
bar is pulled away from it. The film then falls into the delivery hopper
and the clip bar is returned overhead by the endless chains to the storage
ramp on the darkroom side of the processor, ready for further use.

The Processing Cycle

The complete processing cycle of the unit described occupies about 8
minutes. An unalterable feature of it is that the film is bound to spend the
same period of time in each processing compartment. However, the
length of this period can be varied by means of the interval timer already
mentioned.

This timer is calibrated between zero and 120 seconds and is adjusted
to suit the sensitometric needs of a particular installation; for example, it
might be set at 50 or 60 seconds. This facility to alter the length of the
processing stage means that the unit is suitable for any of a number of
departments, whose needs may be as different, for instance, as one which
is processing mainly chest radiographs relative to another which is using

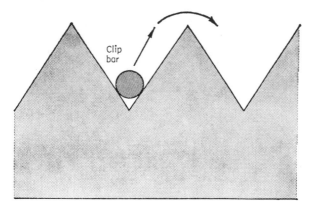

Fig. 9.6. Diagram to show how a film hanger or clip bar can be moved
horizontally through a processing tank by means of a notched ramp fitted
along each side of the tank. The transport mechanism operates to push the
clip bar upwards. When the bar reaches the summit of the peak it will slide
by itself into the next notch.

industrial film. The timer is *not* intended for repeated adjustment by radiographers intent on obtaining an automated equivalent of sight-development.

The unit described and depicted of course is not the only dunking processor available and designs vary in detail. In some processors it is possible to alter not only the length of the processing stage as already described but the number of stages—and therefore the time—which the film spends in a particular section. This is done by means of a notched bar mounted on either side of the processing tanks (Fig. 9.6). The transport mechanism is designed so that instead of being collected by a pair of hooks the film hanger is given an upward push which takes it over the top of an adjacent notch. It slides down the other slope and thus is moved horizontally through a tank of solution. The number of notches which it traverses determines the number of cycles—and therefore affects the length of time—spent by the film in the compartment concerned. It is practicable to extend development, fixing and washing times in this way.

Replenishment of solutions

When radiographs are processed by machinery, this machinery must not only receive, transport and deliver films: it must also provide for the replenishment of solutions if processing is to be standardized.

In Chapter VI the need for both volumetric replenishment and chemical regeneration of a developing solution was discussed. We noticed the problems in manual processing associated with inevitable variations of the drainage time given to films by different operators. These inconsistencies in drainage time are the largest variable affecting the developer's fall in level in the tank.

In automated processing, on the other hand, the drainage time is no longer even a small variable: it is not a variable at all. Processors working on the immersion principle provide a drainage time which is an automatically controlled interval and usually longer than any operator would allow in manipulating films by hand. Furthermore some of these processors—for example the one of which the processing scheme has just been described—pass the film between squeegee rollers after it leaves the developer and these ensure the efficient removal of surface fluid. Consequently the carry-over rate is much reduced and is consistent in quantity.

Because of these facts it is to be expected that the chemical work performed by solutions in automatic processors will be disproportionate to their loss of volume. Adequate chemical regeneration may not be obtained if fresh developer or fixer is added only when it is necessary to restore a solution level. It is therefore usual to arrange that a specific quantity of fresh chemicals shall be injected into both developer and fixing tanks every time a film is taken through the processor. The surplus escapes over a weir which keeps the solution levels constant (see Fig. 10.2 for the use of a weir for this purpose in a wash tank).

The injection of fresh chemicals is made by means of a small pump associated with each tank. The functioning of these pumps varies in different types of unit. One method of their operation is described below and another in the next chapter (see p. 222).

REPLENISHMENT BY METERED PUMPS

In the dunking processor which has just been described the replenisher pumps are of the metered variety; that is, they deliver a fixed amount of fresh solution every time a film is passed through the processor. Thus, the solution's replenishment is irrespective of:

(a) the size of the film processed;
(b) variations in the chemical demand due to these size differences;
(c) similar variations in the amount of solution lost by absorption in the gelatin.

However, this does not matter very much. In a general department, using all sizes of film, the large and the small sufficiently balance each other. One film = 1 sq. ft. of emulsion is as reasonable a working equation here as it was in respect of manual processing (see Chapter VI, p. 130).

In Chapters VI and VII we recognized that the area—or numbers of sheets—of processed film is not the only factor in assessing the replenishment needs of developing and fixing solutions. Other factors of equal importance relate to the type of radiography done and the type of emulsion predominantly used. Because of these variables between different categories of X-ray departments, it is essential in an automatic processor that one should be able to alter the actual quantity of fresh solution which the replenisher pumps inject. This is an adjustment normally made at the time of installation in terms of an assessment of the department's usual processing pattern. It is not a control which the operator is expected to vary and usually will be altered only if the replenishment rate is found to be unsatisfactory. Replenishment rates and tests related to replenishment in automatic processors are further considered in the next chapter (see p. 222).

In the particular immersion processor which we have just described the replenisher pumps operate through the agency of the clip bars. As it is pulled away from the dry film on the completion of processing, each clip bar triggers a microswitch. The microswitch in turn operates the replenisher pumps which automatically deliver a measured amount of solution to the developer and fixer tanks. Because the triggering agent is the clip bar, the replenisher pumps will operate even if there has not actually been a film in transit. In fact operators of this particular processor are advised on starting the unit at the beginning of the day to ensure that solutions are up to correct levels by passing through three empty clip bars.

Replenishment by Fluid Dynamics

A fluid dynamic system has sometimes been employed to provide replenishment of the developer and fixing tanks. This is better known as the *chicken-feeder* method and in contra-distinction to the points made in our earlier discussion its operation depends on a fall in level of the developer solution. The chicken-feeder system is less popular than one

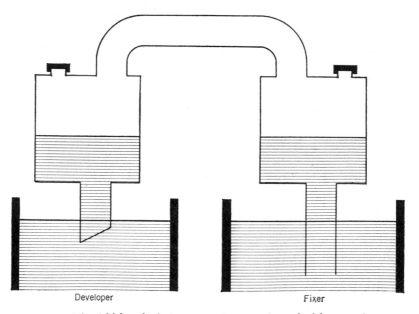

Developer   Fixer

Fig. 9.7. The 'chicken-feeder' system of automatic replenishment of processing solutions. Its operation depends on there being a fall in the level of the developer.

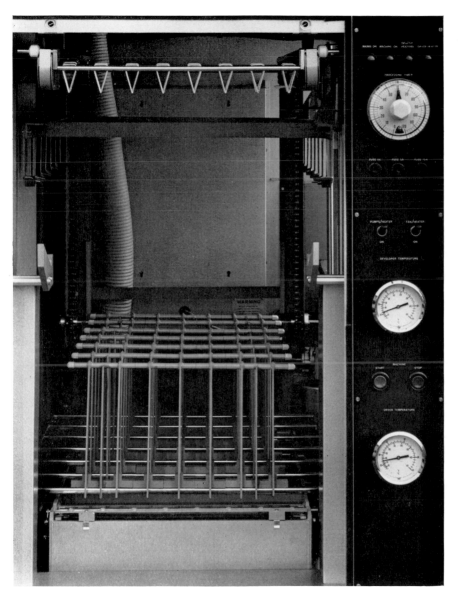

PLATE 9.10. The interior of the processor to which Fig. 9.5 refers. It is seen from the darkroom aspect. *By courtesy of Ilford Ltd.*

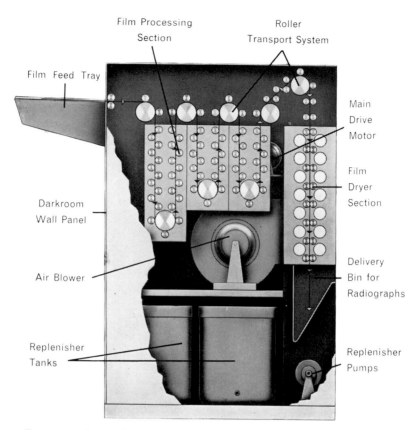

Film Processing Section

Roller Transport System

Film Feed Tray

Main Drive Motor

Film Dryer Section

Darkroom Wall Panel

Air Blower

Delivery Bin for Radiographs

Replenisher Tanks

Replenisher Pumps

PLATE 10.1. Sectional diagram of X-Omat M.4 Processor employing a roller system. In this case, a number of small rollers off-set to each other are used in the processing sections. The drying section is vertically arranged. *By courtsy of Kodak Ltd.*

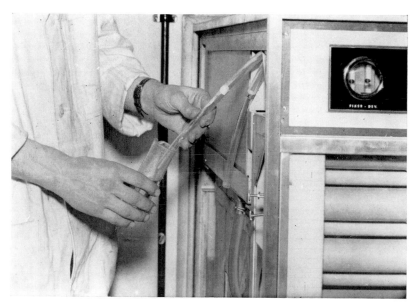

PLATE 10.2. Measuring the replenishment rate in an automatic processor. A 14 inch length of film is fed into the unit, and the additional solution normally supplied to the processing tank by the replenishment pump is collected in a measuring glass. *By courtesy of Kodak Ltd.*

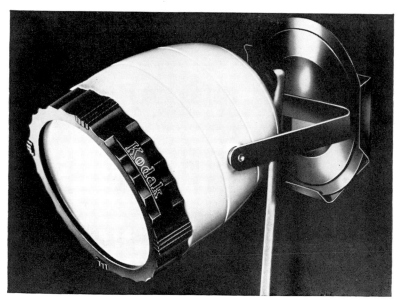

PLATE 11.1. A safelamp for direct lighting. It is suitable for wall fixture or ceiling suspension. *By courtesy of Kodak Ltd.*

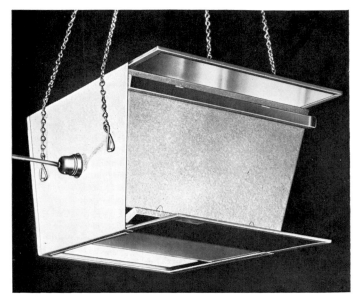

PLATE 11.2. A safelamp which provides indirect and direct illumination at the same time. The filters can be easily removed for cleaning or replacement. *By courtesy of Kodak Ltd.*

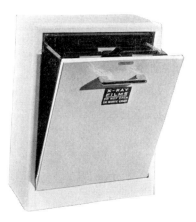

PLATE 11.3. A typical film-hopper for storage of unexposed film in the dark-room ready for immediate use. *By courtesy of Cuthbert Andrews.*

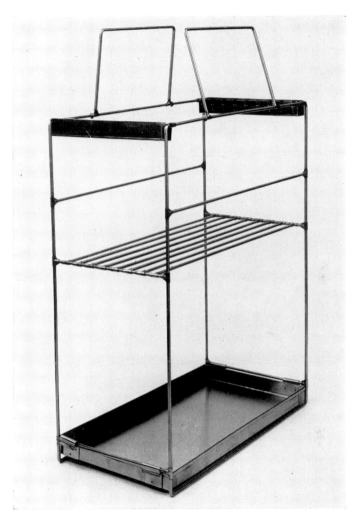

PLATE 11.4. A carrier for transport of wet films from the darkroom. *By courtesy of Ilford Ltd.*

| 40 | 50 | 60 | 70 | 80 | 90 | 100 |

PLATE 12.1. A step-wedge of 17 different thicknesses of aluminium exposed at 7 different kilovoltages. *By courtesy of Kodak Ltd.*

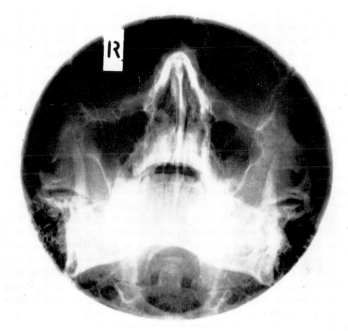

PLATE 14.1. Occipitomental projection illustrating use of a small anatomical marker when a localizing cone is employed.

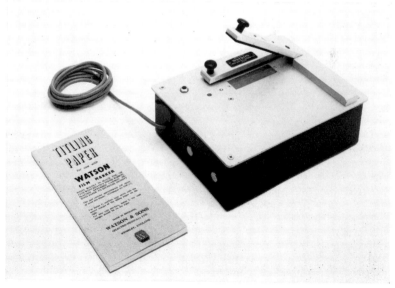

PLATE 14.2. Photographic marker. Closing the pressure pad illuminates the window from below for a fixed interval. *By courtesy of Watson and Sons (Electro-Medical) Ltd.*

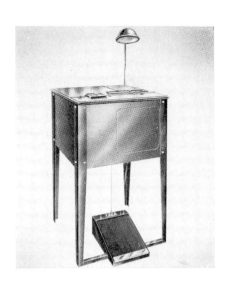

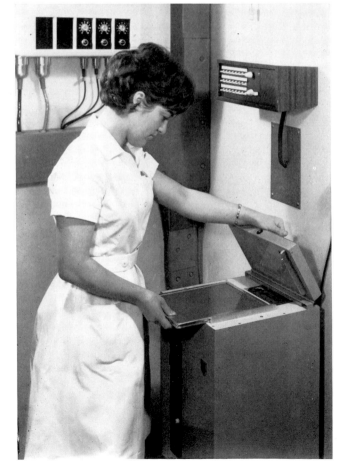

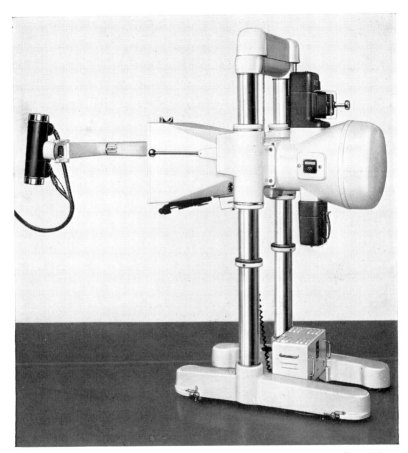

PLATE 17.1. A unit for fluorography, employing 100 mm cut film. The X-ray tube is linked by a side-arm to the fluorescent screen and its optical system, these being supported on a pair of columns; the anode-screen distance is 36 inches and the tube is centred to the fluorescent screen. Both move together vertically on the column by operation of the lever seen at the side. *By courtesy of Watson and Sons (Electro-Medical) Ltd.*

PLATE 14.3. (Upper left) External appearance of the photographic marker to which Fig. 14.3 refers. This marker essentially is a camera. *By courtesy of Theratronics Ltd.*

PLATE 14.4. (Lower left) Radiographic marker. Closing the lid energizes an X-ray tube within the unit; this exposes on the cassette an area corresponding to the rectangular panel in which are placed the marker plates. The exposure interval is predetermined and the unit fully protected against radiation leakage. *By courtesy of Philips Electrical Ltd.*

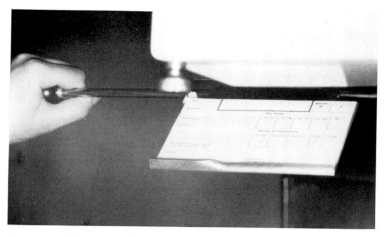

Plate 17.2. The card-holder of a 100 mm fluorographic unit. It is situated beneath the camera tunnel and is seen here in the open position with an identification card *in situ*. When the operating lever is pushed to the right, the tray containing the card moves upwards, and the card's outlined central section is illuminated within the camera tunnel. Details printed in this section will be recorded on the fluorograph. The closed (or exposure) position of the card-holder can be observed in the general view in Plate 17.8.

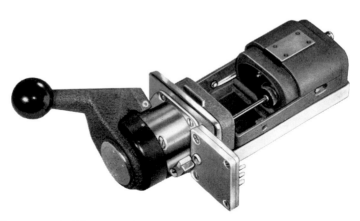

Plate 17.3. Serial cassette for fluorography. This cassette accepts 3 metres of 70 mm roll film. It is hand-operated by the large turning handle at the side. *By courtesy of Watson and Sons (Electro-Medical) Ltd.*

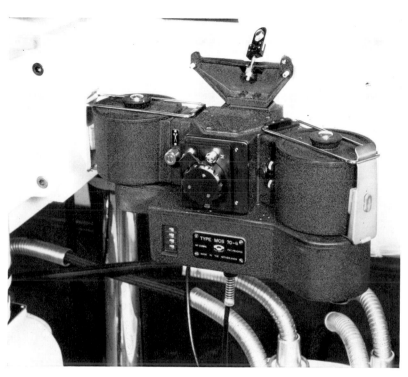

PLATE 17.4. M.C.S. cassette for fluorography. This cassette accepts 30 metres (100 feet) of 70 mm roll film. It is automatically operated. The take-up spool is in the magazine on the left of the photograph; the feed-spool is on the right. The small knob surmounted by the scissors motif indicates a cutter which can be used to shear the film at any point, permitting removal of the magazine. *By courtesy of Watson and Sons (Electro-Medical) Ltd.*

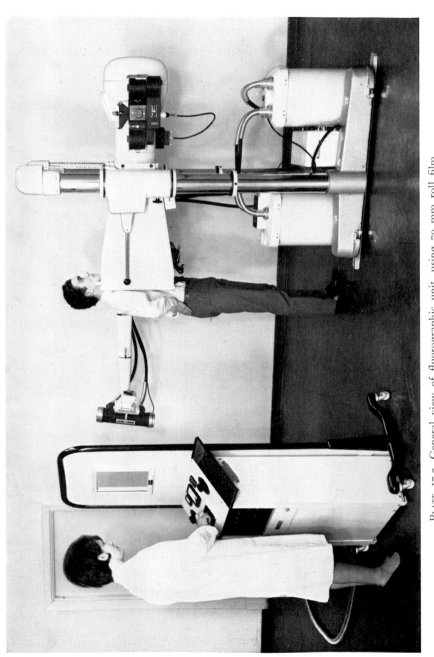

PLATE 17.5. General view of fluorographic unit, using 70 mm roll film. The M.C.S. cassette can be seen in position at the side of the camera tunnel. *By courtesy of Watson and Sons (Electro-Medical) Ltd.*

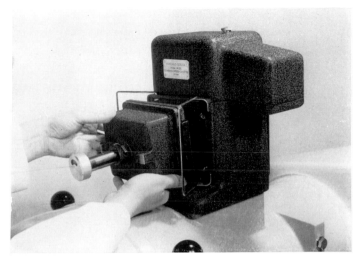

PLATE 17.6. A separator cassette for fluorography suitable for 100 mm cut film. The supply magazine is being withdrawn from the cassette; both are temporarily closed by dark-slides. *By courtesy of Watson and Sons (Electro-Medical) Ltd.*

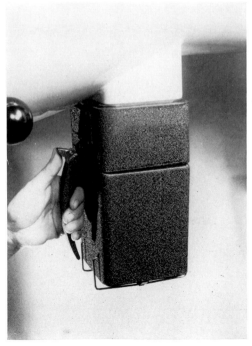

PLATE 17.7. The take-up magazine being withdrawn from a fluorographic separator cassette for 100 mm cut film. *By courtesy of Watson and Sons (Electro-Medical) Ltd.*

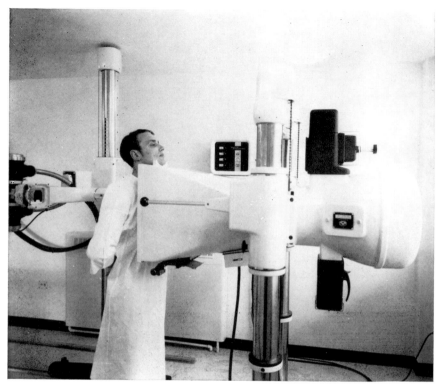

PLATE 17.8. General view of fluorographic unit using 100 mm cut film. The supply magazine of the separator cassette can be seen above the camera tunnel and the take-up magazine below; this should be compared with the appearance of the M.C.S. cassette in Plate 17.5. The card-holder is seen below the fluorescent screen just in front of the patient; it is in the closed or exposure position. The shape of the diaphragm on the X-ray tube should be noted; it is adapted to the general radiographic contours of the lung fields. *By courtesy of Watson and Sons (Electro-Medical) Ltd.*

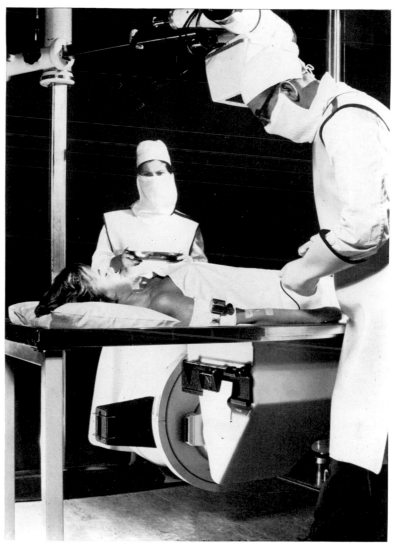

PLATE 17.9. Fluorographic unit employing 100 mm cut film in use for angiography. The magazine of the separator cassette is parallel to the floor. The screen and optical system are at 90 degrees to each other; this arrangement is shown schematically in Fig. 17.8. *By courtesy of the N.V. Optische Industrie de Oude Delft.*

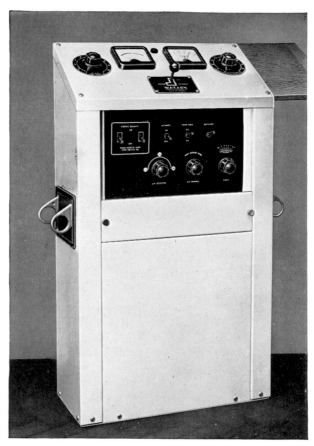

PLATE 17.10. Control panel for mass radiography unit. Its general features are designed for compactness and manoeuvrability. Carrying handles can be fitted through the rings at each side, and the extended portion on the right provides a writing surface. *By courtesy of Watson and Sons (Electro-Medical) Ltd.*

which employs pumps and it is tending to become obsolete. However, a brief description of it is given below.

From Fig. 9.7 it can be seen that the apparatus for replenishment consists of a tank of developer and a tank of fixer mounted above the tanks which are to be replenished, and that these two have at the top an air-communication between them formed by a length of plastic piping. At the outlet of each tank, a relatively short feed pipe connects the supplementary supply of developer to the main body, while a greater length is associated with the fixer system. The developer pipe ends just below the surface level in the processing tank.

In the processing tank the level of the developer falls in proportion to the area of film put through it and as a result of absorption by the dry emulsion and the carry-over of solution: for the reasons already discussed this last factor is minimal. The level will fall to a lesser extent in the fixing tank since the film is already soaked on entering it and absorption is very much less. When the developing solution becomes so low that the aperture of the feed-pipe is exposed then air will enter the replenishing tank and displace an appropriate quantity of developer into the processing tank to bring the level again just above the aperture of the supply pipe.

However, owing to the upper communication between them, air which has entered the system via the developer replenishing tank must affect equally the level in the fixer replenishing tank; these two solutions are bound to be always at the same level and to drop at the same rate. The result of this is the injection of a certain quantity of fixer into the processing tank for every addition of developer; and consequently the overflow of some used and partially exhausted solution, which may be allowed to run to waste but is more likely to be collected in a tank for silver recovery.

Rinsing and Washing

In some automatic processors which employ the dunking method of operation, washing—and rinsing if it is done at all—may be performed at atmospheric temperatures. In this case no special provision need be made for controlling the temperature of the water. However, washing is more efficient and takes place more rapidly in warm water. For this reason, a processor of this type may have its washing tanks fed with water from an externally mounted mixing valve (see p. 175) which maintains a supply at a constant temperature; a typical value for this temperature is $78°F$ ($25°C$).

17

Consumption of water by automatic processors may be considerably greater than when processing is performed manually. This is a point which should not be overlooked by hospital engineers when automated equipment is purchased and installed, particularly if it is to occupy an old building which may have an elderly water supply. The operation of automatic processors in such circumstances has been known to deprive the rest of the department of water for any other purpose.

The amount of water required depends on the processor chosen. The unit earlier described has two 8-gallon (36-litre) wash tanks and needs 1½ gallons (6·8 litres) per minute. This is less than a typical figure.

Automatic processors are sensitive to changes in water pressure. Washing is certainly less efficient and may not be archivally permanent if the water pressure falls. However, the pressure required is not necessarily high and in the data of an automatic processor the minimum figure given is likely to be equivalent to a normal tap supply. If the supply is poor a booster pump may have to be fitted. The immersion type processor which we have here considered needs a pressure of only 4 lbs. per sq. in. (11·7 kg/cm²); this is less than many.

In some units—where there is an insufficient rate of change of the water for the capacity of the tank—washing is a two-stage process. In this case the water is usually fed initially to the *second* section of the wash and from there passed into the washing bath which is *first* in order of the film's progress. If the unit employs a rinsing stage between developer and fixer, water from the first wash may then be fed into the rinse. Here any acquired acid content from the fixing solution actually assists its effectiveness in functioning as a stopbath to the action of the developer.

Recirculation of Solutions

It is essential for automated processing equipment to maintain a continuous recirculation of solutions. The reasons for this will be considered in the next chapter. Processors operating on the immersion principle here make a significant departure from the tradition and practices of manual processing: they include a recirculatory system in the course of which both developing and fixing solutions can be heated to processing temperature and filtered. Heating of the solutions is performed by passing them through conditioning boxes in which are thermostatically controlled immersion heaters.

CHAPTER X

Automatic Processing: Roller Processors

GENERAL ASPECTS

The introduction of automation into medical X-ray darkrooms has had an impact on radiology proportionally as great as that of the industrial revolution on English history. A radiograph which is automatically processed is never handled *wet*. The film, unloaded from its cassette and containing the latent image, is fed in the darkroom into the processor and taken out at the other end of the unit, as a rule outside the darkroom, within a matter of minutes, developed, fixed, washed and dried: it can be put into an envelope and made ready for immediate diagnosis.

The effect of this has been not only to alter the practical realities of processing technique but to require major re-organization of the work necessary on a radiograph after it leaves the darkroom and before it reaches those who originally requested its aid; that is, the procedures of sorting, documenting and reporting of films. The presence in the darkroom of an automatic processing unit must affect the working routines not only of darkroom technicians but also of clerical, radiographic and radiological staff.

Darkroom planning in relation to automation should be such that the processor functions as a pass-through unit: that is, one wall of the darkroom should straddle the processor so that films fed into it in the darkroom will be ejected and can be collected and sorted in normal lighting in an adjacent room or other suitable area. When a unit is arranged in this way, usually only a small section of it—the loading table or ramp—need be on the darkroom side of the wall and servicing can be performed externally from the lighted adjacent room. Some units provide flexibility of installation, inasmuch as the area required by the processor may be mainly in the lighted room, or mainly in the darkroom, or divided equally between the two depending on what seems to be the best disposition of the available space.

It is doubtful if any of these aspects of automation occurred to the originators of mechanical processing systems, inasmuch as their immediate aim was to *standardize* processing technique and that only. The first automatic machine available to medical radiography was devised by Dr Hills of Guy's Hospital and did not include a drying section. The total processing time was 50 minutes divided as follows: developing 5 mins.; fixing 5 mins.; washing 25 mins.; drying 15 mins. The machine provided exactly what was intended—a mechanization or standardization of the conventional manual processing technique.

In the light of further developments and of growing experience with automation, we may now list its advantages over a wider spectrum but among these we should still place first its original asset.

(1) Improvement of radiographic quality.

Radiographers who have no experience of automation may be disposed to argue this point with the contention that repeat films must become more frequent since there is no possibility whatsoever of adjusting processing technique to offset an error in exposure selection. It has been said elsewhere that the majority of radiographers, while owning theoretical adherence to time-and-temperature methods of processing, in practice modify theory to a greater or lesser extent and inspect their radiographs during development. Nevertheless, while this habit of tampering with its processing may produce a useful radiograph on many an occasion, it is doubtful if it is in the interests of consistently high radiographic quality or concomitant with a minimum number of repeat examinations.

(2) Improvement in departmental capacity.

In many busy X-ray departments the manually operated darkroom can constitute a considerable block to the rapidity of a patient's progress. The time spent by the radiographer in making the X-ray examination may often be less than the interval which follows before the films are available for viewing and checking. Patients waiting to have their films seen continue to occupy space which desirably should be free for new arrivals. Increasing the rate of turnover implies an improved use of the department's facilities and may render adequate, waiting space which formerly was scarcely so.

(3) Economy of money and activity.

The initial cost of an automatic processor is very high compared with any manually operated unit, although some are less expensive than others. However, the immediate outlay is not the only one to consider. Automation in the darkroom may reduce the number of technicians required and effect a long-term economy. Any system in hospital which saves the time and effort of anyone, including the patient, is also saving money.

The high cost and big capacity of many automatic processors make them likely occupants of large general departments where several hundred radiographs are handled per day; they constitute furthermore a strong argument for the possible centralization of processing facilities for several departments, geographically separate within one hospital. This aspect is discussed again from the point of view of darkroom planning in the next chapter.

The place of the automatic processor in the small department has received the attention of designers and there is at present a certain trend in favour of the smaller less expensive unit, which would appear to offer three selling points at least:

(1) it is suitable for small hospitals which need only a relatively low through-put of films per day;

(2) it can be employed as a stand-by unit in a larger department for the processing of a few films, for example during the night;

(3) it can be duplicated, so that servicing may be more easily performed with less disruption of work. The department which needs a single large unit, for example, might consider the installation of two smaller ones.

CHEMISTRY AND SENSITOMETRY

Whatever may have been the original aim of those who introduced automation into X-ray darkrooms, it is now true that automatic systems of processing can release a dry finished film within a few minutes of entry into the machine. Indeed the speed with which any particular unit can do this is an important factor in the advantages which it offers. No doubt the student may wonder how processing can be completed within intervals which vary from $1\frac{1}{2}$ to 11 minutes and satisfactory image quality still be maintained. In its general principles, what is different in automation compared to manual operation?

To achieve the now desired rapidity of action every stage of the processing cycle must be accelerated. Below is set down each phase of procedure, together with a note of those factors in automatic systems which permit completion within intervals so short that they are recorded and discussed more usually in seconds than in minutes. It will be seen that the rinsing stage has been omitted. This is possible in most automatic units owing partly to a squeegee action which rollers provide between development and fixation: the action of the rollers reduces the amount of developer carried over into the fixer as compared with manual processing. A secondary factor is found in the increased buffer capacity of the fixer which arms it against the presence of added developer. A third factor is the inclusion of inorganic compounds in the developing solution which inhibit its absorption by the gelatin.

DEVELOPMENT

Development periods vary between different units; the shortest time is 25 seconds and the longest time 140 seconds. It is possible to complete development within these intervals because of:

(1) elevated temperature;
(2) circulation of developer;
(3) movement of the film;
(4) regular replenishment of developing solution for a specified area of film processed;
(5) in some cases the use of a specially modified developer of higher energy;
(6) in very rapid processing systems (90 seconds), the use of a modified, thinner emulsion with a high degree of hardening.

FIXING

Fixing periods vary in a similar way between approximately 15 seconds and 131 seconds. The rapid action of the fixer depends on:

(1) a squeegee process between developer and fixer to remove the developing solution from the emulsion surface;
(2) in roller processors, a developer which has a lower pH than X-ray developers used in manual processors and contains inorganic compounds to reduce swelling of the gelatin;
(3) a fixing solution which is well buffered;
(4) circulation of the fixer;
(5) movement of the film;
(6) regular replenishment for a specified area of film processed;
(7) elevated temperature;
(8) in the case of very rapid systems, a modified, thinner emulsion which absorbs the developing solution to a minimum degree.

WASHING

Again we find that washing periods vary greatly depending on the particular unit considered and that the range is approximately 15 seconds to 131 seconds. That washing can be effectively performed with this rapidity is due to:

(1) a squeegee process in some cases between fixation and washing;
(2) rapid circulation of the water, which in one unit at least is changed at the rate of 40 times in an hour;
(3) in some cases extreme agitation of the water in a small tank;
(4) movement of the film;
(5) sometimes elevated temperature;
(6) in very rapid systems, a modified, thinner emulsion to keep fluid absorption to a minimum;
(7) the fact that only one or two films are washed at one time.

DRYING

The drying times given by differing units also vary. The minimum period is about 25 seconds and the maximum period is 280 seconds. We can list the factors on which such rapid drying depends as:

(1) a squeegee process which removes surface fluid as the film enters the drying section;
(2) movement of the film;
(3) elevated temperature which increases evaporation;
(4) in some cases a reduction of relative humidity by means of controlled air jets directed on the film surface;
(5) in the case of very rapid systems, a modified, thinner film emulsion with adequate hardening properties.

Cycles, Chemicals and Films

CYCLES

A variety of roller processors for medical X-ray film are available. It is convenient to divide them into categories which relate to the length of the processing cycle: that is, to the duration of the interval between feeding an exposed film into the machine and obtaining from it a dry, processed radiograph. This is commonly called the dry-to-dry cycle time.

On this basis we can divide roller processors into the three groups specified below.

(a) Full cycle (dry-to-dry period: 7 min.).
(b) Half cycle (dry-to-dry period: 3½ min.)
(c) Rapid (dry-to-dry period: 1½ min.)

Some examples of roller processing machines give the user the choice of operating on any one of these cycles. This is not to say that it would be practicable to vary the cycle time between film and film. However, it permits a change of mind about a department's processing technique in any special circumstances, without difficulty or extra cost, and obviously the shorter times mean a faster throughput of work and the ability to view processed radiographs more quickly.

CHEMICALS

The developer. We have already seen (Chapter VI) that one method of obtaining a reduction in processing times—specifically in development time—is to raise the working temperature of the developing solution. However, this alone would not meet the full demand of automatic processing: developers used in roller processing machines must have special chemical formulation in addition to their temperature elevation. Chemical activity is increased by:

(1) a higher content of reducing agents;
(2) adjustment of the ratios between the active reducing agents;
(3) adjustment of the pH of the solution and of the amount of restrainer present—both significant factors, as we know, in the energy of any particular developing solution.

Elevated temperatures are inherent in the operation of all roller processing machines. The lowest processing temperatures (78°F–82°F) (25°C–26·5°C) are used by the full cycle machines and these temperatures are increased to between 102°F and 105°F (39°C–40·5°C) in the case of those units which utilize the rapid cycle. Drying temperatures are also raised and vary from 90°F (32°C) to 145°F (63°C), depending on the machine and the cycle time.

In addition to these higher temperatures which it must withstand during processing and drying, the emulsion is at the further risk of mechanical damage from abrasion by the rollers which effect the film's transit through the processor. To protect the emulsion from damage resulting from these causes it is essential to include in both developing and fixing solutions a gelatin-hardening agent.

The hardening agents normally found in acid fixing solutions—aluminium salts and chromium salts (see Chapter VII)—are not effective in the alkaline developer and consequently those employed in developers formulated for automatic processing are organic hardening agents (dialdehyde type).

Unfortunately one processing complexity leads to another. Developers which work at high temperatures more readily oxidize and must therefore be provided with greater antioxidant properties than a normal solution possesses.

Furthermore, higher working temperatures and the inclusion of hardeners both result in an increased tendency of the developer to fog. Consequently special attention must be given to antifoggants or restrainers present in the developers used in roller processors.

Modern X-ray developers contain at least two of these restraining substances:

(1) potassium bromide which inhibits the developer's action on both exposed and unexposed silver halide grains;

(2) an organic compound, such as benzotriazole, which has a selective influence on unexposed grains. It is by adjustment of the ratios of the restrainers present that fog can be controlled in the developing solutions used in automatic processing machines.

The developing systems employed in roller processing machines are characterized by an important change in the roles of the developer and replenisher, compared with the way in which they function during manual processing. Reference was made to this in Chapter vi (p. 119) but it may be helpful at this point to summarize the situation in the following table.

Manual Processing	Developer which is rich in restrainer is used initially.	Replenisher — more active solution—is added to augment the activity of the working bath as this declines.
Automatic Processing	When the bath is first charged its activity is reduced by the use of a separate starter solution containing most of the restrainer.	Replenisher is the working solution.

The fixer. The fixing agent employed in the fixing solutions used for automatic processing is ammonium thiosulphate (see Chapter vii) and in this respect these solutions do not significantly differ from those found in manual processors.

However, the fixer has problems of its own which are associated with the passage of the film from the developer into the fixer, the intermediate rinsing stage being omitted from roller processing machines. Its omission raises two points of significance.

(1) The rapid change in pH between the two solutions causes the gelatin to swell, nullifying the effect of the hardener contained in the developer. If the emulsion is to be successfully dried in the shortened periods implicit in automatic processing it must be re-hardened in the fixing solution.

(2) The pH of the fixer will rise owing to the carry-over of developer and this rise may be sufficient to cause the hardener to be thrown out of the solution. It is therefore necessary to buffer the fixer particularly well (see Chapter VII, p. 137) in order to prevent an undue rise in pH from occurring. High buffer capacity is an essential characteristic of the fixers associated with automatic processing.

When any fixing solution is used, silver thiosulphate complexes accumulate in it (see Chapter VII); these (a) retard fixing action, (b) prevent or at least inhibit the rapid removal of fixer by the wash water. In the case of manual processing a gradually slowing fixing rate—within certain obvious limits—probably does not matter very much. In automatic processing, fixing must be completed and adequate washing given within rigid and very short periods of time. For these reasons there are certain recommended levels above which the silver concentration in the fixing tank should not be allowed to rise. They are:

10 grammes of silver per litre in full cycle and half cycle machines;
6–7 grammes of silver per litre in rapid cycle machines.

Machines in the 90-second category require chemicals which are specifically formulated for them, owing to the highly exacting processing conditions which the rapid cycle implies; chemical changes which are made to occur very quickly are proportionally and inevitably more difficult to control. Preparations intended for full cycle processors as a rule cannot be expected to obtain the best results from 90-second machines, although in the U.S.A. 'universal' roller processing chemicals are presently available. In the half cycle units either type of chemicals may be successfully employed.

FILMS

Normal medical X-ray film at present available—which is intended for exposure with intensifying screens—may be processed in either full cycle or half cycle machines without trouble. In the case of fluorographic film and film of the direct exposure type there is the possibility of fixing being incomplete and such films are probably better not processed by these means.

If a normal X-ray emulsion is put through a 90-second processor the film emerges both foggy and damp. Rapid cycle processing must have specially manufactured emulsions which differ significantly from a normal emulsion in the following respects:

(a) the gelatin coating is of lower weight so that drying may be successfully accomplished within a period of 35 seconds;

(b) the emulsion has further special treatment to keep fog at a reasonable level in spite of the high temperature of the developer. As a rule films designed for rapid cycle processing may be satisfactorily put through the slower machines.

Roller processing, whether in a full cycle, half cycle or rapid machine, is necessarily a more rigorous experience for the film than is manual processing. We can summarize the physical features of emulsions suitable for roller processing in the statement that such an emulsion must possess two important characteristics:

(1) it should be hard;

(2) it should be thinly coated on the base so that both penetration by chemicals and subsequent drying are rapid.

THE MECHANICS OF ROLLER PROCESSORS

It is convenient to consider the mechanical aspects of processing by means of roller equipment in terms of the several operative systems which such a processor requires. We may think of these systems as components which are necessary to the total construction and use of the processor. Between particular examples these systems may and do differ in minor ways but this need not affect the student's understanding of the function and necessity of each. In roller-operated automatic processors we shall find incorporated the several systems listed below.

(1) A film-feeding system.

(2) A film transport system which will mechanically convey radiographs through the processor.

(3) A system of air circulation in the drying section of the unit.

(4) A system which provides for automatic replenishment of the developer and fixer.

(5) A water system which is used (a) for washing; (b) to assist in maintaining processing solutions at the correct temperature.

(6) A system or suitable combination of systems which will give temperature control of processing solutions, particularly of the developer but sometimes in fixing and washing sections as well.

(7) A recirculation system for both the developer and the fixer in order to keep fresh solution always in contact with the film and to obtain even mixing and uniform temperature of these solutions.

Film-feeding Systems

When a film is fed into an automatic processor some interval of time must elapse before another can be accepted. The output of these processors is usually stated in terms of the number of films processed per hour but this figure can be misleading for two reasons.

(1) While it is clear that this statement is derived from the processor's ability to handle a certain area of film in that time, it may not be apparent whether the number making up this area refers to large films only, small films only, or to the mixture which more usually occurs in a general X-ray department. One processor, for example, is said to work at a rate of 100 films per hour, but these are of assorted sizes; the figure for 14 × 17 in. radiographs is 80 per hour, and for small films proportionally greater than 100. It is perhaps most satisfactory if statements of this nature are confined to the number of 14 × 17 in. films which can be processed, since this represents the unit's minimum rate for the hour; the user in a general department may then be confident that in practice its speed will be rather greater.

(2) From the operator's point of view the number of films processed per hour may not be a particularly realistic figure. It is much more important that we know how well the processor can cope with the busiest 5 or 10 minutes within that hour. We may imagine, for example, a situation in which the darkroom rapidly receives two 14 × 17 in. films from an X-ray room where intravenous pyelograms are being performed; a mixed group of 5 or 6 *statim* radiographs from the fluoroscopic room; a single film from the chest room and a further set of 5 or 6 cassettes from the skull room where an examination of the nasal sinuses has just been completed. This or a similar occurrence might not happen again for a further 10 or 15 minutes and the number of films considered over the hour could thus appear misleadingly small.

Of greater value is knowledge of the interval required by a particular processor from the moment when one 14 × 17 in. film is fed into it and another is accepted. This varies from 16 to 56 seconds depending on the unit considered. Even 16 seconds may be more than is needed by the technician to reload the cassette, take a film from the next and possibly mark it as well, if this operation is part of the darkroom's responsibilities. To avoid delay occurring at this moment nearly all these processors incorporate a mechanical feed-system of some kind: that is, a number of films can accumulate in a suitable magazine and each will then be taken up automatically by the processor as it becomes ready to accept it.

Variations in the design of these systems occur between almost every unt. Films may be stacked in a magazine horizontally or vertically—toast on a plate as opposed to a toast-rack arrangement. To take the film from the magazine into the processor the following diverse methods are found:

(a) a pivotted tray which tips under the influence of gravity just enough to bring the top film in the tray level with a pair of rollers;

(b) the force of gravity alone used to push films down a ramp;

(c) a suction device which lifts the top film from a pile;

(d) a system of rotating spiral arms which successively flick stacked films from one position to another.

Since the equipment has such individual characteristics, to describe its working detail is not of marked value in the present context. The student should note the importance of an automatic feed-system if automation in the darkroom is to be fully efficient; indeed the trend at present is towards the provision not only of a film-feed but even of methods for mechanically unloading and reloading cassettes.

A significant and desirable feature of any automatic feeding system is access to it which will permit an urgent radiograph to 'jump the queue'. Most of the methods at present employed afford this facility; a film can be inserted appropriately into the magazine at any time and will be taken next by the processor. The capacity of these magazines generally is for 5–12 films, although the loader described under (a) above in fact will accept a total of 60.

Film Transport Systems

Roller systems employed in automatic processing units move the film between rollers in either of two ways: (a) vertically through a series of deep tanks or sections of the unit; (b) horizontally through a number of shallow trays. Among units using the roller system, vertical transport is the commoner method.

VERTICAL ROLLER TRANSPORT

Fig. 10.1 is a schematic general diagram in side elevation of an automatic processor, showing the principles of the system. It can be seen that the unit is divided into three sections, one each for developing, fixing and washing. These are an integral part of the unit, but virtually they are

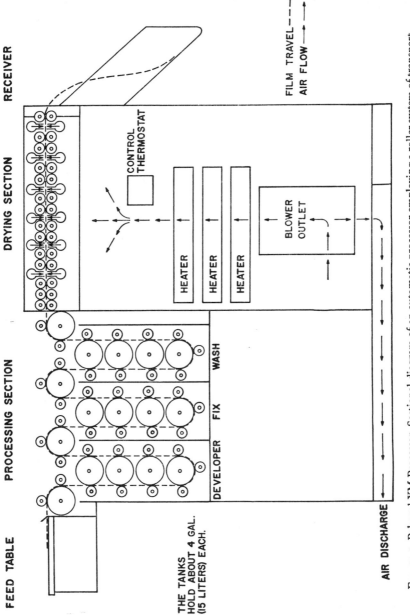

Fig. 10.1. Pakorol XM Processor. Sectional diagram of an automatic processor employing a roller system of transport. (*By courtesy of the Pako Corporation.*) It may be compared with Plate 10.1.

tanks and usually made of stainless steel. The rollers are arranged in a rack in each processing tank and this can be lifted out for cleaning; in most units the raising operation can be performed by hand fairly easily but in one case it is done by means of a light mechanical hoist. In most instances the transport rollers are of synthetic composition, for example a combination of synthetic resin and polyethylene; sometimes the entry rollers at the beginning of the processing section may be of stainless steel.

In the diagram a number of large rollers work in association with a pair of small guide rollers, one on each side of their big companion. In practice the guide rollers are slightly canted in relation to the large one; that is, a pair of lines drawn horizontally through their centres would lie slightly above and slightly below a similar line on the big roller. This provides a more positive feed of the film.

Variations in design naturally occur. Another unit, diagrammatically depicted in Plate 10.1, following p. 206, uses a number of small, 1-inch diameter rollers offset to each other; that is, they are arranged so that they do not oppose each other. In a third unit the rollers are constructed so that the film follows a continuously S-shaped track. However, these differences do not affect the general principle. The action of the rollers in each case both transports the film and provides uniform and vigorous surface agitation.

It may be noticed that in the unit depicted in Fig. 10.1 the film travels horizontally through the drying section, whereas in Plate 10.1 its movement is vertical. Again the difference is not materially important in affecting understanding of essential principles. As the film passes through the drying section, a number of slit tubes direct a forced jet of heated air at high velocity over both surfaces: twelve of these vents can be seen in Fig. 10.1, six on either side of the film. It has already been noted that the characteristics of the emulsion have been adapted to inhibit its absorption of water and this fact together with the squeegee action of the rollers in removing surface fluid enable the film to be rapidly dried in this way without the necessity to use very high temperatures. In the two units described, the temperature in the drying sections is normally in the range 105°F to 120°F (40·5°C to 49°C).

HORIZONTAL ROLLER TRANSPORT

The main difference to be noticed here is that the unit is not arranged as a group of deep tanks. Instead the film travels through a shallow layer of liquid in a series of trays. These are made from a suitable thermoplastic, such as P.V.C., which can be moulded in a concave contour adapted to the traverse of the film. We may think of this as dish development. Rollers arranged horizontally in parallel pairs pass the film into each 'dish', take it up again on the far side and convey it into the next one. In a typical unit of this type there are six such trays, two for developing, two for fixing and two for washing. When a large film traverses such a system it is possible for different parts of the one film to be each in a different processing section; that is, one end of the film is being washed while the other is being developed. Guide plates assist in the direction of the film.

In the drying sections of these units the principles employed are similar: heated air is directed through narrow slots or nozzles at both surfaces of the film as it passes through the chamber.

Replenishment of Solutions

In roller-operated processing systems the squeegee action of the rollers in removing surface fluid from the film significantly reduces the carry-over of the solutions. Chemical exhaustion occurs without a corresponding depletion in volume. It is therefore necessary to revitalize both the developing and fixing tanks by the regular addition of fresh replenishing solutions, even although there has been no appreciable fall in their level; as additional fluid is introduced some solution is run to waste.

It is inherent in this sequence of events that both developing and fixing solutions in theory may continue in use indefinitely without its being necessary at any one time completely to empty and replace the contents of either tank. In practice of course tanks should be regularly drained and cleaned.

The replenishment method to be considered here is the same for both developer and fixer. It depends in each case on the function of a small pump, which injects a pre-determined quantity of the appropriate replenishing solution into each main circulatory system and it relates the volume of additional solution to the area of film going through the processor.

The operation of the replenisher pumps is controlled by a micro-switch which is attached to the centre of the first pair of rollers between which the film passes as it enters the unit. These rollers are known as *detector* rollers: while the film is between them the micro-switch is activated and in turn energizes the replenisher pumps for a period of time which depends necessarily on the length of the film.

It is to enable a detector system of this kind to function efficiently that radiographs fed into some automatic processors of the roller type must usually enter it with the same dimension leading; that is, depending on the unit concerned, either the short edge or the long edge of the film should be consistently presented first. We may notice that normally the micro-switch is so adjusted that it does not operate when cine film, which has a very thin emulsion, is put through the rollers. If it were to do so, extreme over-replenishment would occur.

Thus, we have a replenishment rate which is proportional both to the number of films processed and to their area. Strictly in the case described it is proportional to their length, if we define this as the dimension going through the rollers. It is mainly because cine film has length without great width that it would be so misleading to the detector system. In practice the replenishment rate is nearly enough related to the square footage of film if the smaller sizes, whenever possible, are fed into the unit side by side.

However, this cannot always be done and some automatic processors monitor the width of the film as well as the length. Suitable micro-switches are fitted at each end of the detector rollers as well as the centre for this purpose; their use will avoid the possibility of over-replenishment when a number of narrow films are fed singly to the unit. Not all roller processors use a monitoring system of replenishment. Some employ electronically controlled metered pumps which deliver the same pre-determined amount of solution for every film. These were discussed in Chapter ix (p. 205).

It has been shown elsewhere (Chapters vi and vii) that other factors besides the area or number of processed films influence in some degree the quantity of replenisher required in respect both of the developer and the fixer. These factors include the type of emulsion and the type of radiography, and because of such variables it is important to be able to alter the actual amount of replenisher provided by the pumps during a given interval or for a given size of film, the two being equivalent expressions. This is an adjustment which is performed by the manufacturer at the time of installation in terms of an assessment of the particular conditions in which the unit will operate. This assessment can be and is regularly checked, by processing control strips of film and sending these for sensitometric analysis in the manufacturer's laboratory.

The rate of replenishment in a given instance can be found by feeding a 14 inch length of film into the processor and measuring the amount of additional solution pumped into the tank, in the manner shown in Plate 10.2, following p. 206. Normally the excess solution resulting from the

18

injection flows into a weir, the developer running to waste and the fixer to a silver recovery system. Very often a flow meter is provided—usually a ball in a glass tube which gives visual indication of the occurrence and rate of replenishment.

In the experiment it should be emphasized that the quantity which arrives in the measuring jar corresponds to that supplied by the pumps and is irrespective of any carry-over which may occur: for the reason given earlier this is minimal. The results of the experiment are influenced by the amount of solution which may be present in the replenisher tank. If this is nearly empty, the quantity of solution injected will be less than if the tank is full. It is advisable to test replenishment rates always at one level of the replenisher tanks, ideally when they are half full as this will give a mean rate. Average replenishment rates might be as follows:

35–40 ml of developer replenisher per 14 × 14 in. area of film.
50–60 ml of fixer replenisher per 14 × 14 in. area of film.

It will be noted that the quantities of added developer and fixer are not the same. If we can consider such a hypothetical entity as the 'average' radiograph in a general X-ray department, about two-thirds of its area after exposure is still unchanged silver halide; under these 'average' conditions the demand on the chemical activity of the fixer is greater than in the case of the developer, and consequently, in a general department at least, its replenishment rate should be higher.

The Water System

In processors which depend on roller systems of transport washing is performed at elevated temperatures in the range 68°–80°F (20°–25°C). The question of temperature control will be considered in the next section which deals with this aspect of automatic processing.

Depending on the processor the consumption of water varies considerably. Figures are found which range from 90 to 280 gallons per hour (408–1260 litres per hour). It is more important that the student radiographer should notice the general sensitivity of automatic processors to any fall in water pressure. Roller systems require a sustained water pressure. However, while the pressure of water is significant, it should not be thought that as a rule a particularly high value is needed. 9 lbs. per sq. inch (0·6 kg/cm^2) is a typical figure and this is equivalent to a normal tap supply. Booster pumps can be employed if necessary to augment the pressure of a poor supply. In many roller units, the water is

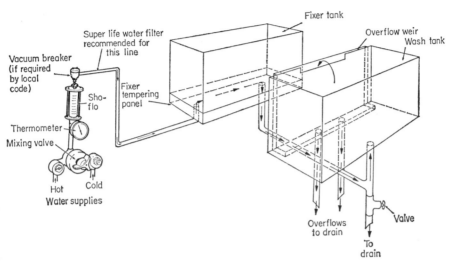

Fig. 10.2. Schematic representation of the wash-water system of a roller processing unit. Warmed water from the mixing valve is fed into the bottom of the wash tank at one side and leaves diagonally opposite by means of an overflow weir. The route to the wash tank takes warmed water underneath the fixing tank and heats this solution to processing temperature. *By courtesy of Pako Corporation.*

filtered on entry, or its filtration may be recommended if this is not an integral feature of the equipment.

Fig. 10.2 is a schematic representation of the wash-water plumbing of a typical roller-type processor. In this particular unit washing water is obtained at the stipulated temperature directly from an externally mounted water mixing valve which feeds tempered water at a rate determined and shown by means of a flow meter ('Sho-flo'). The water is used in this instance to heat the fixing tank, on its way to the site of washing operations. This is one way of providing temperature control of the fixer, although not the only one (see the following section).

The student is asked to note the presence of the filter in the output line from the mixing valve: dirt in the washing water is a common cause of films having a dirty appearance and this filter should be renewed periodically. Also to be noticed is the diagonal direction of flow in the washing tank from an inlet pipe in the floor to an overflow weir on the other side.

Systems of Temperature Control

Automatic processors employ certain types of device for controlling the temperature of processing solutions; this may include the temperature of the washing water. These devices may work in combination and are of the following kinds:

(a) Immerson heater, thermostatically regulated.
(b) Water mixing valve.
(c) Heat exchanger.

The operation of the first two of these we have already considered in earlier parts of Chapter ix relating to manual processing. The heat exchanger is described below.

HEAT EXCHANGER

This device is shown schematically in Fig. 10.3. It can be used either to raise the temperature of solutions or to make them cooler.

The heat exchanger consists of an outer tube which is filled with warmed water and surrounds a number of much narrower tubes through which the solution for temperature control is made to pass. The water in the outer jacket is obtained from the mixing valve which provides hot water for the washing tank. In some processors the tempered supply from the valve passes first to the heat exchanger and then to the wash; in others, the reverse occurs.

When the processing solution enters the narrow tubes, which pass through the much larger volume of water in the jacket, it will either lose heat if the jacket is cooler or gain heat if the jacket is hotter than is the processing solution itself. To give a practical example, in one rapid cycle processor the developer is initially and rapidly heated by an immersion heater to a temperature of 106°F (41°C), while the tempered water in the heat exchanger's jacket is at 101°F (38°C). The heat exchanger thus has a cooling effect on the developer and is used to maintain an accuracy of ±2F° (±1°C) in the developer's temperature; it is estimated that this accuracy would be of the order only of ±6°F (±3°C) if the heat exchanger were not present in the temperature control system.

Study in detail of individual processors reveals a considerable variety of application of these devices. For instance, we find that the temperature of the developer may be controlled by any of the following.

(1) Immersion heater with thermostatic regulator.
(2) A heat exchanger alone.
(3) A combination of an immersion heater and a heat exchanger.

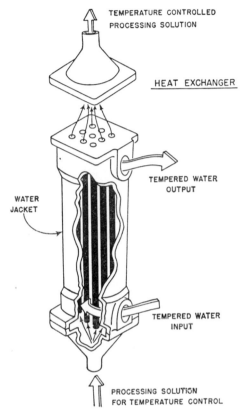

TEMPERATURE CONTROLLED
PROCESSING SOLUTION

HEAT EXCHANGER

TEMPERED WATER
OUTPUT

WATER
JACKET

TEMPERED WATER
INPUT

PROCESSING SOLUTION
FOR TEMPERATURE CONTROL

FIG. 10.3. Schematic diagram of a heat exchanger used in automatic units for controlling the temperature of processing solutions (usually the developer but sometimes also the fixer). The warm water fed into the water jacket of the exchanger is obtained from a water mixing valve, either directly or via the washing section of the unit; the output water runs to waste. The solution to be warmed is fed into a number of narrow pipes which traverse the water jacket. *By courtesy of X-ray Sales Division, Eastman Kodak Co., Rochester, New York.*

In regard to the fixer, exactness of temperature control is less stringent than for the developer; the following methods are used in various units.

(1) An immersion heater with thermostatic control, possibly in association with an underlying water bath; horizontal roller system.

(2) A water mixing valve (see Fig. 10.2).

(3) A heat exchanger.

As washing is performed at elevated temperatures, temperature control must extend to the washing section of the processor. It is usually obtained by means of a water mixing valve which feeds to the wash tank a blend of the hot and cold water supplies, as shown in Fig. 10.2. We may note again that if the atmospheric temperature is high and the cold water as a result is at or very near to the required temperature of the blended water, then it must be refrigerated before entering the mixing valve.

Recirculatory Systems

It is usual for automatic processors to have a circulatory system for both the developer and fixer: this sometimes applies to the wash water as well, although not in the processor of which the plumbing system is depicted in Fig. 10.2.

Recirculatory systems may vary in some minor respects and close knowledge of them is hardly possible and certainly unnecessary to student radiographers. Basically they consist of a circuit of pipes and a pump for each main processing tank. It is common practice to filter solutions in the recirculatory systems, particularly the developer.

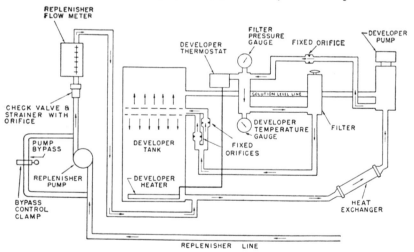

FIG. 10.4. Schematic diagram of the recirculatory system of the developer in a unit employing the roller transport system. The recirculatory pump is seen in the top right-hand corner; also seen are the immersion heater and thermostat and the heat exchanger for temperature control of the developer. The pump which feeds replenisher into the system is seen towards the left of the diagram. *By courtesy of X-ray Sales Division, Eastman Kodak Co., Rochester, New York.*

Fig. 10.4 shows the recirculatory equipment for the developer in the case of one roller processor. Perhaps the main point to be appreciated in any such system is that the circulatory system and the pump or motor which operates it are not to be confused with the replenisher system of the unit. These are separate entities, different in function and intention. The purposes of the circulatory systems for developer and fixer are:

(1) to afford better thermal control, particularly of the developer;
(2) to obtain more even flow and distribution of the solutions;
(3) to allow solutions to be filtered before re-entry into the processing tanks and thus to ensure the removal of any accumulated particles.

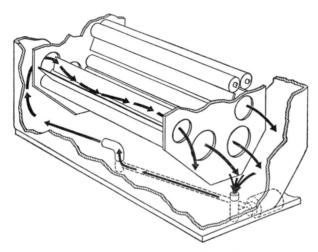

FIG. 10.5. A roller processing machine in which baffles are used to create a strong flow of solution and agitation at the film surface. *By courtesy of Du Pont Company (United Kingdom) Ltd.*

In addition to a recirculatory system, roller units may employ a system of positive agitation as well. What is known as a solution distributor tube is located in the developer or fixer rack near to the inlet of the recirculating fluid. Through ports in this distributor tube, the solution is forced upwards and downwards in the processing tank. These tanks are of relatively small capacity—compared for example with those of a dunking automatic unit or a manual processor—and very effective agitation can be provided in this way. Fig. 10.5 shows a method of obtaining solution agitation by means of apertures in steel baffles at the sides of the rollers.

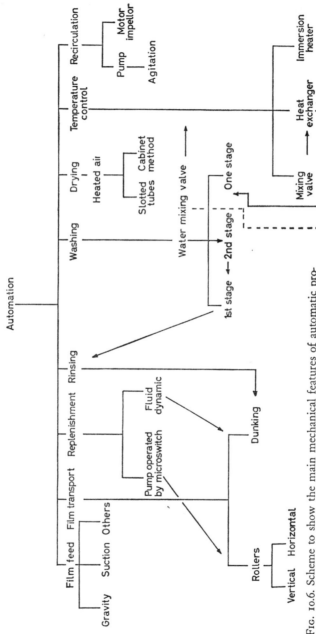

Fɪɢ. 10.6. Scheme to show the main mechanical features of automatic processing equipment. The broken line passing from the water mixing valve to the wash and then to the heat exchanger indicates that the progression is sometimes in this direction. In other units the sequence follows the diagram from the heading *temperature control*; that is, water is fed by the mixing valve to the heat exchanger first.

By way of summary Fig. 10.6 tabulates the important mechanical features of automatic processing which we have discussed in the previous pages. The table presents visually as far as possible the main systems involved in the construction of these units. To this we may add that in the fullest sense automation includes and depends on:

(1) mechanical equipment;
(2) physical and sensitometric characteristics of film;
(3) chemistry, in order to obtain optimum processing in a few minutes and a long replenishment cycle.

Care of Automatic Processors

Like other darkroom apparatus, automatic processors require regular cleaning. This is precision equipment and a faithful routine of cleaning and inspection is the basis of preventative maintenance. The recommendations of manufacturers' instructional manuals should always be observed.

Some units in this respect are more demanding than others. For example, in certain of the roller type, the upper or cross-over rollers which carry a film into succeeding adjacent sections of the unit must be wiped clean at the end of every working day: this is to prevent the formation on them of a crystalline deposit of dried solution which, if present, will give rise to marks on the next film processed when operation of the unit is renewed. However, a unit of this kind which is switched off at the close of the day can be re-started during the night to process emergency radiographs. After use it can safely be left without further cleaning until the following day's regular session, provided less than 100 sheets of 14 × 17 in. film are processed during the night.

Most automatic processors require a warming-up period, although a stand-by setting of temperature and other controls usually permits this interval to be brief, for example 10 minutes. In the case of a unit which is used again within two hours of closing down, 1–2 minutes' preparation may suffice, particularly of course if the surrounding room temperature is not too low. In normal circumstances a radiographer who switches the unit to full operation on reaching the department, may expect to find it ready for processing by the time the first X-ray examination has been completed.

For more information the reader is referred to Appendix 1.

CHAPTER XI

The X-Ray Darkroom

A dental surgeon was once heard to remark that three dentists together constitute five opinions. Possibly this is applicable with equal truth to those who are associated with the planning and operation of radiographic darkrooms. The ideal design of these to some extent is a matter of opinion and individual experience. For instance, the capacity of the department and the type of work which it handles must affect the organization of processing procedure. What would be good planning for one hospital might be unsatisfactory for another.

However, in this book we can consider certain basic practical features and from among these students no doubt will recognize some which are similar to the arrangements within their own hospitals.

There is no doubt at all of the importance of the darkroom and of the work for which it provides. Bad processing technique affects every radiograph taken in a department and will spoil its products more readily and insidiously than any other source of misadventure. The aim of radiographic darkroom practice is to standardize and maintain without variation a sound processing procedure, whether processing is by automation or by the manual method. This is the reason for the darkroom's existence. All aspects of planning, equipment and organization are directed towards the production of clean, unblemished radiographs, and if at the same time this can be achieved easily and simply then it is more likely to be obtained with consistence.

LOCATION OF THE DARKROOM

To this question of the correct siting of the darkroom in the department, the quick answer is that it should be central. Since every radiograph must be processed, the best position for the darkroom would appear to be the one which is close to as many X-ray rooms as possible.

Application of this principle results in the darkroom being adjacent to a single radiographic room in a small department, or placed between two radiographic rooms in a rather larger one. In each case the common wall or walls are likely to be provided with a hatch, through which cassettes may be passed on their way to and from the processing room. This system clearly saves time for radiographers as well as such wear and tear as may be associated with walking further than they need while carrying cassettes.

It is obvious that this type of planning is sensible and correct for many small departments and that in the larger one a natural extension of it might be to provide a darkroom for every two or three radiographic rooms, in the manner sketched in Fig. 11.1.

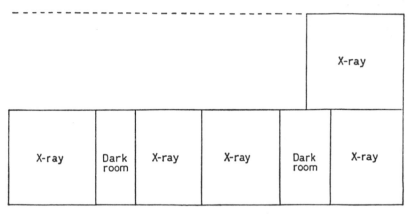

Fig. 11.1 Central siting of two darkrooms to serve five X-ray rooms.

However, this is not the only method of planning. Whether it is the one of choice or not, may be influenced significantly by certain related factors. These include both the type of work which is undertaken in the darkroom and the method of processing. We will consider at present the first of these points.

In the simplest radiological department which consists of one X-ray room and generator and is staffed probably by only one radiographer, the likelihood is that, apart from its actual radiographic exposure, all other work on the film will be done in the darkroom. This means that cassettes will be unloaded, reloaded; films developed, rinsed, fixed, checked, washed, dried, and possibly even sorted in the darkroom. This is perfectly satisfactory for the type of department just described.

However, if we imagine this situation scaled two or three times larger, then it becomes obvious that delay will occur because parts of the work cannot be done simultaneously.

Films may not be checked for quality and sorted by one group of people, while others are unloading cassettes or chemically processing, since the first activity requires white light and the second depends on a reduced specialized illumination to which the film is not sensitive. It becomes necessary when the volume of radiographs in a department is above a quite limited level, to break down darkroom procedure into stages of the work which need safelighting and those which do not. This means—if processing is manual—that films are developed, rinsed and fixed, or at least partially fixed in the darkroom; they are then passed by means of a special tank through the wall, into an adjacent room where they are assessed for quality, fixation is completed if this has still to be done, and washing, drying and sorting subsequently undertaken.

The last part of the procedure implies linking each set of films, where necessary to those of a previous examination, and certainly to an envelope and the requisition form and index card of the patient concerned. We see this particular activity becoming allied to the work of the department's record-keeping office and thus the sorting room should be within easy reach of the office. A new factor has entered our original idea of correct darkroom planning and if we wish to have several darkrooms we must consider, with *their* position, the situation of sorting areas in relation to the functions of radiographic documentation and of radiological reporting.

In the sketch in Fig. 11.1, both darkrooms could feed into a common viewing and sorting area placed where the dotted line indicates and this no doubt would be an acceptable arrangement. In other cases, one darkroom with its viewing facilities might have to be relatively remote from another and the real efficacy of the arrangement should then be given careful thought.

There is an argument for the decentralization of special groups of films: for example, angiographic studies, or those taken during surgery, all of which may well be more effectively handled by a small self-contained unit. However, the present trend towards automation in the darkroom must make very attractive the principle of a single processing centre to serve the whole department, as far as possible in all branches of radiological work. The initial costs of automatic processing systems largely prohibit their multiplication within most hospitals. To use fully their advantages of speed and consistency, consideration at the present time is more often given to methods of transporting films from wherever they are exposed *to* such a unit, than to planning a number of processing points close to radiographic or surgical rooms.

SYSTEMS OF FILM TRANSPORT

Methods of film transport are available and in operation in some X-ray departments. One of the conveyor belt type can be suitable for taking cassettes to and from the darkroom. Alternatively the system may have to carry only films for processing, if use can be made of dark cubicles within each X-ray room for the purpose of unloading and reloading cassettes. This feature is briefly described below.

The Loading Cubicle

A general design suitable for a loading cubicle is sketched in Fig. 11.2. No scale is given but essentially it is a small place, no bigger than it need be to allow one person to work in comfort; perhaps about 20 sq. ft.

A feature of significance is to give adequate protection to the walls and door against radiation: preferably the door should not be in the line of the primary beam at any time. A sliding door would economize on space.

The provision of effective ventilation is also important. For the sake of freshness it is better if the inlet of air can be taken from outside the X-ray room. A cassette hatch is shown but is inessential, and only useful if it is in direct communication with the processing room or is a source of transport.

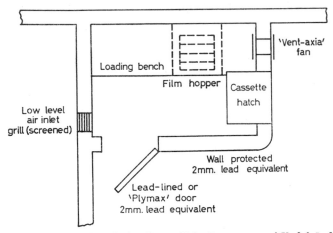

Fig. 11.2. Sketch plan of a loading cubicle. *By courtesy of Kodak Ltd.*

The use of these dark cubicles is discussed from another point of view in Chapter xiv and a reference to their equipment is made in a later section in this chapter (Darkroom Equipment and Layout).

A transport system which is appropriate for cassettes will be capable of conveying any other type of container which might be associated with the release of films from the loading cubicle of an X-ray room; for example, some variety of light-tight portfolio or sealed box.

An air-tube system is in use in certain hospitals for the transport of records, reports and memoranda and it would seem possible to adapt this to the carriage of films. The documents, or similar material to be conveyed, are placed in cylinders about 5 in. × 14 in. in size. These are then air-driven through a system of tubes to a designated station, which in this case would be the X-ray darkroom. The dispatch points can be placed anywhere in the hospital and by this means radiographs could rapidly reach the processing room from theatres or other specialized units which might be situated quite remotely from the main X-ray department, even on another storey of the building.

Clearly this system is applicable to films only: it cannot by any means cope with cassettes. Consequently in one respect departmental planning cannot be quite so flexible as when a conveyor belt is used; in the latter case some of the X-ray rooms might have their own loading cubicles and others none, depending perhaps on their size or other architectural features. The first would feed films only to the darkroom and the second would feed cassettes with equal facility.

There are difficulties in adapting this system to radiographic use. For the larger sizes of sheet film, 5 inches is rather a sharp radius of curvature, and equally there is an upper limit to the dimensions of a container which can move easily through the system of tubes and successfully negotiate bends. Unlike the similar case of a long road-vehicle faced with a sharp corner, there is no opportunity here for manoeuvre.

Apart from the chance that the emulsion might be physically damaged by making the film into a tight roll, the formation of a static electric charge seems possible as a result of friction between opposing surfaces. Such a charge will fog the film, producing a characteristic flaw of zig-zag design. Pressure marks are a more likely result even than this. Furthermore, the cylinder has to be securely light-proof yet capable of being easily opened and closed. However, in principle the air-tube system is more compact and, as it runs overhead without difficulty, is out of the way and can be concealed from sight.

DARKROOM CONSTRUCTION

In the darkroom many features of equipment and layout must vary with the dimensions of the room, the method of processing and the division of the work. These will be considered in later sections. Certain structural aspects are important for all darkrooms. These include the nature of floor, walls and ceiling; the ventilation and heating; the type of entrance.

Floor, Walls and Ceiling

Many X-ray departments have suffered from darkrooms which are too small, as well as having other faults no doubt: but it is equally possible for a darkroom to be too large for maximum efficiency, if technicians must cover a wide area between, say, the point at which a cassette is unloaded and the processing unit.

To give some 'ideal' size in precise figures is not helpful, for a general assessment cannot take into account the number of people likely to work in a particular darkroom, or the number of examinations made in the department which it serves. Another factor is the type of processing: automatic units make large darkrooms less desirable. Thirdly significant is whether processing is completed in the darkroom or in an adjacent room. All these aspects should be considered when planning the size of a new darkroom. We can say, however, that no processing room which is in constant use should be smaller than 100 sq. ft. in area. The ceiling should not be less than 8 ft. 6 in. in height, and preferably not greater than 11 ft. if ceiling reflector lamps are to be used.

The nature of the floor's material should be such that:

(1) it is non-porous;
(2) it is resistant to staining by chemicals or other liquids;
(3) it does not become slippery when wet.

An absorbent floor covering cannot easily be cleaned. Chemicals spilled upon it not only will stain the surface but as they remain in the floor's material may possibly contaminate the surrounding air when dry.

Not all impervious materials are equally resistant to stains and some may easily become slippery when wet. Semi-vitreous and non-vitreous tiles are unsatisfactory from the first point of view, and concrete, terrazzo or ceramic tiles have a tendency to the second disadvantage; this can be improved by the inclusion in them of a small amount of abrasive, granular material. Satisfactorily resistant substances are those of a composition which has a high proportion of asphalt: porcelain and natural clay tiles also are good, as well as some varieties of hard rubber and rubber sheet.

Any adhesive material employed to fasten down a floor covering must of course be waterproof, as also should be the floor itself.

In general the previous recommendations apply as much to the walls as to the floor, particularly of course to areas in the neighbourhood of sinks and wet processing equipment which should be protected to a height of at least 4 ft. 6 in. A rear splash panel for this purpose is a common accessory to processing units. Alternatively, or even in addition to it, ceramic or plastic tiles or sheets of Formica or similar material can be applied to adjacent wall surfaces.

Elsewhere on the walls, a durable, good quality paint should give adequate protection if tiling cannot be used throughout. Untreated brickwork which is exposed to constant chemical contamination may undergo a gradual process of destruction which is difficult to arrest.

The decor chosen must not be dark in colour. In fact a gloomy environment is insiduously depressing and unnecessary. A glossy cream or white paint on the walls, for example, would do very well. Orange, yellow, or green, are to be avoided since they will reflect very poorly the light from safelamps of a similar colour.

Modern practice is to obtain as much reflected light as possible in a darkroom. Reflection of the available light provides throughout the room a diffuse illumination which often can be maintained at a surprisingly high value and gives little impression that the place actually *is* dark. Reflected light does not differ in wavelength from the incident light which causes it and consequently offers no greater risk to sensitive materials. It may in fact decrease the number of lamps required in the room and certainly lessens strain on those who must work there.

Paints are sometimes said to be acid-resistant. It is worth noting that, while this description may testify to their behaviour when under fire from fixing solutions, it is no indication at all of what may happen should the splashes be of an alkaline nature; that is, should they have come from the developer and not the fixer.

The type of paint on the ceiling is also significant since it should not be of a character to produce flakes which are likely to fall on sensitive materials or on open cassettes below. It is bad practice to leave cassettes lying open. For the same reason plaster is to be avoided. A good quality, modern emulsion paint is probably a satisfactory material from this point of view. To avoid a similar risk from falling particles, any water pipes, electric conduits or air ducts preferably should be enclosed above a false ceiling. This provides a smooth, intact surface overhead which can easily be kept clean.

Some of the foregoing observations are directed towards the protection of the darkroom from the effects of contact with chemicals. While others remain important, this aspect has less significance if processing is by automation. In this case the darkroom, unless it contains as well a stand-by unit for hand processing, becomes virtually a dry working area in which chemicals are not prepared, solutions changed, or wet equipment cleaned.

However, the problem has been moved rather than removed. Resistant materials which we have mentioned as suitable for a darkroom are appropriate also for the adjacent viewing room, whether this is intended for the completion of manual processing or contains the major part of an automatic unit: in the latter case, servicing and cleaning of the equipment and the preparation and storage of chemicals are likely to be conducted in this immediate area. The wet-viewing/film-sorting room will be further considered in a later section.

RADIATION PROTECTION

Darkrooms, or rather the personnel and sensitive materials associated with them, require protection from ionizing radiation, usually—although not necessarily—X rays from adjoining radiographic rooms. Existing situations should be re-examined when new installations are made, particularly when a minor diagnostic unit is replaced by one of high voltage output. The arrangement of X-ray apparatus in any case should be such that the primary beam is never directed at a wall of the processing room.

Walls are mainly affected but ceilings and floors also should be considered if X-ray generators, or equipment employing radio-active isotopes are in operation on another storey of the building. These remarks apply also to storerooms where reserve stocks of film may be kept, and in this connection some attention should be given to the route along which films are normally taken, either from their point of delivery to the store room, or from the latter when they are moved to the position of current stock in the darkroom.

The structure of a room in which film is stored or handled should have a lead equivalency of 2 mm. For this purpose the following are appropriate materials:

(1) A 1 inch layer of high quality barium plaster. (1 part fine barium sulphate; 1 part coarse barium sulphate; 1 part Portland cement.)
(2) A single brick wall; that is, 9 inches of *solid* brick.

19

(3) A wall which is half a brick in thickness and has in addition a half-inch layer of high quality barium plaster.

(4) A 6-inch thickness of concrete.

(5) A 10-inch thickness of coke-breeze blocks.

(6) Lead 'Plymax' boards with 2 mm of lead.

In using protective materials attention particularly should be given to obtaining an overlap at points of discontinuity in the wall; for example at the site of a transfer hatch for cassettes.

It is an accepted regulation of the Code of Practice that the Physics Department should monitor any new rooms, or modified existing rooms, in or near to which ionizing radiations are being handled: this rule naturally will include the processing room. In the absence of a more accurately made check, the entry of ionizing radiation into a darkroom can easily be proved by placing a coin on an envelope-wrapped film and fixing the latter to the suspect wall of the room; the coin should lie between the film and the surface of the wall. This can be left for some time, for a week perhaps but the period certainly should be longer than that for which any film would remain in the vicinity during the normal occurrences of work: in this connection the susceptibility of stored film materials should not be overlooked. In a room which is not sufficiently protected, a faint image of the coin will be apparent on the test film after processing.

Ventilation and Heating

Owing to its enclosure for many hours of the day adequate ventilation of the darkroom is extremely important. The space considered necessary for a patient in a hospital ward is given as 1,000 cu. ft. and this would seem a fair recommendation for each technician in a darkroom. Unfortunately much lower figures are sometimes stated and applied. During intermittent use an allowance of 400 cu. ft. upwards might be tolerated but in most X-ray departments which employ technical darkroom staff it is unrealistic to suppose that these people are not subjected to a confining environment continuously throughout the day.

It is very often recommended that darkrooms should have large windows which can be opened after working hours or at any other convenient time. Experience suggests, however, that in a busy department there is hardly a convenient time, and even the phrase 'after working hours' is found in fact probably to signify those of the night between 12 and maybe 8.0 a.m. Perhaps a better direction of energy is to provide the darkroom with a fully efficient system of air-conditioning rather than expend concern if planning is such that it cannot possess a window.

The air in a darkroom should be completely changed at least 3 times per hour; some authorities have been found to state even up to 10 times in the same period. The most usual way of doing this is to obtain cross ventilation by means of an extractor fan or fans situated at a high level in the room, while air is drawn in from some outside source at a low level. While many darkrooms possess the amenity of an extractor fan, sometimes insufficient attention is given to the air intake of the room, reliance being placed simply on what may be drawn through its entrance, perhaps from a reception area or corridor. The air intake preferably should be from the outside and ideally would be filtered to remove dust and other particles.

Suitable apparatus for the intake of air may be either a blow-in fan, or else non-mechanical in kind: that is, a light-proof baffle with a variable aperture which can be fitted in a wall, window or door. Any device which communicates from the darkroom must be light-trapped: this applies equally to a simple louvre and to 'intake' and 'extract' fans. Ideally intake and extraction would be from diagonally opposite points, both open to fresh air. In practice this situation can seldom exist.

An intake fan situated on an outside wall will lose efficiency if the temperature of the room is much greater than that outside; the tendency of the air is to move outwards then, rather than inwards. This will be improved if the incoming air can be warmed by passing it through a radiator. Some fans have a heater attached for this purpose. It is also helpful if the extractor fan or fans can be given greater power than their intake companions. Fans placed outside the building should, as far as possible, be situated in places sheltered from prevailing wind pressures and they must have a cowl for light-proofing and to protect them in bad weather. Many fans have switches which permit adjustment of their speed.

The installation of a good air-conditioning system would be more efficient than cross ventilation by fans and perhaps not enough use is made of it. Certainly it is not found in older institutions.

Darkroom temperatures should be maintained between 65°F (18.3°C) and 68°F (20°C). The relative humidity of the atmosphere should be ideally 40 to 60 per cent.

Proper heating of the darkroom is a lesser problem as a rule than its ventilation. Whatever system is employed in other parts of the hospital is likely to serve also the darkroom. Hot water radiators are very common. If electrical heaters are used they should not be of an open filament type which are dangerous to personnel and an added fire risk to sensitive materials. Furthermore attention must be given to the brightness of any pilot lamps associated with electrical equipment in the darkroom: the light emitted may be of a colour or intensity which will fog X-ray or fluorographic film handled in its neighbourhood.

Type of Entrance

It is of course possible to employ as a means of entering or leaving the darkroom a simple, single door. If only one person is using the room there is unlikely to be any difficulty from lack of access to it during processing procedures.

The door should have a lock to avoid mishaps from attempted entrance when sensitive materials are being handled. It should be sound in structure, well fitting and completely light-proof. To this end it may be necessary to fit round the edges a sealing strip of a type sold commercially for the exclusion of draughts. This is better than the suggestion sometimes made of hanging a curtain across the door: to be effective such a curtain must reach and overlap floor level and it becomes inevitably not only a light trap but one for dirt and dust as well.

However, if a number of people have to use a darkroom it is helpful to provide an entrance able to function independently of any processing needs. The outlook on the design and choice of darkroom entrances in recent years has been completely altered by the introduction of automatic processing into nearly every X-ray department in the United Kingdom. Traffic to and from the darkroom has diminished because of:
(a) shorter processing periods;
(b) the impossibility as a general rule of viewing radiographs during automatic processing;
(c) the increased use of mechanized methods of film transport between X-ray rooms and darkrooms.

For all these reasons a light-lock at the entrance to a darkroom is unlikely at the present time to be more elaborate in form than a simple pair of double doors arranged one on either side of a small vestibule. It is as important for double doors as for a single one that each should be sturdy in construction and well fitting. Figure 11.3 shows two possible schemes for the use of double doors.

The double door system is economical of space. If the door nearer to the darkroom opens into the room and the outer door opens outwards, the dimensions of the vestibule between them can be—and sometimes are—very small indeed: the space may be no larger than is required to accept one adult of average build (while breathing out?). However, it has the disadvantage of being not fully foolproof since there is certainly a chance that someone may emerge from the inner door simultaneously with the entrance of someone else through the outer. An electrical interlock can be fitted which prevents either door from being opened unless its fellow is closed. Such a sophistication inevitably is subject to failure at some time or another and the occasional disaster to films can occur.

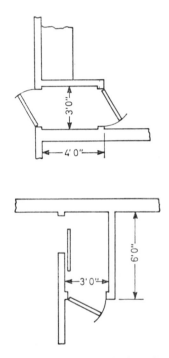

FIG. 11.3. Two examples of the use of double doors in a darkroom entrance. In the lower one, space is saved by making the inner door of the sliding type *By courtesy of Kodak Ltd.*

A darkroom of which the door is locked and which is inaccessible from the windows might be hazardous in certain circumstances: it would be very difficult to bring help to someone alone in the room who had become suddenly ill and collapsed. Because of this it is desirable and proper to provide some means of overriding an electrical interlock or of using a master key to obtain entrance from outside the darkroom.

DARKROOM ILLUMINATION

Electric shock is a potential hazard in the darkroom owing to the proximity of electrical equipment to water and the likelihood that persons using this equipment may have damp hands and be standing on a floor possibly wet.

Any light or illuminator situated near the site of wet manipulations, and preferably *all* lights in the darkroom should be operated by a pull-cord switch. Electrical points should be of the three-pin shuttered type and both these and any hand-switches of insulating material should be waterproof. Non-current-carrying metallic items, such as the case of an electric interval-timer, should be earthed.

Darkroom illumination is in two categories. These are:

(1) general white light;
(2) safelight.

To this we may add in some instances:

(3) viewing equipment.

General White Light

Usually this will conform with normal hospital practice. It should be placed close to the ceiling to avoid strong shadows and 5 to 10 lumens per sq. ft. at 3 ft. above floor level are recommended average values of illumination.

White light is necessary to the darkroom to enable work which does not involve sensitive materials to be properly performed; for example, cleaning of the room and processing equipment, and the inspection of intensifying screens. A reasonable strength of light obviously is required but if it is dazzlingly bright technicians may suffer loss of visual accommodation which will be disadvantageous to them.

If the room is large enough to warrant more than a single central ceiling fixture, one should be placed over each main working area.

Safelighting

A darkroom's safe illumination need not—and consequently should not—be less than the maximum level of brightness permitted by the most sensitive material which is being handled in it.

The term 'safe' to some extent is misleading in so far as it is not absolute: it implies only a degree of safety. No emulsion is completely insensitive to light, even to a darkroom lamp of the colour described as safe for its handling. We can say (a) that its response is related predominantly to wavelength or colour, but that also significant are (b) the intensity of the light and (c) the duration of the exposure.

In the X-ray darkroom (a) is a readily established factor if the correct colour of safelight is chosen; (b) is controlled by attention both to the wattage of the lamps used and their distance from any point at which sensitive material is handled; (c) is bound to be a variable, depending on the technician's method and speed of work. Overlong exposure to safelight is a possibility which is always present and no one responsible for any processing should permit sensitive materials to remain unprotected: it is very bad practice to unload a large number of cassettes and stack their contents along a bench prior to putting all the films simultaneously into the developer. If films must be accumulated in this way, a fitted lighttight drawer or container, deep enough to allow hangers to stand vertically within, should be provided.

In a general radiographic darkroom there is no necessity to work in a red light. Fluorographic materials require special consideration and are discussed in Chapter xviii. Apart from these the spectral sensitivity of X-ray film, whether it is to be used with intensifying screens or intended for direct exposure, does not extend beyond the blue bands of the spectrum. It can therefore be manipulated for a limited period in brown or olive-green lighting and one of these is generally employed: they represent the region of the spectrum for which we have greatest visual sensitivity at low levels of illumination.

Lacquered bulbs or those of coloured glass are not a satisfactory form of darkroom lighting. The first are very likely from wear to suffer cracks in their coating and become unsafe for sensitive materials; the second do not provide a sufficient range of colour to be useful.

Safe illumination commonly takes the form of a lamp fixture of special design. In this an ordinary pearl bulb of not more than 25 watts is used and a coloured filter placed in front of the bulb will tint the light to the required hue. This makes it quite simple to alter the colour of the safelighting should it become necessary, or to renew any filters that are damaged. Safelighting can be either direct or indirect.

DIRECT SAFELIGHTING
Direct illumination is local in nature. A lamp of this kind is shown in Plate 11.1, following p. 206.

The lamp has a circular filter 5 ½ in. in diameter and it may be either suspended from the ceiling or fixed to the wall above a bench, processing unit or other working point. It should be placed so that sensitive material is normally handled no nearer to it than 4 feet and it should be situated 4 feet from any similar lamp placed in another working area of the room.

Films should not be held close to safelamps. To do this is to expose them to an uncontrolled intensity of light to which quite probably they are sensitive. This situation is most likely to arise if the radiographer attempts to assess a radiograph's quality during processing by removing it from the developer and holding it against the light from a neighbouring safelamp. Because in these circumstances a film cannot readily be brought very near to it, overhead lighting is much safer than wall or bench mounting and is to be preferred.

It is often stated of X-ray darkrooms in general that, wherever else in the room safelamps may be situated, one is required near the processing unit; the implication sometimes is that this lamp is needed for the inspection of films during development. Whether or not this is its intended purpose, it is often unfortunately the use to which it is put. There *are* arguments for placing lamps near the processing unit: it is a major working area and may not otherwise be adequately illuminated, but in principle these safelamps should always be suspended overhead.

The use of any direct illumination is not recommended for fast orthochromatic or panchromatic materials.

INDIRECT SAFELIGHTING

Indirect safelighting is intended to provide general illumination of the darkroom. In this case the safelamp directs the light towards the ceiling which reflects it back into the room. When lighting is used in this way some standardization of the reflective abilities of the ceiling clearly is needed. It should not have a dull surface but should be painted a glossy pale cream or white. Its height should be within 9 to 11 feet. If a high ceiling cannot be avoided then it is necessary to hang white reflectors at least 3 feet square above each safelamp and these are more efficient if their surface is convex.

Plate 11.2, following p. 206 shows a safelamp which has filters on both its upper and lower surfaces and is thus suitable for providing both indirect and direct illumination simultaneously. One of these may be allowed for every 70 sq. ft. of floor space. The lower edge of the lamp should be not less than 7 feet above floor level.

SAFELIGHT FILTERS

The filters used in safelamps are usually a sheet of gelatin dyed to the appropriate colour and for protection sandwiched between two sheets of glass. The glass incidentally also helps to diffuse the light but this is a minor function.

The gelatin will deteriorate if it is subjected to extremes of heat and moisture. Assuming that the design of the lamp is efficient in keeping it cool, the most likely cause of overheating of the gelatin is the use of an electric bulb of too high a wattage. It is very tempting to try to improve darkroom illumination by replacing a 25 watt lamp with another of greater power but this must never be done.

If the level of safe illumination appears to have diminished in a darkroom it may well be because cleaning is overdue. Safelamps and filters require regular attention in this respect: they readily attract dust and loss of efficiency from this cause can be insidious and unnoticed. The suspension of hanging lamps should be such that they can readily be taken down if necessary. There is usually provision for easy removal of the filters.

SAFELIGHT TESTS

Safelights should not be trusted implicitly or indefinitely. From time to time tests are necessary to ascertain that the illumination employed in fact is safe. These may be required in any of the following circumstances.

(1) The darkroom is a new one.

(2) Safelights have been changed or additions made to them.

(3) A technique or method of work has been altered. For example, the introduction of a faster type of emulsion, or of a multi-film cassette such as that of the Schonander rapid changer, both may entail intervals of exposure to safelight which have become unsafe; the first because the emulsion is more sensitive and the second because the time required fully to load a cassette is naturally longer.

(4) A particular lamp is suspect as the cause of fogging, perhaps because of deterioration of the filter, or less probably erosion of metal parts.

There are several ways of making a check on the safety of darkroom illumination. The following is one recommended procedure.

(1) If the intention is to examine only one particular safelamp all other illumination should be extinguished. Otherwise the normal safelighting of the room should be used for the test.

(2) A film of some convenient size is given a slight X-ray exposure: for example, 0·5 mAs at 50 kVp and an anode-film distance of 6 ft.

Exposed emulsions are rather more sensitive to light than those which have had no exposure and thus our test of the darkroom lights is more stringent if we use for the purpose a previously exposed material. For the same reason this film should be in the fastest category which the department employs and the darkroom processes.

(3) All illumination in the darkroom is extinguished.

(4) The exposed film is placed at some customary working position on the loading bench.

(5) A row of opaque objects, coins for example, is placed on the surface of the film.

(6) An opaque card is laid over the film; in the first instance it covers all the coins.

(7) The lamp or lamps to be tested are switched on.

(8) The card is withdrawn in a regular series of steps to expose each time an additional strip of film with a coin on it. It is suggested that the card be moved perhaps every 10 or 15 seconds.

(9) The film is processed in the normal way and examined.

Let us suppose that we have used an 8 × 10 in. film, arranged on it a row of 8 halfpennies and moved the card at intervals of 15 seconds. We will have made altogether 8 moves and each strip of film will have received the following successive exposures: 120 secs.; 105 secs.; 90 secs.; 75 secs.; 60 secs.; 45 secs.; 30 secs.; and at the last 15 secs.

If we now examine this film, any fog on it which is caused by the exposure is readily detectable on comparison with the areas protected by the coins and therefore completely unexposed. The longest exposure which produces no visible image of the coin is the longest interval during which we may safely handle that particular sensitive material in these particular conditions. If even the last strip, which in this case was the result of 15 seconds' exposure, shows evidence of fogging the test must be repeated so that the minimum exposure of the previous experiment becomes the maximum period of the new. In any case selected values of exposure should have some relation to the time normally required for the manipulation of films. This no doubt will vary but half a minute is perhaps a fair estimate since most operations would be completed within that interval.

Viewing Equipment

In a small department where the darkroom must contain all stages of manual processing provision is necessary for the assessment of wet radiographs.

For this the minimum requirement is a single illuminator wall-mounted above the processing unit, possibly on a shelf but preferably attached directly to the wall. In principle this illuminator should be situated above the washing compartment of the processing unit. In practice the tendency of radiographers and others is to try to examine films as soon as they are cleared in the fixer—sometimes before they are cleared. Films taken from the fixer and held over the washing tank are likely to contaminate the latter: films taken from the wash and examined above the fixer may lead to its dilution. In either position, the illuminator is almost certain to be wrongly situated at least some of the time and in any event it is very susceptible to splashing: rust and corrosion of metal parts are bound to develop sooner or later.

As far as possible an illuminator used in this way should be protected. A wet film attachment is helpful. This is a sheet of clear Perspex which has the same area as the illuminator and can be suspended in front of it by special fixtures at the top; the free lower end is formed into a curved drip tray. The efficacy of this arrangement will be increased if the illuminator can be supported at a very slight forward angle to bring its lower part out of the line of falling drops.

A special design of illuminator for darkroom and other wet use is wall-mounted in a completely enclosed shell of translucent plastic material. This is very serviceable. Any illuminator employed for wet viewing must be operated by a pull-cord switch. It is bad practice to use in the darkroom an illuminator discarded from elsewhere and operated by the usual form of toggle or variable control rotary switch.

Switching of Light Circuits

White-light switching should be arranged to reduce the possibility of its being switched on accidentally while films are under manipulation. If the safelight and normal light circuits are separately controlled at wall points in a 'dry' area of the room, the switches should be placed at very different heights, the one for the white light being put out of normal reach: for example the safelight switch might be 4 ft. 6 in. from the floor and the whitelight switch 6 ft.

It is recommended practice to have a cord-operated master control for both circuits positioned near the door of the darkroom. This is often combined with a cord-operated change-over switch which will give either white or safe lighting and this should be situated near a working area: there can in fact be more than one switch for this purpose, for example near the loading bench and another above the processing unit. If the room has several white lights this arrangement may operate only the central light or all of them, if desired.

The situation of pull-cord switches in the vicinity of working areas needs to be considered. They should not be in a position where they are likely to become entangled with stored hangers and thus accidentally pulled on when these are lifted from a rack.

Another system sometimes used is to provide a separate pull-cord switch for every white light and to situate this near the light. The method does not exclude the provision of a master control near the entrance but there seems little to recommend it from the point of view of convenience.

A drawer- or door-operated switch in series with the white lights is a useful safety device which can be fitted to a hopper or container used for the storage of unexposed and largely unprotected sensitive materials. Should it be opened when the white lights are on in the room this switch will operate to extinguish them.

Another common practice is to fit an indicating lamp, usually red or orange, outside the darkroom door. This is wired in parallel with the safelights and provides visible warning whenever they are in use. Such a device becomes less desirable, and no doubt is unnecessary if the entrance to the darkroom is by means of a continuous light-trap without the use of doors. Safelamps placed in the latter type of entrance for guidance preferably should not be associated with the safelights of the room. They are better operated by a master control switch for all circuits placed near the point of entry, from which one at least of these lamps should be visible.

DARKROOM EQUIPMENT AND LAYOUT

The work to be done in an X-ray darkroom involves (a) the handling of dry film materials and (b) processes which depend on chemical solutions and consequently are wet in nature. Cassettes, intensifying screens and unexposed film—all costly items—become unserviceable when damaged by stains and splashes. A radiograph contaminated similarly prior to processing, or during or after drying, may be useless because of lost image quality. It is clear that overlap between the wet and dry operations in a darkroom should be avoided.

If this important consideration is remembered it will be seen that certain other desirable features are involved with it and probably will follow from its application. A well planned darkroom should have these associated characteristics.

(1) Effective separation of the wet and dry sides of the work.
(2) Orderly sequence of successive stages of the work.
(3) Neat layout of the equipment in adequate space.
(4) Clear 'traffic lanes' so that technicians are not in each others' way if more than one is working in the room. We will return later to these four points, having some knowledge of the appliances concerned.

In broad terms we can say that the equipment necessary to an X-ray darkroom is (a) a bench upon which to unload cassettes, prepare films for processing and reload cassettes; (b) apparatus in which processing is performed; (c) certain essential accessories. When we examine these headings in more detail we find that some of their practicalities depend closely upon whether the method of processing is manual or automatic. These methods and the instruments for each have been described in the previous chapter and need not be discussed now. We will consider for the moment what else is required in a darkroom where the processing equipment is for manual operation.

The Darkroom with Manual Processing

Perhaps the first requisite of a darkroom's loading bench is that it should provide enough space. It should be long enough to allow 3 or 4 of the largest cassettes to be placed upon it side by side without an overlap if they are opened. At least 8 feet per operator is the recommended allowance in length and 2 feet the minimum width of such a bench. It should be not less than 3 ft. high and preferably mounted on a plinth which will allow the operator a 3-inch toe space.

The top of the bench should be a hard wood, such as teak. Very often now it is covered with some material which can be easily cleaned. Thick linoleum is a very good choice. Formica is another substance which is sometimes used. Theoretically any such covering should be of a kind which will not readily acquire a static electrical charge, such as linoleum. Formica is *not* non-static and consequently as a rule is not recommended. However, in practice it appears to give little trouble under general working conditions, if technicians devote reasonable care and do not handle film with haste and roughness.

Unless the unloading and reloading operations have been done in a dark cubicle in the X-ray room, the work bench of the darkroom requires storage space for:

(a) hangers;
(b) cassettes;

(c) unexposed films ready for immediate use;

(d) a further stock of unexposed materials for use in the near future, perhaps a week's supply.

If the X-ray department is provided throughout with a system of dark cubicles and no cassettes are ever taken to the processing room, then storage space for these and for films becomes unnecessary in the latter. However, such provision is then essential to the equipment of the dark cubicles, although on a smaller scale. In either case the observations which follow are valid.

HANGER STORAGE

The most usual arrangement is to provide wall brackets above the loading bench on which a supply of clean, dry hangers can be hung ready for use. One type of bracket in common supply projects about 9 inches from the wall, holds a minimum of 12 hangers and is angled at the far end to lessen the risk of hangers falling and damaging intensifying screens or films on the bench.

Hangers commonly are grouped on the wall according to their size, a pair of brackets being necessary for every category of hanger. The brackets should be spaced 14½ in. from each other, with an allowance of 3 to 4 inches between each pair. A height of 30 inches above the bench is quite suitable for a single row, but if restriction of space makes a double row necessary the low one should be 24 inches and the upper one 40 inches above the bench top. Alternative to a bracket a simple wooden rod might be used in a similar manner but perhaps offers greater risk of hangers falling if they are accidentally knocked.

Sometimes hangers are suspended, from points situated *underneath* the loading bench. This removes their potential hazard to other materials but occupies space which may be regarded as better put to another purpose. Possibly they are also rather more difficult to reach since the operator must either stoop for them or else pull out a drawer; if the latter arrangement is employed the hangers must be *hung* in the drawer and not simply stacked horizontally.

CASSETTE STORAGE

A feature in design of darkroom benching which is often mentioned as essential is the provision of compartments to house cassettes. In some circumstances perhaps they are desirable but experience leads to the suggestion that in many their practical value is not very great.

The reasons for this are as follows:

(1) The number of cassettes which can be stored under the benching is very limited, perhaps 10 to 20 all told.

(2) Cassettes under a darkroom bench are relatively inaccessible to radiographers in X-ray rooms. Either those who need them must enter the darkroom to fetch them or the cassettes must at some time be moved by darkroom staff to a transfer hatch or film transport system. In the latter circumstances there seems little point in storage space which is only for some intermediate stage: a better arrangement would be to provide a greater number of transfer hatches or more adequate accommodation in X-ray rooms for unexposed materials.

In a 'single-handed' department in which the X-ray room and darkroom inter-communicate, perhaps no transfer hatch is fitted and the number of cassettes in circulation is very small, the radiographer no doubt may find it convenient to store cassettes in the darkroom. In this event the provision of compartments for them under the loading bench is sensible and desirable.

These compartments should consist of a number of vertical slots. Each slot should have no greater width than will comfortably contain one cassette. This will prevent cassettes falling sideways when some are removed from the ranks; possible damage to cassettes will be avoided and their withdrawal made easier in this way. To prevent small cassettes from sliding out of reach, the depths of the compartment as well as their heights should be graded in a suitable range to allow a number of each size to be stored.

Cassette hatches are intended primarily to allow cassettes and films to be passed between radiographic rooms and the processing room without the necessity for staff to come and go. The hatches should open on the loading bench and are most conveniently fitted on a communicating wall when X-ray rooms and darkroom can be adjacent. However, if the darkroom serves several X-ray rooms it obviously cannot be next door to all of them. In these circumstances and if no mechanical system of film transport is available, hatches placed in a wall accessible from a corridor or hall-way and near to radiographic rooms are beneficial. They enable work to flow easily into the darkroom and provide lodging for cassettes which have been reloaded and are ready for use.

In simplest terms a transfer hatch is an opening in the wall, of similar design to the domestic pattern so often found between dining room and kitchen. However, a cassette hatch, if it is to be practical, must have certain special features as follows.

(1) An interlocking device is necessary in order to prevent both doors of the hatch from being simultaneously opened and thus admitting white light to the darkroom at some unwanted moment.

(2) The hatch must be light-proof in structure.

(3) If its situation is between radiographic room and darkroom, the hatch must be proof also against X rays; this is usually ensured by incorporating lead in its composition. Some hatches are all metal in construction and others are made of plywood on either side of a layer of lead.

(4) There must be some means of distinguishing beyond doubt between exposed films entering the darkroom for processing and reloaded cassettes passing from the darkroom. This most commonly takes the form of a division into two compartments, one being labelled 'Exposed' and the other 'Unexposed'. Each legend must be repeated so that it is apparent from either side of the hatch.

Various slightly different designs of cassette hatch are in general use and students may be acquainted with a number in their own departments. One type, for example, consists primarily of a vertical drum which can be rotated. Another pattern may have a lower horizontal compartment for exposed materials and two vertical sections above for outgoing cassettes. Alternatively, perhaps in a large department, the whole of a hatch may be allocated to arrivals and other separate hatches to departures: in this case it is probably wise to give a rather larger number to the outgoing reloaded cassettes than is required for materials entering the darkroom for processing.

FILM STORAGE

Hopper. Unexposed films intended for immediate use in reloading cassettes are most conveniently kept in a hopper under the loading bench. This device roughly is a cone shaped drawer hinged at its lower edge. Its appearance is shown in Plate 11.3, following p. 206.

Usually the hopper has about four compartments, the first and deepest of which will accept the two largest sizes of film, for example a box of 14 × 17 in. and another of 14 × 14 in.; the next slot may house the 12 × 15 in. films; the third compartment will have 10 × 12 in. and 8 × 10 in. together; and the last space may be occupied by 6 ½ × 8 ½ in. and perhaps narrower films, such as 6 × 12 in.

Whatever the particular sizes or varieties of film in use in a department, or their actual dispositions in the hopper, it is clear that this is a useful piece of equipment in providing orderly storage with ready access. Each box of films should be opened. The contents should be unpacked down to their folder wrappers, if any, and replaced in the box so that the folded edge of each covering is uppermost; that is, in the position it usually occupies when dispatched by the manufacturer. The box itself is then put into the hopper, both as a protection to the films against dust and to prevent the likelihood—particularly as depletion occurs—of films becoming curved under their own weight when standing vertically in a free space.

It is suggested that in reloading the hopper, the new box should go in with the new supply of films. This will assist determination of the emulsion serial numbers should any of a batch of films be found to be technically faulty. Manufacturers' representatives consulted about such occasional defects are in a poor position to give assistance if the films are in the wrong box.

The hopper must be well made and completely light-tight. It frequently includes the following additional features.

(1) On the outside a prominent printed warning that it should not be opened in white light. It is well to keep this notice fresh and readily visible.

(2) A lock of the 'Yale' type to enable the hopper to be left secure in the absence of trained staff.

(3) A switch which breaks the white light circuit should the hopper be opened.

(3) is often considered as alternative to (2) though it is not necessarily so: if the darkroom has a window only the lock may save the films from exposure to daylight.

Drawers. In place of a hopper a number of shallow light-tight drawers could be used; one is needed for every size and variety of film required in the department. Preferably these drawers should be plainly labelled in regard to their contents. While singly they require less space, their sum demand—if an adequate number are to be provided—is perhaps greater than that of a hopper. They would appear to be less convenient and of course locks and other safety measures have to be multiplied. For all these reasons, they are rarely used.

Cupboards. Cupboards in the loading bench are intended to stock a small current supply of films for the replenishment of the hopper. Their dimensions should allow boxes to stand upright. Three inches more height than that of the film are needed, and 3 inches more depth; that is, a space 20 inches high and 17 inches deep is required for a box of 14 × 17 in. material.

20

A good design of cupboard has vertical divisions to prevent boxes tipping sideways as the stock becomes diminished. A run equivalent to slightly more than a third of the benching has been estimated as adequate for a darkroom of moderate size. It may be noted that a 6-inch run will usually accommodate the following permutations of boxes of interleaved film.

$$2 \times 75 + 1 \times 25$$
or
$$5 \times 25$$
or
$$1 \times 75 + 3 \times 25$$

Planners mathematically inclined can make their own calculations, on the basis of this information and the units in which they normally purchase their film.

Cupboards in a darkroom which may be opened in diminished illumination, for safety should be fitted with sliding doors.

It is quite common practice to provide under a loading bench a bin for waste paper which can be reached from the work-top by means of a slot with a hinged lid. This is not so convenient in use as would appear, generally because the aperture allowed is too small. A large bin, free standing at one end of the loading bench or at some other handy point, is often the better arrangement.

ACCESSORY EQUIPMENT

Sink. A major item of accessory equipment required in a radiographic darkroom is a general purpose sink. With the processing unit itself, this will constitute the 'wet' section of the room. While there may not be a completely free choice of site for equipment which requires a water supply, it is of course of first importance not to place the sink, or processing unit, in a position contiguous with the loading bench. The 'wet' and the 'dry' should be along opposite walls.

The sink should be deep, about 9 inches, and about 30 × 18 in. in its other dimensions. For comfort the top of the sink should not be less than 30 inches from the floor. Hot and cold water should be supplied, the taps being placed at least 15 inches above the sink to allow the introduction under them of a two-gallon bucket or Winchester bottle without difficulty. An anti-splash device should be fitted to each tap.

Draining boards are useful on either side of the sink if space allows. Good quality stainless steel or teak are suitable materials for these. It is sometimes suggested that a drainage area for wet films can be formed by placing the sink between the processing unit and the drier but this space is seldom large enough to be really useful in a busy darkroom. Furthermore racks over a sink for the drainage of films are above eye level in order to be out of the way: this results in water running down the technician's arms when hangers are put in position and naturally the arrangement is unpopular. A reasonable supply of wet film carriers with adequate drip trays, of the kind shown for example in Plate 11.4, following p. 206 are more likely to be used than are draining racks in the neighbourhood of the sink.

There are of course other good reasons for placing the sink and the processing unit adjacent to each other. Such a situation makes for compactness in the wet section of the room and facilitates cleaning of the processing unit, since a hose can readily be run from the taps to the latter.

Cupboards under and near the sink should be provided if possible. They are useful for the storage of any equipment for cleaning and for mixing chemicals, and of chemical stocks.

Drier. There are various types and sizes of equipment available for drying processed radiographs but all use the same simple commodity— hot air. Moist air exhausts from all driers and it should not do so into the darkroom. If the unit is situated there, a duct must be provided for the air's removal.

The traditional form of drier is a free-standing metal cupboard, usually finished in enamel or lacquer. In this, films of assorted sizes can be hung in their hangers, or by means of suspension bars and clips, from slotted racks; generally a double row of racks is fitted but if the cabinet is small it may have only a single one. A drip tray is often provided beneath and sometimes an interior safelight to facilitate use of the drier in the darkroom.

The cabinet has a fan for circulating the air and heater elements to warm it; these are sometimes separately switched. Doors should not be kept open when the heater is on and some units have a thermo-switch which will break the heater circuit in these circumstances and prevent excessive rise of temperature in the electrical elements.

The operation of the drier is often thermostatically controlled to maintain the air temperature at a level considered optimum for drying radiographs, that is from $110°-118°F$ ($43.3°-47.7°C$). Sometimes a thermometer is provided to record this. Power consumption varies very much, depending on the size of the unit, and may be from 800 watts up to about 2.5 kW. A large drier of this type would accept about fifty to sixty hangers and offer a drying time of between 20 and 45 minutes. An installation equipped with two such driers could pass through films at a consistent rate of about 100 per hour.

A variation from the cabinet design is an otherwise similar unit in which the hangers are suspended in a deep drawer. The drier is 35 inches in height and the top is finished with linoleum to make it suitable as a working surface in a darkroom. This is a handy characteristic, particularly in a cramped department where space must be used with maximum economy.

Certain rapid driers are available which depart altogether from the older washing-day conception of hanging films to dry in hot cupboards. Basically, these driers are the drying section of an automatic processor.

The operator feeds the film to an input tray whence it is taken through squeegee rollers and so through other assemblies of rollers. As it travels, hot air is blown on to the film through tubes directed at both emulsion surfaces. The air is filtered to ensure that it is clean and warmed by a 1 kW heater and fan, the temperature being electronically controlled.

In a manner similar to the assemblies of complete automatic processors, the rollers can be easily removed for cleaning; the filter is accessible for replacement. The materials used in the construction of the drier are mainly stainless steel and modern chemically resistant substances such as PVC (polyvinyl chloride); the bearings on the unit are nylon.

The drier is compact in design, its base occupying less than 3 sq. ft. and thus it is suitable for bench or table mounting. It can be operated from a 13 ampere or 15 ampere wall socket. A drip tray receives the small amount of water discharged during use of the drier and this can be drained by means of a clamped tube.

A drier of this kind is very much more rapid than any of the cabinet type and its maximum rate of operation represents a through-put of ninety 10 × 12 in. films per hour.

The Darkroom with Automation

The darkroom which has an automatic processing system is equipped at much greater expense but in one sense much more simply than that in which the method of operation is manual. The effect of the processor is to take the 'wet' section of the work from the darkroom altogether; in most cases the only part of the unit which actually is within the darkroom is a feeding table or loading aperture which will project perhaps about 18 inches into the room.

Consequently our ideas of how such a darkroom is to be equipped are very different. The loading bench should have transfer hatches in its vicinity and—assuming cassettes are in circulation—film storage; but it need not provide for hangers. No viewing equipment, sink, wet film carriers, draining racks or driers are required. Even an interval clock for timing processing procedures becomes unnecessary. In these circumstances darkroom planning is a matter of adequate, well fitted, well illuminated benching arranged so that a free work flow is obtained between the film's reception point and the intake of the processor.

By way of summarizing this discussion of darkroom equipment the student is referred to Fig. 11.4 which shows an outline plan of what we have taken as a basic unit; the room which uses a manual system of processing and includes all stages of processing.

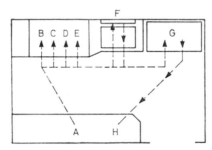

FIG. 11.4. Simple plan of a small darkroom. *By courtesy of Kodak Ltd.*
A ... H   Dry bench.
B,C,D,E   Processing.
F   Sink with draining-rack above.
G   Drier.

The student should look at this in relation to the four points which we first considered. These were:

(1) effective separation of wet and dry sections;
(2) orderly sequence of events;
(3) neat layout;
(4) clear traffic lanes.

THE VIEWING AND SORTING ROOM

A film-viewing and sorting room is necessary to most X-ray departments. Usually this will be the room or area into which films are delivered by an automatic processor—or processors—fed from an adjacent darkroom. If the film-reporting room also can be near at hand this is obviously helpful. The viewing room itself is seldom suitable for reporting purposes, owing to the distractions of noise and staff movements.

The area required for an efficient sorting room is difficult to define since there are several variable factors, of which perhaps the most significant is the number of films which the department usually handles during the day. The Ministry of Health in the United Kingdom suggests 125 sq. ft. for a sorting room but this figure does not seem realistic in many cases and indeed none can be correct for every situation. In general it is desirable—and necessary in busy hospitals—that the room should be spacious. Its work is essential and exacting and it is appropriate to regard this as an important nerve centre in any X-ray department. Efficient operation of the viewing and sorting room greatly affects the efficiency of the whole radiological service.

The functions required of a film-viewing and sorting room comprise (a) checking processed radiographs for quality, (b) preparing radiographs for report. The marking, trimming and documentation of radiographs which are implicit in (b) are further discussed in Chapter xiv, together with small items of equipment which may be needed for this work. The features of the room itself must vary, depending partly on the space available and the quantities of radiographs handled but much more upon whether processing is automated or manual.

Processing by Automation

An area in the immediate vicinity of the output end of an automatic processor must allow for two separate categories of activity:
(1) the reception, viewing and sorting of dry films;
(2) the maintenance and cleaning of processing equipment, the mixing of chemicals and usually the housing of large replenisher tanks which contain developing and fixing solutions.

Whenever possible, the room should be well demarcated into separate areas, for (2) essentially is the wet section of the darkroom's work although it is now outside the darkroom.

Equipment for Viewing and Sorting
Radiographs can be checked for quality upon wall-mounted illuminators placed conveniently to the delivery hopper of the processor. The number of illuminators employed is dictated by the space available, the quantity of films going through the processor and the numbers of people attempt-

ing to evaluate radiographs at any one time. The allowance should be as generous as possible for to do this work in cramped and difficult conditions is usually to do it badly.

Depending on the dimensions and scope of the room a central bench is appropriate and it is advantageous if the surface of this can have an illuminated middle section. Some types of corner cutter are suitable for fitting flush with a bench top and while this is not necessary it gives a more stylish appearance to the equipment. Suitable stools and a few cupboards for storage are obvious assets.

Over the sorting bench a vertically partitioned shelf is helpful. Some of these sections can be alphabetically indexed and used to house envelopes or radiographs until their appropriate partners are linked with them in the due courses of the process. Others intended for outgoing radiographs on completion of sorting and documenting might have designations relating them to a particular category of work: for example, the name of a consultant radiologist would be a means of gathering together for report a group of gastro-intestinal or angiographic examinations made by him. It is quite helpful in fact if the labelling of these partitions is not of a permanent nature. A surface on which a legend can be written temporarily makes for greater flexibility of the system.

Depending on the methods of their own departments students are likely to know of various ways of organizing this essential work. It is impossible here to detail several systems when they are often so individual in nature; nor would it be helpful to do so.

In the wet section of the room, floor and wall surfaces should be treated accordingly and a sink and hot and cold water supply are needed. Chemicals in reserve should be stored somewhere near at hand. Depending upon the variety of processor in use, accessory equipment may be fitted; for example, the hoist used to lift rollers from the large X-omat unit.

Manual Processing: Wet Viewing

In a department where either all or some processing is manually performed, arrangements are often made to remove from the darkroom those stages of processing which do not require safe lighting and to use an adjacent room or area to view wet films as they are washed—or even when they have been partially fixed. As many departments at present employ automatic processors, the wet viewing room is very much less common than it was a few years ago.

This system of wet viewing—whether it is done at the fixing or washing stage—depends on the use of a pass-through tank. This is a large, deep tank which is designed to be fitted through the wall between the darkroom and the viewing room; its contents are accessible from either side. The pass-through tank has two light-tight lids, only one of which can be opened at a time. This is necessary to prevent light from the viewing room entering the darkroom. Rails which run from one end of the tank to the other carry cradles and from these the radiographs in their hangers can be suspended. The films can be lifted from the cradles and examined wet as each batch is pushed through to the viewing room by a technician working from the darkroom end of the tank.

Such a viewing room requires adequate facilities for illuminating wet films and for the subsequent completion of their processing, including their sorting when dried. In the last respect its needs are similar to those of the dry sorting room already discussed.

CHAPTER XII

The Radiographic Image

The student now understands how a radiographic image is produced by radiation transmitted in varying amounts through the subject to activate silver halide grains in an emulsion and produce black deposits of silver. The action of the X rays (or of the X rays in combination with the light from intensifying screens) is amplified many times by chemical development, the object of the processing cycle being to produce a permanent image which can be viewed by transmitted light. In the present chapter certain features of this image and factors affecting it are further considered.

The sole object in producing the image is that it should be *seen*. In order that it may be seen, it must have (i) sufficient sharpness of outline and (ii) sufficient radiographic contrast. Radiographic contrast is the difference in brightness between various parts of the image, these areas in the image corresponding to areas in the subject of different X-ray absorption. A structure in the subject will not show if the image has no sharpness of outline, and if there is insufficient radiographic contrast between it and its surroundings.

Three important features of the image are therefore to be distinguished. These are:

(i) Sharpness of outline.
(ii) Radiographic contrast, or differences in brightness.
(iii) Distinctness with which the image is made visible and can be seen.

The subject consists of a number of elements which form it—for example the trabecular structure of bone is a series of small bone elements. These structural elements are the *detail* of the subject. The distinctness with which the detail of the subject is made visible in the radiograph is known as the *definition* of the image.

The distinctness with which the detail is made visible depends both upon its sharpness of outline and upon differences in brightness. Definition is therefore a function of sharpness and contrast. However sharp in outline, a black cat in a dark cellar will not be defined since it has no contrast; however high the contrast, a man in black on a snowfield will be without definition if he is going past on skis at a speed which makes all his outlines into a blur. Where images are of equal sharpness, the one with the greater contrast is better defined; where images are of equal contrast, the one which has sharper outlines has also the better definition.

What does the expression 'sharpness of outline' mean? It is the breadth of the boundary between two areas of different density, and it can be measured by means of a special densitometer known as a microdensitometer.

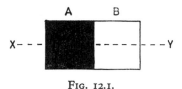

FIG. 12.1.

Fig. 12.1 shows two areas of different density, A and B. A recording densitometer can be used to record the densities measured along the horizontal line XY, and a graph can be made in which density is plotted against points on the line (millimetres). If the boundary between the two areas is sharp in outline, the graph will show a vertical drop between A and B as in Fig. 12.2. If the boundary between A and B is not sharp but is diffuse, the graph will show a sloping fall between A and B as in Fig. 12.3. The breadth of the boundary indicates the degree of unsharpness.

From what has been said, we can give here the following statement concerning these features of the radiographic image so far discussed:

(i) Sharpness of outline is the breadth of the boundary between two areas of different density.

(ii) Radiographic contrast is the difference in brightness between two areas of different density.

(iii) Definition is the distinctness with which the detail of the subject is made visible in the image, and it is a function of both (i) and (ii).

In reading textbooks the student may meet other statements concerning the term definition, and may find that it is used to mean sharpness of outline. Many people do use it in that sense, and others use the term *objective definition* to mean sharpness of outline, and *subjective definition* to describe the distinctness which the detail of the subject has for an observer of the image. These several definitions may for the student define despair. We can only recommend that the student should keep firmly in mind the three statements made above, and use the terms with these meanings, eschewing others.

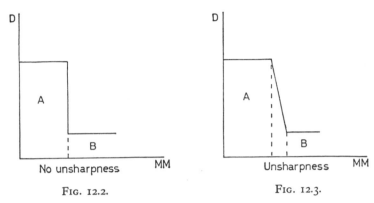

No unsharpness MM

FIG. 12.2.

Unsharpness MM

FIG. 12.3.

The curves shown in Fig. 12.2 and 12.3 are sketches and not actual graphs obtained. (Unsharpness curves obtained are shown in Plate 5.1 following page 94.)

THE SHARPNESS OF THE RADIOGRAPHIC IMAGE

The radiographic image is a shadow image. It is made by a body intercepting radiation, as an image can be put on a wall by a body intercepting rays from the sun. In the ideal radiographic image there would be complete sharpness of outline of the shadows which form it. In practice these shadows always possess some diffusion of outline, and the total degree of diffusion is a composite of several factors. We will consider three main groups.

(i) Factors connected with the geometry of shadow formation, known as *geometric factors.*

(ii) Factors connected with the subject and its movement, known as *motional factors.*

(iii) Factors connected with the recording of the image, known as *photographic* or *intrinsic factors.*

Geometric Factors of Unsharpness

Geometric unsharpness in the shadow image has three origins. These are (i) the size of the X-ray source, (ii) the distance between the X-ray source and the recording surface, which is the film, and (iii) the distance between the film and the subject being radiographed. The total degree of geometric unsharpness is determined by the relationship existing between these three factors when the image is made.

THE X-RAY SOURCE

The importance of the size of the X-ray source or the focal spot of the X-ray tube can be demonstrated by a simple diagram of the geometry of image formation. In Fig. 12.4 diagram A represents image formation from a point source. It shows that the shadow cast by the object, although larger than the object's true size owing to the spread of the image-forming rays, is nevertheless sharp in outline.

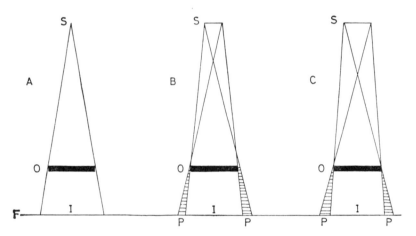

FIG. 12.4. Geometric unsharpness
S X-ray source
O object
I image or true shadow of the object
P penumbra or half-shadow surrounding the image
F film

Diagram B shows an image formed by a source which has a certain size; radiation now reaches the object not from a point but from an area. Each part of the object intercepts radiation from all parts of the focal spot, and as a result of this points in the image cease to be points, and become blurred by areas of half-shadow round them. This area of half-shadow is called the *penumbra*, and as the penumbra increases in size the true shadows in the image become more and more diffuse in outline. In diagram C is shown the increase in penumbra resulting from a larger X-ray source. Sharpness of outline is therefore influenced by the size of the X-ray source in this way: the smallest source gives the least penumbra (if other factors are constant).

It is perhaps worthwhile to consider in more detail the implications of the expression 'the size of the X-ray source'. What is its meaning? In the X-ray tube, X rays are produced over the area of the target receiving electron bombardment. The size of this area covered by the electron beam is determined by the shape and size of the filament, and the measurements of the focusing slot in the cathode in which it is set. This area of electron bombardment is termed the actual focus of the X-ray tube, and is the real size of the X-ray source.

In the formation of the image the 'size of the X-ray source' refers not to the real size, but to the size that the source *appears* to be when it is viewed from the film. This apparent size of the source is the projection of the actual focus and is called the effective focus of the X-ray tube. The earlier statement might more precisely be reworded: the smallest effective focus gives the least penumbra.

The actual focus of the X-ray tube is foreshortened by angulation of the target face. A rectangular area of electron bombardment projects as a square when viewed from a point directly below the centre of the anode at 90° to the long axis of the tube. If an observer imagines himself looking up at the anode from this point (A in Fig. 12.5), he will perceive the focal area as a square. If he then moves from his vantage point, goes

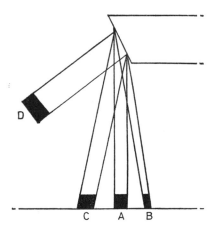

FIG. 12.5. Variation in the apparent size of the focal spot along the long axis of an X-ray tube.

A, B, and C are three apparent focal areas.
D is the actual focal area.

a little towards the anode end of the X-ray tube, and looks up from there (B in Fig. 12.5), he will find that the focal area is now further fore-shortened, and its vertical dimension appears smaller than it did from the first viewpoint. If he takes another walk back to the first viewpoint, and then an equal distance away from it towards the cathode end of the X-ray tube, he will find on looking up from there (C in Fig. 12.5) that the focal area is now less foreshortened, and its vertical dimension appears longer than when he viewed it first. This series of viewpoints and their effect on apparent size of the X-ray source are shown in Fig. 12.5.

This means that in the image less penumbra is produced in parts of the subject under B than in parts under A, and in parts of the subject under A than in parts under C. The image is not equally sharp in outline at all points along the long axis of the tube. This effect is demonstrable in special conditions and is likely to be most noticeable with large focal spots when the X-ray beam is used to cover a big film area at a short distance. In general departmental practice it is usually disregarded, being not perceived when radiographs are viewed.

THE TUBE-FILM DISTANCE

The penumbra produced by an effective focus of a certain size becomes smaller as the distance between the X-ray tube and the film is increased. This is shown in Fig. 12.6, where diagrams A and B should be compared The effective focus is the same in both, but in B the tube-film distance is greater and it can be seen that the resultant penumbra is less in size. It can therefore be stated that long tube-film distances reduce penumbra.

THE SUBJECT-FILM DISTANCE

The effect of the distance between the film and the subject being radio-graphed is shown in diagram C in Fig. 12.6. Here the effective focus is again the same size as in A and B and the tube-film distance is the same as in diagram B, but the subject is much closer to the film. It can be seen that the penumbra is again reduced in size.

These dimensions which contribute to geometric unsharpness are closely related to each other and to penumbra in the image in this way.
(i) The smaller the effective focus, the smaller the penumbra.
(ii) The longer the tube-film distance the smaller the penumbra.
(iii) The shorter the subject-film distance the smaller the penumbra.

The increase in penumbra resulting from a larger effective focus, a shorter tube-film distance, or a longer subject-film distance can be offset by adjustment of the other two factors to reduce it. The principles appear

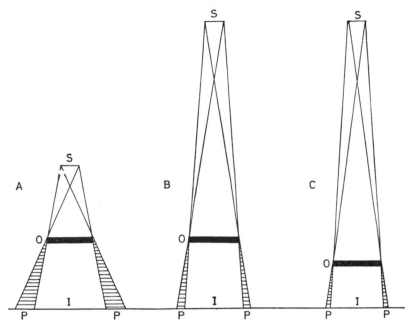

Fig. 12.6. Geometric unsharpness.

S   X-ray source
O   object
I   image or true shadow of the object
P   penumbra or half-shadow surrounding the image

simple, but their application to medical radiography involves compromise. This will be discussed in detail when other sources of unsharpness in the image have been examined.

Motional Factors in Unsharpness

So long as the subject is alive some degree of movement during the exposure is always a possibility, with certain types of subject it is a probability, and with certain fields of examination it is a certainty if the exposure lasts long enough. It must be remembered that, apart from the patient's capability in stopping voluntary movement, there are involuntary movements over which he has no control. Peristaltic action in the abdominal viscera and the heartbeat are examples.

A sufficient degree of motion blurs the shadow outline. A point within the subject is recorded not as a point in one place on the film, but in more than one place on the film and therefore as a blur. The degree of unsharpness produced by motion depends on the rate at which movement has taken place, the extent of movement, and the length of time the exposure lasts. If the exposure time is sufficiently short and the movement is sufficiently slow in relation to it or small in extent, unsharpness in the image will be minimal.

It is common knowledge that photographs of moving objects can be made with cameras allowing short exposure-times. Horses can be shown going over obstacles on a racecourse, golfers can be shown at the height of their 'swing' with all motion apparently arrested. This principle can be applied in radiography. By the use of short exposure-times satisfactory radiographs can be made of body parts where movement is likely or certain.

Some estimate can be made of the probability of subject-motion in regard to any radiographic examination. The radiographer's first assessment will be of the type of subject and his degree of ability to co-operate, taking into account age and physical and mental state. The next assessment takes note of the field of examination, and the presence or absence within it of involuntary movements which it is beyond the patient's will to stop.

This informed assessment is a part of radiographic technique and detailed discussion of it not within the scope of this book. Here it may simply be said that unsharpness due to subject movement is more likely in some instances than in others; it will vary in degree with the rate of movement, the extent of the movement, and the duration of the exposure; it can be reduced by the use of short exposure-times. There are other factors which influence degrees of motional blurring—for example whether the moving part is near the film or remote from it, near the X-ray source or remote from it, moving transversely or otherwise in relation to the beam. These factors are somewhat theoretical and beyond the practical sphere of the radiographer, so they will not be discussed. Difficulties connected with the use of short exposure-times will be considered again in a later section when all the factors of unsharpness are related to each other.

Photographic or Intrinsic Factors of Unsharpness

INTENSIFYING SCREENS

The most significant photographic factor in unsharpness of the image is the use or absence of intensifying screens. Such screens are fully discussed in Chapter v. The salt screens commonly used are made of crystals, each of which fluoresces as a separate entity under the action of X rays. The image is therefore produced by many separate sources of light. These separate light sources result in images with a certain diffusion of outline. The extent of this diffusion depends on the size of the light-emitting crystal, and also upon the distance of the crystal from the film since there is divergence of screen light.

Screens made of larger crystals and consisting of deeper layers of crystals are faster than screens made of very small crystals spread in thin layers—that is they allow of greater reduction in exposure-time. They inevitably result in greater screen-unsharpness in the radiographic image. Screens of very fine grain, that is made of a thin layer of small crystals, are usually termed 'high definition' to draw attention to the fact that they are designed to give a minimum amount of screen-unsharpness. They cannot be expected to be fast enough to allow of very short exposures, since the two qualities—speed and minimal unsharpness from crystal size and distribution—are incompatible.

Where screens are not used at all this factor of unsharpness of course does not exist in the image. Students can see this for themselves by radio-

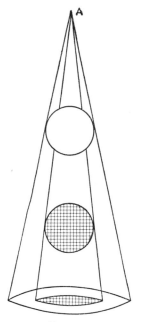

FIG. 12.7.

graphing a specimen bone both by direct exposure and with the use of screens, and then comparing the results.

When screens are used it is extremely important that both screens in a cassette should be in close and complete contact with the film situated between them. This contact must be evenly maintained over the whole area of the surfaces in apposition. Where the contact is poor a marked degree of unsharpness appears in the image.

PARALLAX

This term refers to the fact that when near and distant objects are seen from different viewpoints, their relationship to each other seems to change and is not perceived as it truly exists.

Fig. 12.7 shows a dark circle immediately beneath a light circle, and when viewed from position A they are seen to be superimposed. In Fig. 12.8 they are seen from two other positions. An observer in position B would find the dark circle towards his left hand and the light circle towards his right. An observer in position C would find the dark circle

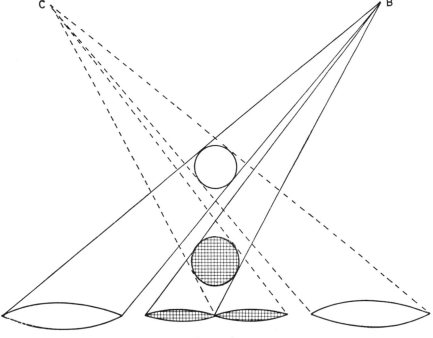

Fig. 12.8.

to his right hand and the light circle to his left. This apparent change in relationship is called parallax.

X-ray film has an image produced on both sides at once, and thus there are really two separate images at a distance from each other which is the thickness of the base plus the thickness of each emulsion layer. When the film is wet and the two emulsions are swollen by moisture, the images have appreciable separation. As they are viewed by an observer, one is closer to him than the other; the one image might be termed a near object, the other a more distant one.

This separation of the images gives rise to a parallax effect or an error in superimposition of the two images. As a result the final image viewed does not have outlines as sharp as those seen in an image which is truly a single one. This degree of unsharpness is greatest when the film is wet and it is negligible when the film is dry. Even in a wet film it is not necessarily noticeable, but it is one of the reasons why radiologists prefer not to make final reports on radiographs which they have not viewed dry.

EMULSION SOURCES OF UNSHARPNESS

When photographic materials were discussed in Chapter 11, reference was made to a phenomenon known as *irradiation*. This was described as a sideways spread of light in the emulsion, and it is a source of unsharpness in the image. A similar effect occurs in radiographs, a sideways spread in the emulsion both of X radiation and of the fluorescence of intensifying screens. In the case of X rays there is scattering within the emulsion not only of the X-ray quanta but also of electrons released in absorption processes. These electrons can make developable silver halide grains which have not been reached directly by an X-ray quantum. The contribution of these effects to the total unsharpness may be regarded as very small indeed in most diagnostic radiography on medical subjects.

With very high energy X rays the film unsharpness resulting from electron scattering will be greater, since the more energetic quanta can energize more electrons. It has been said that for X rays produced at 1,000 kV each quantum absorbed accounts for 80 grains being made developable. The unsharpness resulting from these effects would be measurably greater in a radiograph taken with a supervoltage therapy set than in radiographs made at conventional diagnostic kilovoltages.

In regard to the resolving power of photographic materials, grain size was mentioned in Chapter 11 and the phenomenon of graininess was discussed. The size of the grains in emulsions used for radiography makes no significant contribution to the unsharpness of the image. It has been shown that there are many factors resulting in such degrees of unsharpness that grain size and its effect on resolving power can be neglected in conventional radiographic images.

Geometric, Motional and Photographic Unsharpness in Relation to the Radiographic Result

Consideration of these factors together, and of the degree of unsharpness actually present in a radiograph, leads straight to the heart of the radiographic problem. Students can soon appreciate the dilemma if these groups of factors are taken in turn, and thought is given to making the contribution of any one of them absolutely minimal.

What would reduce geometric unsharpness? Clearly the answer is short subject-film distance, long tube-film distance, and small effective focus for the X-ray tube. Very short subject-film distances may be impossible to obtain. The heart, for example, is lodged within an incompressible thoracic cage and the patient's measurements may provide additional distance beyond the radiographer's control.

It may be easy to arrange for the X-ray tube to be remote from the film, but if this is done exposure factors must be increased. This requires long time-intervals or greater electrical loads on the X-ray tube, and perhaps a combination of both. The greater electrical loads require larger focal areas because of the heat generated, so the use of small effective focus becomes impossible. The longer time-intervals may increase motional unsharpness. If it is decided to use the smallest possible focus, then long tube-film distances cannot be used for the reasons shown above.

What would reduce motional unsharpness? The use of short exposure-intervals. This requires high electrical loads, which demand large focal areas; or less electrical load combined with shorter tube-film distances. Both these factors increase the unsharpness of geometric origin.

What would reduce unsharpness from photographic factors? The most significant improvement would be given by refusal to use intensifying screens. This would demand for thick body parts exposures many times greater than those in use with screens, longer time-intervals would be necessary (with increase in motional unsharpness), higher electrical loads (with need for larger focal areas), and shorter tube-film distances; both these last would increase geometric unsharpness. So perhaps it might be decided to use screens, but to keep their unsharpness minimal by using only those giving high definition. These are inevitably slow, and the disadvantageous conditions outlined previously would still apply with some force.

It is thus clear that any attempt to make one source of unsharpness minimal in its effect can succeed only at the price of increasing the unsharpness arising from one or both of the other groups. This can occur to an extent that invalidates any gain. At this stage the student may be wondering wildly how it is possible to obtain any radiographic image with outlines acceptably sharp. The answer is in compromise. It has been shown that the *total* unsharpness is least when the geometric, motional and photographic factors make *equal* contributions to the whole. This forms the basis for selection of technical factors in any given radiographic examination.

The thickness of the body part, the probability or certainty of movement, the rating of the X-ray tube, the size of the focal spot and permissible levels of electrical load, the radiographic output required to give adequate film density at a given tube-film distance—all these are balanced and selected to give an optimum result in each case. The radiographer may be said to work with an informed empiricism. If the student will mentally review familiar radiographic techniques, and consider fully the effects on unsharpness of changing one or more of the factors, it will doubtless be possible to appreciate how the contribution from each of the sources is made equal so that the total unsharpness shall be as small as possible.

Certain examinations naturally present little difficulty. For example, when X-raying one finger the radiographer has every assistance in trying to obtain a sharp image. The body part is small, the subject-film distance is short, total immobility can be secured in most cases, little radiographic output is required from the X-ray tube so small effective focus and short time-intervals can be used, and screens are not necessary. In obstetric radiographic examinations, the problem is very much greater and is solved only by accepting some elements of unsharpness in order to prevent others from producing intolerable diffusion in the image.

THE CONTRAST OF THE RADIOGRAPHIC IMAGE

It was explained in Chapter III that radiographic contrast is a function of radiation contrast in the subject and the gamma of the material being used. This is true, but as well as these important factors there are others which influence the contrast of the image. The topic will now be given fuller consideration.

The contrast of the radiographic image can be distinguished as having two separate elements. These are:

(i) Objective contrast. This can be calculated and given numerical form since it is the difference in density in various parts of the image. As shown in Chapter III, density can be measured with instruments. If a certain area of the film has density D_1 and another area has density D_2, then the objective contrast between them is $D_1 - D_2$.

(ii) Subjective contrast. This is visual contrast, the difference in brightness between areas of the film as it seems to an observer. It is clearly not measurable since it is an individual assessment, variable between observers and for one observer at different times.

Factors affecting objective contrast influence also subjective contrast, but there are factors affecting the contrast as it seems (for example, viewing conditions) which have no effect on the computable objective contrast. In the present section subjective contrast will not be considered, since its proper place is in relation to the distinctness with which the image is made visible—that is the definition of the image as it was earlier stated. Subjective contrast will therefore be discussed again under the heading of definition.

While it can be stated that the outlines wanted in a radiograph are simply the sharpest possible, it is by no means so easy to express what is wanted in contrast. Radiographs are produced to be viewed and used by all too human observers, and radiographers soon learn that variations are possible in individual judgements on what constitutes a 'good radiograph'. These individual judgements turn on differences in density and contrast, not upon differences in sharpness about which everybody is agreed.

It can be said that the highest possible contrast is not the most useful diagnostically, and very low contrast can fail to make structures visible. Between these two extremes is a level of contrast which is satisfactory and gives good visibility of structures. This 'satisfactory' contrast will not be the same for all types of radiographic examination. The student can appreciate this by comparing as examples a barium meal study, a cholecystogram, a plain film of the renal area, a posteroanterior view of the skull. It may be difficult to be content with these vague statements, but it is a fact that no one can give a simple and quantitative answer as to what satisfactory contrast will be.

The factors which influence objective contrast can be divided into three main groups. These are (i) radiation factors, (ii) film factors, and (iii) processing factors.

Radiation Factors in Objective Contrast

Radiation factors altering contrast are twofold and result from (i) the quality of the primary radiation and (ii) the scattered radiation reaching the film.

QUALITY OF THE PRIMARY RADIATION

The student is by now familiar with the facts that the quality of primary radiation is altered by change in the kilovoltage across the X-ray tube and that raising the kilovoltage makes the beam more penetrating. A change in penetration by the X rays alters radiation contrasts within the subject.

If a certain step-wedge is radiographed at low kilovoltage there will be a big difference in the intensity of radiation transmitted through its two ends; this means greater image contrast. The same step-wedge radiographed at higher kilovoltage gives a changed picture. There is less difference in absorption between the two ends of the wedge, the harder beam being better able to penetrate the thick end of the wedge, so that more radiation than previously is transmitted through this part.

Plate 12.1, following p. 206 shows a step-wedge radiographed at seven different kilovoltages, and the picture obtained with 40 kV on the left edge of the figure should be compared with that given by 100 kV on the right edge. It can be seen that at 100 kV there is less difference in density between the two ends of the wedge, and every step in the wedge is recorded. This is the picture of low radiographic contrast. At 40 kV there is greater difference in density not only between the ends but between all the steps of the wedge that can be seen; it should be noted that not every step of the wedge is recorded. This is the picture of high radiographic contrast. What is true of the step-wedge is true of all radiographic subjects; higher kilovoltage as illustrated in Fig. 3.14 on pages 54–55 levels out absorption differences in the subject, and results in lower image contrast. Low contrast records a long scale of intensities (every step in the wedge); high contrast records a short scale only.

A certain value of objective contrast is not, however, the first aim of radiographers selecting radiation quality since other factors limit choice of tube voltage. Leaving aside 'high kilovoltage techniques', it may be said that radiographers select kilovoltage for particular radiographic examinations with adequate penetration of the subject as the basis for selection; the alteration in radiographic contrast is an accompanying effect which is accepted. In certain cases when selecting kilovoltage the radiographer *does* use knowledge of the resultant changes in radiation contrast within the subject. For example, in an anteroposterior projection of the dorsal spine choice of higher kilovoltage (by flattening absorption differences) enables the relatively radiolucent upper parts and the relatively radio-opaque lower parts of the subject to be successfully recorded together.

Choice of kilovoltage, whether based on the need for penetrating the subject or consideration of radiation contrasts within the subject and their effects upon the image, is not an exact process. It is made empirically by the radiographer on the basis of experience.

EFFECTS OF SCATTERED RADIATION

The student has learned by now what happens to X radiation when it passes through the human body; some is transmitted, some is truly absorbed, some is scattered. In diagnostic radiography a proportion of scattered radiation can reach the film if no preventive measures are taken. On the film it creates a density which in the main is not image-forming. This has a most significant effect on the contrast of the resultant radiograph.

When it is remembered that objective contrast is difference in density, and that density is an expression of the light-transmitting ability of areas of the film, then it can be seen that an overall added density which decreases light transmission over the whole radiograph is bound to affect contrast. Since the scattered rays do have some projective action, their effect is also to decrease slightly the sharpness of the recorded detail, but it is their effect on contrast which is most significant in the general deterioration of the image.

When the kilovoltage across the X-ray tube is increased, there is less production of scattered radiation but at the same time the scattered radiation becomes more penetrating than that produced by a primary beam generated at lower kilovoltage. These changes in scattered radiation and the greater chances of its reaching the film by reason of increased penetration are most important results from the use of higher kilovoltage.

If no measures are taken to control the effect on the film, the loss of contrast is most marked. Since thick body-parts require higher kilovoltage for adequate penetration and give rise to more scattered radiation by reason also of the greater volume of tissue irradiated, loss of contrast will be most severe in these cases. It is a fact that without means to control scattered radiation it would be quite impossible to secure good radiographs of thick parts of the body; the images would be entirely unacceptable because of the low level of contrast.

In practical radiographic technique this loss of contrast is controlled through two approaches. These are (i) to reduce the formation of scatter, and (ii) to prevent scattered radiation from reaching the film.

Reduction in the formation of scatter. This will result from (i) the use of lower kilovoltages and (ii) limitation of the volume of irradiated tissue. It has been explained that the need for adequate penetration of the subject determines choice of kilovoltage, so this is not available as a method of controlling scatter. Much more important and useful is the reduction in scatter made by limiting the volume of tissue which the beam irradiates.

Compression of compressible body parts and the use of beam-limiting cones and diaphragms achieve this limitation. The student may be assured that the improvement in contrast which follows is not just a piece of textbook theory. It really works, as will be evident by comparison of radiographic results. The student should take opportunity to compare any of the following examples: a cholecystogram on a corpulent subject done with and without compression and a small cone, an anteroposterior view of the lumbar spine of a similar subject in the same conditions, a lateral pelvimetry projection taken with and without a cone, or any similar examinations where the part to be demonstrated is very thick. (This is *not* a suggestion that such radiographs should be produced experimentally with a view to comparison.)

Preventing scattered radiation from reaching the film. This is done by the use of a secondary radiation grid interposed between the patient and the film. Lead strips which compose part of the grid absorb oblique scattered rays, while the useful image-forming primary rays pass through radiolucent elements in the grid. Modern grids perform very effectively their task of screening the film from scattered radiation, and are an essential accessory for X-ray examination of thick parts of the body. They provide the means to obtain radiographic contrast which is not merely adequate but can be brilliant.

Since the grid inevitably absorbs some primary rays as well as the scattered radiation, exposures must be increased when a grid is used. This means increase in dose to the patient. This increase in dose is insignificant when it is realized that to make the radiograph without a grid would result in a valueless film, and thus exposure of the patient to a dose of radiation which would certainly be smaller but also quite useless.

As well as being scattered by the patient's body, radiation is scattered from other structures such as the X-ray table. Some effort can be made to prevent access to the film by this radiation. It is therefore common practice to make the backs of cassettes and exposure-holders radio-opaque. When direct-exposure film is used in its paper envelope, a piece of lead-rubber can be put behind it to absorb radiation scattered back towards the film from the table; this takes the place of the radio-opaque backing to a cassette.

Film Factors in Objective Contrast

The most important of these is the inherent contrast of the film material —its gamma in the conditions of development being used. It was explained in the last section of Chapter III that two important factors in radiographic contrast are (i) radiation contrasts within the subject and (ii) the film gamma. If the film gamma is low, the radiation contrasts within the subject are not amplified and the resultant contrast in the radiographic image is poor. Radiation contrasts in the subject are often very slight and film of low gamma cannot give good results. On the other hand film material of high gamma amplifies radiation contrasts in the subject and results in an image of good contrast which is acceptable. Films used in radiography now have a gamma which rather more than doubles the radiation contrasts within the subject when they are recorded in the radiographic image.

The gamma of the film material is not a factor in the control of contrast which can be manipulated by the radiographer. It is inherent in the material, is characteristic of it in the conditions of development used, and is standardized in manufacture. It remains a most important factor in the contrast of the image. Images seen on fluoroscopic screens not only are markedly less bright than those viewed on radiographs, but are much lower in contrast. The lack of contrast results from absence of the help given to radiographic images on film by the gamma of the materials in present use.

Faster materials tend to have lower contrast, and screen-type film exposed to direct radiation has less contrast than when exposed between screens. This is a fact demonstrable by D log E curves and plain observation of results, but perhaps it is not of much importance to a radiographer who is not driven by some failure in supply to make the experiment. Certainly in emergency screen-type film has been used without screens to radiograph extremities, when the marked loss of speed is immaterial, with results that were acceptable though slightly lacking in contrast.

Processing Factors in Objective Contrast

These relate almost solely to factors of development. The effect of photographic reduction by chemicals will be considered also; this is not a feature of the standard processing cycle but it can affect objective contrast when it is done, and must for completeness be included in this section.

There are many aspects of a developer and the technique of its use which can influence the contrast obtained. These may be listed as follows:

(i) Type and constitution of developing solutions.
(ii) Temperature of developer and time of development.
(iii) Freshness of developer.
(iv) Agitation of the film in the developer.

The aim in radiographic processing is to standardize as many of these as possible, and one of the benefits of automatic processing is that standardization of all can be achieved.

TYPE AND CONSTITUTION OF DEVELOPING SOLUTIONS

A great number of different developing formulae have been devised for general photography, even although the number of basic solutions is relatively small. Different formulae achieve different results, and the composition of the developer markedly influences the time required to reach a given contrast. The limit on the contrast which can be achieved is set by the film material used, but the time taken to arrive at the maximum obtainable contrast depends on the developer.

The number of available X-ray developers is small, and they are all Metol-hydroquinone or Phenidone-hydroquinone solutions. These function to give good contrast in the standard development time at a given temperature.

The various ingredients in developing solutions have different functions to perform, and the developer will vary in performance if its ingredients are not all present, or are present in proportions which are not correct. Thus the amount of actual developing agent present, the Metol-hydroquinone and Phenidone-hydroquinone ratios, alterations in the amounts of alkali and of restrainer present, and the concentration of the solution as a whole, are all factors which influence the length of time required to reach a given contrast.

TEMPERATURE OF DEVELOPER AND DEVELOPMENT TIME

A family of D log E curves is shown in Fig. 12.9. These are the result of developing X-ray films for different lengths of time in a developing solution at a standard temperature. It can be seen that the slope of the straight-line part of the curve at first increases rapidly with development time but does not appreciably change after 5 minutes' development.

This demonstrates that the gamma of the film increases as development continues through its early stages, but that soon a point is reached beyond which gamma does not increase although development time is extended. As was seen in Chapter III, from this group of curves a new curve could be made showing the growth of gamma with time of development—a time–gamma curve; the point of no increase in gamma is called *gamma infinity*, and development carried beyond this can result in fog and consequent decrease in contrast.

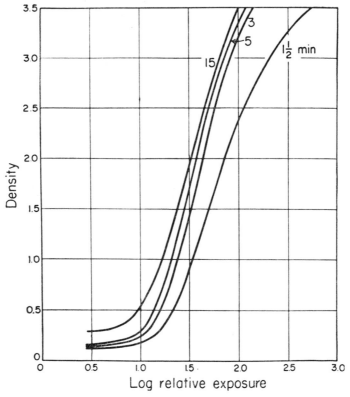

Fig. 12.9. Characteristic curves of a typical screen-type X-ray film, developed for a series of times at 68°F. *By courtesy of X-ray Sales Division, Eastman Kodak Company, Rochester, New York.*

Fig. 12.10 shows another family of D log E curves made to demonstrate the effect of developing films for the same length of time at different temperatures. Such curves show an increase in contrast between about 55°F and 68°F and later (80°F) a reduction in contrast. There is a point around 65°F beyond which no increase in contrast is achieved by increasing temperature.

In conventional manual processing the standard conditions of time and temperature have been set at 4 minutes (in the U.S.A. 5 minutes) development at 68°F (20°C). In automatic processing the technique of development is different, and development times are much shorter. Success depends on the use of special developing solutions suitable for working at a raised temperature, together with other factors. Whether

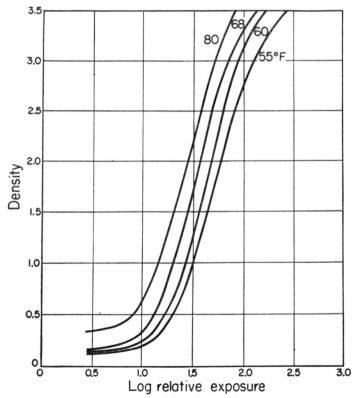

FIG. 12.10. Characteristic curves of the film of Fig. 12.9, but developed for 5 minutes at a series of development temperatures. *By courtesy of X-ray Sales Division, Eastman Kodak Company, Ltd.*

manual processing or automatic methods are used, the object of the standardized technique is the same—to provide an image of satisfactory contrast in a period of time which is short enough to avoid fogging by action of the developer on unexposed silver halide grains. The effects of time and temperature may be summed-up by saying that slight prolongation of time increases contrast, but that long extension decreases contrast, and that in general development at extremes of temperature (50°F and 86°F) results in impaired contrast (10°C and 30°C).

Exhaustion of the Developer

As seen in Chapter vi, developing agents exhaust through use, when their reaction with silver bromide results in oxidation of the agents; and also through standing, when oxidation by air takes place. In use the restraining bromide content of the developer is increased by the release of bromine ions. These changes result in increase in the time required by the developer to produce a given contrast.

Agitation

Agitation of the film during development increases the speed at which the process occurs. If a film not agitated at all during development is compared with a film given agitation and developed for the same period of time, the second one will usually have the better contrast (although with some types of film it has been found that agitation makes very little difference to contrast).

There is an undefined limit beyond which increase in agitation has no effect on contrast. Nevertheless effective agitation remains one of the benefits of automatic processing. It is an important factor in producing radiographs of satisfactory contrast and density in the development times which are used. Manually processed radiographs usually receive an insufficient degree of agitation.

Photographic Reduction by Chemicals

The use of chemical agents to remove metallic silver from the radiographic image in an effort to correct for overexposure or overdevelopment is described elsewhere in this book (Chapter xix). The action of such photographic reducers can be proportional to the amount of silver in the image, removing most silver where most is present. Since this reduces differences in density between various parts, it lowers objective contrast.

THE DEFINITION OF THE RADIOGRAPHIC IMAGE

As explained earlier in the present chapter, this term is used here to mean the distinctness with which the detail of the subject is made visible in the image. The factors which affect definition therefore include all those which govern radiographic contrast (differences in density) in the image. These features are objective and can be measured.

Definition is governed also by factors which are not objective. These subjective factors can be stated, but they are variable and cannot be measured; they include elements which are external to the image, for example the conditions in which it is viewed. It may fairly be said that definition is a visual quality and has more subjective than objective components. While not measurable these components can be listed and their effects assessed; this will be done in the following paragraphs.

Factors Affecting Definition

IMAGE FACTORS

These are (i) the sharpness and objective contrast as already discussed, and (ii) the degree of exposure. Where boundaries are sharp, it is possible to perceive differences in density which are very slight indeed; there is good definition even when the objective contrast is very low. If the difference in density is very great, structures can be clearly perceived even when the boundaries are not very sharp; definition is good even when the detail sharpness is not the best that can be obtained.

The student may care to consider practical radiographic examples of these phenomena. In certain examinations differences in density *are* slight and maximum sharpness of outline results in satisfactory definition; for example the demonstration of foetal parts in early pregnancy, and visualization of the bile ducts in intravenous cholangiography. Equally it is possible to consider instances where the difference in density is very great, and the definition is acceptable even although the outline is not sharp. This fact is sometimes a comfort to radiographers when they view the films of a recalcitrant child with a coin in his stomach. (At the same time it is on record that a straight pin has been made to disappear because it was moving; its image had no sharpness of outline, and definition was not obtained even although contrast existed.) It is clear that definition does not depend upon sharpness only or upon contrast only, but is determined by the two in correlation.

The degree of exposure significantly alters contrast in the image as it seems to an observer. Where overexposure exists, densities overall are increased but objective contrast (unless overexposure is gross), is not altered; differences in light-transmission through various regions of the film are in fact there and could be measured. It is simply that the eye cannot perceive these differences if the densities in general are so great that the light of the illuminator is not transmitted through them. The observer finds therefore that visual contrast is diminished by over-exposure; this visual contrast is subjective contrast and it cannot be measured since it is an impression received by the eyes of an individual viewer.

Underexposure results in lack of density. The developed image does not have the full range of densities produced in it, and there is thus deficiency in contrast both objective and subjective. The light from the illuminator coming through the film diminishes apparent contrast further, for the bright light in areas of low photographic density reduces for the eye small differences that exist.

Viewing Factors

The importance of these to definition in the image is their effect upon subjective contrast. Viewing factors can be considered under two headings. These are (i) those relating to the illumination, and (ii) those relating to the eyes of the observer.

The illumination. The viewing illumination can vary in colour, intensity, and uniformity. Modern X-ray illuminators are fluorescent-strip lighting not groups of electric bulbs, and they give a uniform blue-white light. This colour of light and its uniformity result in an improvement in visual contrast, enabling the range of densities in a well-exposed and correctly processed radiograph to be perceived as they actually exist.

In overexposed radiographs, increasing the brightness of the light improves subjective contrast. It allows the viewer to appreciate differences in density that he could not previously see. For an underexposed image, decreasing the brightness of the light improves visual contrast up to a certain point; there is an obvious limit here, for eventually the light would become too dim to penetrate the denser parts of even a weak image.

Illuminators are frequently equipped with a control for altering brightness so that conditions can be adapted for viewing a variety of radiographs. It is common practice also to have available in the reporting room a source of bright light (this may be just a single light bulb of sufficient wattage conveniently placed) against which regions of high photographic density can be viewed.

The level of illumination in a room where viewing is done also is significant in its effect upon apparent contrast. If the room is brightly lit the subjective contrast will be diminished. The effect of a shaft of sunlight illuminating the radiograph by reflected light can be to reduce to nil the apparent differences in light transmitted through the image from the X-ray illuminator. It is customary for reporting rooms to have their windows covered by curtains or screens so that the illumination in the room is low, and there are no unshielded bright lights when reporting is in progress. It is unnecessary, however, for radiographs to be viewed in a room from which all light apart from that of the viewing illuminators is entirely excluded.

The eyes of the observer. Image contrast as it seems to the eye is affected by the level of illumination to which the eye is adapted, and by the extent to which dazzle is present. An eye adapted to a bright light is unable to perceive differences in the deeper density range, and beyond a certain level all the densities look black, the eye being unable to perceive detail in these regions. If the eye is dazzled by bright light coming through parts of the image which have little density, there is again lack of ability to perceive detail.

It is possible to prevent dazzle by masking areas from which bright light is coming. For example if a radiograph of 12 × 10 size is being examined against an illuminator which is 17 inches by 14 inches, a piece of black card to cover the illuminator with a 12 inch by 10 inch aperture cut in it can be placed as a surround to the radiograph. This will exclude extraneous light. It is customary to view industrial radiographs against very bright illuminators which have a means of confining the light to certain areas of the film.

This importance of the viewing situation to definition in any radiographic image is well recognized by radiologists, who would not consider basing a report on appearances which had been viewed against a window or before a ceiling light. While his clinical colleagues may sometimes regard viewing conditions more casually, the radiologist will give to these so that they may be exactly favourable as much care as he devotes to other aspects of radiographic technique. It is of little value to expend time, effort, and money in the production of first-class radiographs if they are to be viewed in conditions which vitiate their quality.

22

DISTORTION IN THE RADIOGRAPHIC IMAGE

This term refers to incorrectness in the proportions of structures recorded radiographically, and to lack of truth in their apparent alignment and relationship to each other. The most truthful result is obtained when a structure being radiographed rests with its principal planes parallel to the film, and the X-ray beam is aligned so that the central ray is at right angles to these planes and to the film.

The student should compare two such examples as these: (i) a lateral view of the lumbar spine, the patient lying correctly in the true lateral position and the vertical X-ray beam centred at the level of the third lumbar vertebra; and (ii) a lateral view of the same region in a subject with a broad pelvis who has been allowed to sag at the waist towards the table so that the long axis of the spine is not parallel to the table, and the central ray is not vertical to it. In the first case the bodies of the vertebrae are seen as they are, distinct and separate from each other, with radiolucent structures occupying the spaces between them. In the second case the vertebral bodies overlap each other, and do not appear to be separated in space at all. If knowledge of them rested solely on such radiographic appearances, one would assume that in parts they overlay each other. The second image is a distorted one.

In dental radiography it is very easy to produce a similar effect by incorrect alignment, and to cause teeth to overlap each other, thus failing to render truly their relationship. It is equally easy to distort their true proportions, and produce images which are elongated or foreshortened in shape.

In general, radiographic technique is directed to restricting to a minimum distortions due to projection, but in some cases such alterations in apparent alignment and relationship are made with intention. It can be a useful technique for separating from intrusive structures some particular region which is to be visualized. The student can doubtless think of several examples; separation of the two sides of the mandible in lateral-oblique projections; the 30 deg. occipitomental view of the facial bones which by this technique are cleared of structures in the posterior fossa of the base of the skull; displacement of the clavicles from the apical regions of the lungs in examination of the chest.

Exact knowledge of the distortions producible in radiographs is thus part of the radiographer's armoury, whether the effect being sought is their avoidance or their deliberate production.

THE SIZE OF THE RADIOGRAPHIC IMAGE

The X-ray beam diverges from its source, spreading out so that it becomes greater in cross-section. This results in radiographic images which may truly be said to be larger than life (Fig. 12.11).

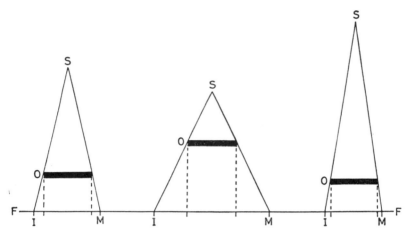

FIG. 12.11. Enlargement in the X-ray image
S   X-ray source (assumed to be a point)
O   object
IM   size of the image
F   film

The degree of enlargement that occurs is not a constant. It is determined by the distance separating structures being examined from the film which records them, and the distance between the X-ray source and the film. Magnification becomes greater for structures which are further from the film and for short source-film distances; it becomes less for structures which are close to the film and for long source-film distances.

With an anatomical structure parallel to the film and the central ray at right angles to the film, the true dimensions of the structure can be calculated from its image size by this relationship:

$$\text{True size} = \frac{\text{Image size} \times \text{Tube-structure distance}}{\text{Tube-film distance}}$$

This inevitable enlargement in the image is the reason why pelvic measurements for obstetricians and bone measurements for orthopaedic surgeons cannot be made on the simple basis of putting a ruler against a conventional radiographic image of the parts concerned. Where measurements are necessary, some method of correction or some means of reducing enlargement must be used.

Long tube-film distances diminish the difference between the true size and the image size because they result in the tube-structure distance and the tube-film distance being more nearly the same. If in fact they could be the same, if no distances separated the structure from the film, then the relationship between them would be unity. The true size of the anatomical structure would then be exactly equivalent to the dimensions of its radiographic image.

Appendix II at the end of this book presents, in table form, factors in the radiographic image which we have discussed in this chapter.

CHAPTER XIII

Exposure Factors in Diagnostic Radiography

Whether a radiographic image is produced by the action of X rays directly, or of fluorescent light from intensifying screens, the result is obtained because the photographic emulsion has absorbed some energy from the X-ray beam. There are many variables which influence this absorption of energy. These variables are assessed by the radiographer in selection of radiographic techniques, and they form a complex which now will be examined in more detail.

The variables involved can be seen to come under two main headings. They are (i) variables which constitute the exposure factors; these amount to statements concerning the conditions of operation of the X-ray tube: and (ii) variables which modify the selection of exposure factors if a correctly exposed radiograph is to result; this group embraces certain factors in the use of the X-ray tube and accessory equipment as well as variations connected with the subject of the radiographic examination.

EXPOSURE FACTORS

These may be listed as below:

(i) The X-ray tube voltage, expressed in kilovolts.

(ii) The X-ray tube current, expressed in milliamperes.

(iii) The tube-film distance, expressed in inches or centimetres.

(iv) The time-interval of the exposure, expressed in seconds.

In the absence of a patient the X-ray beam can be considered as more or less constant over the whole surface of the film. This statement can be made because in practice there is little noticeable difference; in actual fact there is less intensity of radiation at a point of measurement beneath the anode end of the X-ray tube than at a point of measurement beneath the cathode end. The effect is demonstrable on film if very short tube-film distances are used, but in most radiographic examinations it is ignored.

It can be said that the photographic effect (or the amount of silver deposited, or the blackening of the film) depends upon the intensity of the X-ray beam producing the reaction. If the intensity of the X-ray beam is increased the photographic effect is increased, and similarly the two decrease together. The current through the X-ray tube, the voltage across it, and the distance separating it from the film alter the intensity of the X-ray beam reaching the film. The time-interval of the exposure is in effect the length of time during which energy is given to the film, and so the total amount of energy received by the film depends (if all other factors are equal) on the exposure-time. Thus all these factors influence the photographic effect in their several ways as discussed in the following sections.

The X-ray Tube Voltage

Altering the tube voltage alters two characteristics of the X-ray beam—its penetrating power and its intensity. These are two distinct features, as the colour and the brightness are separate characteristics of a beam of visible light.

The effect of a change in ability to penetrate by the X rays, and consequent alteration in the contrast of the radiographic image, has already been discussed in Chapter XII. In this section we are now concerned with the change in *intensity* that follows alteration in tube voltage, and the consequent change in photographic effect.

The change in intensity that occurs when kilovoltage is altered cannot be considered as an entirely simple matter. The basic statement which *is* simple is that when kilovoltage is raised the intensity of radiation leaving the X-ray tube also is increased. Difficulties arise when we wish to know the relationship more precisely, and we ask by what factor is the intensity increased.

It has been said that the intensity of the X-ray beam increases approximately as the square of the tube voltage in kilovolts peak, and that X-ray intensity is proportional to kVp^2 or kVp^3 depending on filtration. These have been used as acceptable statements and student radiographers have been given the exercise of calculations involving the assumption that they are true, though approximate in character. The X-ray intensity reaching the film holder after passing through the patient increases by a higher power, and is proportional to kVp^4 or kVp^5 according to the part being radiographed. This relationship is further modified by the nature of the beam being considered, that is whether it is being produced by a high

tube kilovoltage or a relatively low one and the proportion of long wavelengths to short wavelengths that it contains.

The practising radiographer finds slight application for this knowledge, and is little interested in the intensity of the X-ray beam as it comes
off the anode of the X-ray tube or even as it emerges from the tube housing. Radiographers *use* X-ray beams, and are therefore concerned most
with the results on the film of these physical phenomena. What a radiographer needs is the answer to this question: *Since intensity increases
with increase in tube voltage, if I raise the tube voltage, by how much
should I decrease the time-interval of the exposure to achieve a radiographic result in which film blackening looks more or less the same?*

Here again there is no simple answer which is not an approximation.
If intensifying screens are used, there is alteration in the intensification
factor with tube voltage which theoretically affects the result. An increase
of 10 kVp from, say, 50 kVp to 60 kVp does not have the same effect on
the film as an increase of 10 kVp from 90 kVp to 100 kVp. This can be
appreciated if some numerical examples are worked out on the basis of
the fact that the X-ray intensity reaching the film holder is proportional
to kV^4. For example, a change from 50 kV to 60 kV would require the
time interval of the exposure to be reduced by a factor

$$\left(\frac{50}{60}\right)^4 = 0.48$$

A change from 90 kV to 100 kV would require the time to be reduced
by a factor

$$\left(\frac{90}{100}\right)^4 = 0.66$$

So the change in time required for a change in kilovoltage depends on
the ratio of the kilovoltages concerned. Differences in waveform between
X-ray sets, and perhaps also differences in performance in one X-ray set
when its loading is low or sufficiently high to be near its limit, are other
factors which add to the complexity of the situation.

It can be seen therefore that to provide to this question an answer which
shall be universal and precise is perhaps not possible; perhaps also it is not
necessary. It has been attempted, and nomograms and charts and graphs
have been made which suggest the correction in time-interval required
for changes in kilovoltage through the conventional diagnostic range.
These do not seem to be much used by radiographers.

There is a tradition that if 10 kVp are added to the tube voltage the exposure time may be decreased to half its previous value. This is a comfortably definite statement for the student to accept. While it may appear that this rule cannot bear scientific scrutiny, its satisfactory justification is that it seems to work.

The radiographer selects kilovoltage for a radiographic examination on the basis of previous experience. The following considerations will affect the choice.

(i) Knowledge of what has been used before, of the performance of the X-ray set in use, and of the practice of the department.

(ii) The need for adequate penetration of the subject.

(iii) Recognition of the fact that higher kilovoltage reduces radiation contrasts in the subject, and allows a wider range of tissue differences to be recorded together.

(iv) Knowledge that when higher kilovoltages are used intensity increases and times of exposure can be decreased; this is very marked when 'high kilovoltage techniques' (100 kVp to 140 kVp range) are used.

The X-ray Tube Current

The intensity of the radiation emerging from the X-ray tube can be considered to be proportional to the X-ray tube current as it is indicated by the controls and recorded on the milliampere meter of the X-ray set. This is a direct proportion; for example doubling the tube current increases the intensity by the same factor.

The radiographer is again concerned less with the intensity of the X-ray beam emerging from the X-ray tube than with the effect upon the film; that is to say less with the emergent intensity than with the quantity of radiation that the film receives. This is given by the product of the tube current (mA) and the time for which it flows (S), the result being milliamperesconds (mAS).

When the film is exposed directly to X rays without the use of intensifying screens, a milliamperesconds value of (say) 20 mAS produces the same effect whether it is delivered as a tube current of 20 mA passing for 1 second, of 200 mA passing for 0·1 second, or of 400 mA passing for 0·05 second. Provided that the product of tube current and time remains the same, the photographic effect is unchanged, irrespective of the separate values of milliamperage and time. This interchanging of intensity and time follows the law which is called the Law of Reciprocity. This is valid for X radiation acting on photographic materials.

When intensifying screens are in use the effect on the film is produced mainly by visible light emitted by the screens in response to X radiation. In this case there is reciprocity failure: this means that high intensities of light acting for short times and low intensities of light acting for long times do not produce the same photographic effect with the product Intensity × Time staying constant; at both extremes the effect is to produce less density than a reciprocal relationship leads one to expect. High tube currents passed for a short time and low tube currents passed for a long time may not produce the same result in comparison with each other, and indeed may not compare in effect with intermediate values of tube current and time, even although the milliampereseconds are the same in all these cases.

In practice radiographers regard reciprocity failure as having no practical significance, and assume that milliamperes and time are interchangeable whether intensifying screens are used or not. If 50 mAS has given a reasonable result in a certain examination and it is wished to shorten the time because the patient cannot keep still, then the new time-interval is derived by multiplying the tube current and dividing the time by the same factor; for example it might have been 50 mA for 1 second, and it could become 200 mA for 0·25 second. Here again the justification for such disregard of scientific fact is that the assumption works, perhaps because in any given examination radiographers are not likely to change milliamperage over a very wide range.

As with other factors of exposure, the radiographer selects milliampereseconds on the basis of previous experience. The following consideration will affect the choice.

(i) Knowledge of what has been used before, of the performance of the X-ray set in use, and of the practice of the department.

(ii) The need for adequate film density.

(iii) Assessment of the likelihood of subject-movement, taking into consideration the state of the patient, the nature of the examination, and the body-part involved.

(iv) The assumption that milliamperage and time are in effect interchangeable.

The Tube-Film Distance

Since the X-ray beam is divergent from its source, it covers an area which increases in size with distance from the source. The energy of the beam is therefore spread over a large area and the intensity (which may be defined as the energy reaching unit area in unit time) is thus diminished. The intensity varies inversely with the square of the distance from the source.

The student is surely familiar with this law known as the Inverse Square Law, and doubtless has been taught the conditions in which the law breaks down—namely when the source is not a point and when scattering or absorption occur in the intervening medium. It will be realized from the discussion on geometric unsharpness earlier in Chapter xii (if from no other head of knowledge) that the source of radiation in an X-ray tube is *not* a point. When radiographers are concerned with X-ray beams there is generally a patient of appreciable if varying size occupying *some* of the distance through which the beam travels to reach the film; in this patient's tissue scattering and absorption occur.

It is now easy to reach the conclusion that in diagnostic radiography the law strictly is not valid. Yet radiographers assume that in the conditions of their work the Law of Inverse Squares is sound and applicable. In practice it proves to be a reasonable assumption, once again justified by the fact that it seems to work. When it is realized that the usual tube-film distance is great in comparison with the size of the source, and that the larger proportion of this distance is occupied by air and not the subject's tissue, the apparent validity of the law may be explained.

Radiographers therefore use the Law of Inverse Squares when computing alterations in exposure required by distance changes. Since intensity decreases with increase of distance, exposure must be increased to compensate for this; and at shorter distances must similarly be decreased. The exposure must be altered by a factor related to the *squares* of the distances involved.

This factor is found simply by the ratio

$$\frac{(\text{New distance})^2}{(\text{Old distance})^2} \text{ or } \frac{(\text{Old distance})^2}{(\text{New distance})^2}$$

It is easier to use this ratio if the *greater* of the two distances is placed 'on top' in the relationship. The student should take care *always* to do this and keep firmly in mind the simple fact that (i) increase in distance requires increase in exposure, decrease in distance requires decrease in exposure, and (ii) multiplication by figures greater than unity increases quantities, division by figures greater than unity decreases quantities. Then problems involving the law of inverse squares can be tackled without dismay and with success. If the new milliampereseconds value is required to be greater than the previous one, then simply multiply the old milliampereseconds by the distance ratio; if the new milliampereseconds value is required to be less than the previous one, then simply divide the old milliampereseconds by the distance ratio.

For example: *If 16 mAS give a reasonable radiograph of a chest at a focus-film distance of 4 feet, what milliampereseconds must be used if the distance is increased to 6 feet?*

The new distance is the larger of the two figures so it is put 'on top' and the distance ratio is:

$$\frac{\text{(New distance)}^2}{\text{(Old distance)}^2} = \frac{6^2}{4^2}$$

$$= \frac{36}{16}$$

The new milliampereseconds must be more than 16 mAS (since the distance has been increased), so the new value is:

$$16 \times \frac{36}{16} \text{ mAS}$$

i.e. 36 mAS

If 10 mAS give a good radiograph of the knee at a focus-film distance of 40 inches and the examination must be made in conditions which impose a distance of 30 inches, what milliampereseconds must be used?

The old distance is the larger of the two figures so it is put 'on top' and the distance ratio is:

$$\frac{\text{(Old distance)}^2}{\text{(New distance)}^2} = \frac{40^2}{30^2}$$

$$= \frac{1600}{900}$$

The new milliampereseconds must be less than 10 (since the distance has been decreased), so the new value is:

$$\frac{10}{1600/900} \text{ mAS} = 5 \cdot 6 \text{ mAS approximately}$$

It may be of help to give some correction factors for certain changes of distance and we give a few below. The arithmetic has been done to yield approximate answers, which may be easier to remember and are adequate in use. Without automation, exposure selection is not a precise procedure.

Changing distance:		Multiply mAS by:
From 30 ins. to	36 ins.	1·5
36 ins.	40 ins.	1·25
30 ins.	40 ins.	1·75
48 ins.	60 ins.	1·5
60 ins.	72 ins.	1·5
48 ins.	72 ins.	2·25

		Divide mAS by:
From 36 ins. to	30 ins.	1·5
40 ins.	36 ins.	1·25
40 ins.	30 ins.	1·75
60 ins.	48 ins.	1·5
72 ins.	60 ins.	1·5
72 ins.	48 ins.	2·25

The radiographer selects the tube-film distance for an X-ray examination with the following points in mind:

(i) Knowledge of what has been used before and of the practice in the department.

(ii) Long tube-film distance reduces geometric unsharpness and enlargement in the image.

(iii) Long tube-film distance requires greater radiation intensity from the X-ray tube to obtain adequate film density. This needs greater electrical power input which may impose the use of larger focal spots; these increase geometric unsharpness. Or it may be necessary to use longer exposure times; these increase the chance of unsharpness due to movement.

(iv) Short tube-film distance increases geometric unsharpness. Structures remote from the film are recorded less sharply than those close to the film and if a short tube-film distance is used the differential is increased. This can be useful. For example in an anteroposterior projection of the sterno-clavicular joints a short tube-film distance will 'blur out' the shadows of the upper dorsal vertebrae; in an occipitomental view of the nasal sinuses a short tube-film distance will aid dispersion of the shadows of structures in the middle and posterior fossae of the skull.

(v) Very short tube-film distances imply short tube-skin distances. Where these are less than 6 inches, repeated exposures carry risk to the patient of damage to the skin.

(vi) Where subject-film distances are very short, the tube-film distance can be decreased without the geometric unsharpness becoming objectionable.

As a general rule tube-film distances are standardized for particular examinations in a given X-ray department. For example, chests may be examined at 6 feet, nasal sinuses and extremities at 30 inches, abdominal viscera at 40 inches. This standardization is essential if satisfactory and repeatable results are to be obtained.

The Time-Interval of the Exposure

The total amount of energy received by the film depends on the intensity of radiation reaching the film and the time for which it does so. It may be worth noticing here that the time during which X radiation reaches the film and the time during which the X-ray tube is supplied with electrical energy are two separate quantities.

A four-valve full-wave rectified X-ray set may be considered. On the 50 c.p.s. supply main commonly encountered in the United Kingdom there are 100 half-waves of voltage of sinusoidal wave-form supplied to the X-ray tube in one second. This voltage varies from zero to maximum and back to zero every half-cycle or 100 times in one second, and the X-ray beam is thus being produced at voltages between zero and maximum throughout the cycle. Tube voltages which are less than about 40 kV result in radiation which is not sufficiently penetrating to reach the film; it is absorbed by the tube wall and filter, the patient's body, and other structures. The length of time during which X rays reach the film is therefore limited to those periods during the cycle when the tube voltage is high enough to produce X radiation sufficiently penetrating to arrive there. It can be seen that this is bound to be a shorter period of time than that during which the X-ray tube is supplied with electrical energy.

A 'constant potential' unit supplies the X-ray tube with a voltage that either is truly steady in value or shows a ripple from maximum voltage to some value not far below it (this being called 'constant' by courtesy or tradition). In this case the time during which X radiation reaches the film is closer to the time during which electrical energy is supplied to the X-ray tube. In a true constant potential unit the two quantities are virtually the same.

These facts are mentioned here because they explain why constant potential units give better radiation output to the film per milliamp and kilovolt in comparison with conventional full-wave sets, and allow the use of shorter exposure-times when techniques are transferred between such units. In both types of unit, however, the time during which radiation reaches the film is *proportional* to the time during which electrical energy is supplied to the tube. So from a practical point of view the exposure-time is considered to be the period of time during which the X-ray tube is energized, and the period during which radiation reaches the film is not distinguished from it.

From what has been said in the foregoing sections, the relationship between exposure-time and the other factors of exposure can be appreciated. It can be summed-up as follows.

Exposure time can be decreased when: kilovoltage is raised, milliamperage is raised, tube-film distance is shortened.

Exposure time must be increased when: kilovoltage is lowered, milliamperage is lowered, tube-film distance is increased.

In selecting an exposure-time for an X-ray examination, the radiographer's choice is affected by the following considerations.

(i) Knowledge of what has been used before, of the performance of the X-ray set in use, and of the practice of the department.

(ii) The need for adequate film density.

(iii) Assessment of the likelihood of subject movement, taking into consideration the state of the patient and the nature of the examination and the body-part involved.

(iv) The assumption that milliamperage and time are in effect interchangeable.

(v) Knowledge of the way in which alteration in kilovoltage, milliamperage and tube-film distance modifies exposure-time.

VARIABLES MODIFYING SELECTION OF EXPOSURE FACTORS

The foregoing sections have been a discussion of the way in which the exposure factors modify each other. It is clear that certain features of technique and of the subject alter their selection. The choice of exposure factors will now be considered further.

The student doubtless has realized that the selection of exposure factors in radiography is not a precise process limited by exact definitions. Certain general rules are used for guidance and certain features can be standardized in practice—for example tube-film distances, films, intensifying screens, and processing procedures. Modern methods of automation both in processing and in exposure techniques are an advance in standardization which cannot fail to aid the radiographer by making procedures more exact. The variables that must be considered, and the several quantities that must be assessed by the radiographer on an empirical basis make it almost surprising that in practice a reproducible standard of result has long been obtained.

The following factors modify exposure selection.
(i) Type of unit.
(ii) Use of filters.
(iii) Size of field.
(iv) Use of a secondary radiation grid.
(v) Use of intensifying screens.
(vi) Speed of film.
(vii) Developer and development technique.
(viii) Absorption in structures radiographed.

Type of X-ray Unit

It might be expected that if the controls of two X-ray units are set to give the same factors of milliamperage, kilovoltage, and time they would yield comparable results if the subject and other conditions of operation also are standardized. This is not necessarily so, and in practice it is not possible in transferring factors between X-ray sets to secure precisely similar results in every case. There are various explanations for this.

A distinction has been made between the performance of four-valve full-wave sets and sets in which the X-ray tube is supplied with constant potential. As explained in relation to the exposure-time, the radiation output for every kilovolt and milliamp in the tube factors is improved when the X-ray tube is energized by a voltage which is steady, and not varying in a cyclical manner from maximum to zero values. Truly constant potential should give better output than potential with a ripple, and both should be better than voltage with the waveform of conventional full-wave and half-wave sets.

So for the same values of kilovoltage and milliamperage and the same exposure-time, a constant potential unit should produce greater image density. It may be noticeable that radiographs produced by such units are somewhat flatter in contrast than those given by units in which the voltage is of sine-wave form. The long wavelengths produced by the low tube voltages of the normal cycle are eliminated from the beam, and this results in a beam of which the *average* wavelength is shorter for the same tube voltage. The beam is therefore effectively more penetrating; this levels out absorption differences in the subject resulting in lower image contrast.

Where two X-ray sets seem to be comparable (for example both may be conventional full-wave sets) there can still be differences in radiation output, although the controls are set to give the same milliamperage and kilovoltage for the X-ray tube. Control and measurement of tube voltage and tube current are not direct procedures. There are also complexities of voltage stabilization, kilovoltage compensation at different tube currents, space charge compensation for the X-ray tube, and mains resistance compensation to be arranged. It is hardly surprising that two X-ray sets with the same settings on their controls and meters do not operate with precisely identical values in milliamperage and kilovoltage and precisely identical waveforms. In practice it is not essential that they should. It is much more important for one X-ray set to operate consistently at different tube loads, so that the radiographer may manipulate exposure factors over the full range available from the controls and obtain consistent results.

The Use of Filters

A modern X-ray tube is constructed as a glass insert in a ray-proof metal housing. The insert is smaller than its housing, the space between them being filled with oil both for insulation and for cooling. The X-ray beam coming from the focal spot of the tube therefore penetrates the glass envelope of the insert, the oil surround, and the port of the housing. These materials act as a filter on the beam, removing some of the components of longer wavelength. The total effect is described as the inherent filtration of the X-ray tube.

Current codes of practice require the permanent total filtration of the X-ray tube to be the equivalent of 1 to 2 mm of aluminium. This can be achieved by adding an additional aluminium filter to the X-ray tube so that the combined effect of this filter plus the filtering action of the tube materials is equivalent to 1 to 2 mm of aluminium. Tubes are provided with this level of filtration at the time of installation.

The reason for this requirement is that such filtration removes from the X-ray beam the long wavelengths which will be absorbed by the patient's superficial tissues. They do not contribute to the radiographic image of the parts examined, for they are insufficiently penetrating to reach the film, and their sole achievement is to provide the patient with a dose of unnecessary radiation.

Since radiation being removed from the beam could not reach the film through the patient, the use of such filtration requires no alteration in exposure factors and may be disregarded in selecting them. In some cases, however, there is an appreciable difference to be detected in the *appearance* of radiographs taken with such filtered beams; this is noticeable particularly in the case of extremities radiographed on direct-exposure film. The contrast of the image appears to be less and the radiograph seems much 'flatter'. This may be due less to any reduction in contrast within the image itself as to the fact that the background to the image is greyer in tone. If the soft radiation which the filter removes is left in the beam it can reach those parts of the film not covered by the patient. Being absorbed by the emulsion it serves to enhance the blackness of the surround.

Additional filters, or filters of materials such as copper or iron, may sometimes be added to diagnostic tubes as a special practice. When such filters appreciably reduce the radiation output of the tube to the film they must be taken into account in selecting exposure factors. The increase required will depend on the characteristics of a particular filter and its attenuating action on the beam.

Special filters are sometimes used to solve the problem of subjects which show great differences in radio-opacity—for example the dorsal spine in an anteroposterior projection, and the pregnant abdomen in a lateral projection. In these cases a filter might be used which is wedge-shaped, being thin over those parts of the subject which are thick and thick over those parts of the subject which are thin. Inserted into the X-ray tube or placed between the patient and the film, the filter *plus* the subject ensure a more even absorption of the beam. Exposure factors are then selected with the thick parts of the subject in mind.

Size of Field

Modern X-ray units are invariably equipped with beam-limiting devices in the form of multi-plane or double-leaf diaphragms. Also provided are radio-opaque cones which can be fitted additionally to the tube-head, giving another means of limiting the beam. The use of these is to define the area of irradiated tissue, thus reducing both dose to the patient and the production of scattered radiation.

This reduction in scatter improves the contrast of the image but at the same time lessens its density since less radiation is reaching the film. When a very small field of irradiation is used it is necessary to increase the milliampereseconds factor in the exposure by some amount. The amount required will depend on the restriction of the field and must be determined empirically for the size of diaphragm or cone in use for a

23

particular examination. It may vary from an increase of 25–30 per cent to some much higher value.

The Use of a Secondary Radiation Grid

The functions of a secondary radiation grid are to transmit primary radiation which forms the image on the film, and to absorb scattered radiation which impairs the definition of the image. The efficiency with which a grid performs the first function is known as its transmission efficiency, and its degree of achievement in regard to the second is known as its screening efficiency. The two functions show incompatibility, and a grid with high screening efficiency has less transmission efficiency. When a grid is used exposure factors must be increased, since both functions result in less radiation reaching the film.

The exact increase required depends on the characteristics of the grid being used, the amount of both primary and secondary radiation which it removes, and the kilovoltage range being employed. It is therefore impossible to give precise figures for adapting exposure techniques to the use of grids. In practice radiographers work by somewhat general rules, without making use of detailed information on the characteristics of the grids in their departments.

As a practical procedure, exposures would be increased by a factor of approximately 3 for a stationary grid; and by factors of approximately 3 to 4 for a moving grid of 6–1 or 8–1 ratio. The change in the exposure factors can be made by increasing the milliampereseconds, or by increasing the kilovoltage, or by a smaller increase in both. Very high ratio grids with high screening but reduced transmission efficiency require a greater increase in exposure. High ratio grids are used only with high kilovoltage techniques which involve special selection of factors and make the use of a grid essential in most cases. In these techniques it is unlikely that radiographers will be required to make comparisons between exposures with and without grids.

The Use of Intensifying Screens

Intensifying screens and the difficulties in expressing a factor of intensification as a single absolute value have already been discussed in Chapter v. In practice radiographers are most often concerned with comparing the relative performances of different screens in use in their departments. In doing this they do not undertake any very exact tests, and rely mainly on a simple visual comparison of radiographic results, together with some information from the manufacturer. The radiographs under inspection may be test films made with a step-wedge, or they may be clinical radiographs in examination of a patient. In any case the conclusions reached on the necessary modifications to exposure are neither exact nor inflexible. Some such statement as this might be made: *The new screens are probably about twice as fast as the old, so we can divide the milliampereseconds by 2.* With other conditions of exposure the same, the use of faster screens reduces the milliampereseconds required.

Speed of Film

It is doubtless clear to the student by now that the speed of the film used must alter the selection of exposure factors. Faster materials require less exposure to produce the same film density. The advantages in using them are that shorter exposure-times can be employed, better radiographic results can be obtained with X-ray sets of low output, and a smaller dose is given to the patient. As explained in Chapter iii, the speed of X-ray films is not stated as an absolute value, and in the selection of exposure factors the speed of the film does not appear as a precise quantity.

When using a new X-ray film, the radiographer, aided by information from the manufacturer, compares it with another film the performance of which is already known. For example, it may be said that the new film is twice as fast as the old one; or perhaps that the exposures can be reduced by one-third for the new film. The radiographer then understands that in the first case the milliampereseconds value may be reduced to one-half of that used for a comparable examination with the old film; and in the second case that the milliampereseconds required are two-thirds of the value previously used.

Comparison in performance between the two films may be made by exposures with a step-wedge or based on clinical radiographs. In either case these are usually visual assessments without exact measurements and the required modifications to exposure factors are judged in this way.

Films which differ in speed often differ also in contrast, so that it may be impossible to secure with material of two different speeds results which are exactly comparable. The object of the radiographer's assessment is therefore not so much to decide whether two radiographs are identical, but to determine whether the one made on new film with the new exposure is approximately comparable with the old, and is acceptable in the quality of its image.

Developer and Development Technique

The effective speed of a film material (as well as its contrast) can be altered by the composition of a developing solution and by the technique of development in use. The effect of development time on the characteristic curve of an emulsion was mentioned in Chapter III, processing factors in the contrast of the image were discussed in Chapter XII, and developers and their use were considered more fully in Chapter VI. Here it may be sufficient to sum up the situation with some general statements, and say simply that important factors are: the constitution of the developer and the activity of the developing agents in it, the degree of exhaustion of the solution, the temperature of the solution, the development time, and with some films the amount of agitation given during immersion in the developer.

Since there are so many variables here which alter both speed and contrast, the radiographer would find it quite impossible to select exposure factors in relation to them if they were not standardized as far as possible. In departmental practice features such as the constitution of the developer, its replenishment against exhaustion, the temperature of the solution, and the development time are (or should be) standardized.

In manual processing the amount of agitation cannot be standardized and is usually inadequate. The benefits of automation include complete standardization in agitation, temperature, time, and replenishment. It is found that the installation of automatic processing and the development techniques it imposes may result in an increase in the effective speed of the film material used. It is then possible to decrease exposure factors in use throughout the department.

Adjusting film density by some prolongation of development time in cases of a degree of underexposure, and shortening development time in cases of some degree of overexposure is impossible with automation. This makes selection of exposure factors more critical. In practice, however, the certainty of really standardized processing is not a hindrance but an aid to the radiographer. Any dismay at the reduced margin of error in the X-ray room is usually expressed only by those who have yet to enjoy the benefits of automation.

Absorption in Structures Radiographed

Exposure factors are selected to obtain a good radiographic record of structures under examination. The choice of factors must clearly be modified by the structures themselves, and also by the presence of extraneous materials such as splints and dressings of varying radio-opacity; these may vary from plaster of Paris which is moderately radio-opaque to aluminium or wood which are virtually radioparent.

No attempt will be made here to suggest specific exposure factors for given examinations. This is never an entirely satisfactory process. In any case the student obtains knowledge and practice in the selection of factors through experience in the X-ray department; this is more useful than anything written here.

It is already clear that a considerable number of variables modify exposure selection, and by no means the least of these are variations within the subject. Human tissues absorb an X-ray beam to different extents, matter which has high atomic number absorbing it most heavily. The absorption that takes place depends not only upon the nature of the tissue which is traversed but also upon the wavelength or energy of the X-ray beam, beams of short wavelength and high energy being absorbed less heavily than those of long wavelength and low energy.

In human subjects bone, muscle, fat, and air are all found, and show descending degree of radio-opacity, normal bone absorbing radiation to a marked extent, and air showing virtually no absorption. Different structures therefore need different exposure factors (that is different radiation dose) if a radiograph of adequate density, penetration, and contrast is to be obtained.

Where body parts are of the same composition, thick parts absorb more radiation than thin ones and require more exposure (more milliampere-seconds and/or kilovoltage). Assessment of thickness alone, however, is not an entirely reliable guide; for example two patients whose trunks appear to be relatively similar in thickness may indeed be very different in radio-opacity. One man may have several inches of fat on his torso, and another man several inches of well-developed muscle, the muscular subject requiring greater penetration. Two people of the same weight can be very different subjects radiographically—one may be a healthily developed child, the other a frail old woman in whom age has atrophied muscle and decalcified bone so that little penetration is needed. Even the same subject at different times can show variation. When John Smith is brought into the accident department with a fractured tibia which he has just acquired on the sports field, the structures of his leg absorb radiation much more heavily than they do some weeks later when disuse has atrophied muscle and made the bone osteoporotic. In choosing exposure factors the radiographer applies knowledge of the nature of bodily structures and of disease processes, as well as an understanding of the radiation physics concerned with the absorption of X-ray beams.

CHAPTER XIV

The Presentation of the Radiograph

Correct presentation of the radiograph is an important part of the radiographer's responsibilities, though this is not always apparent to the new student. In the more immediate issues of obtaining correct radiographic positioning and determining acceptable exposure factors we should not lose sight of certain features which can affect the ultimate value of the radiograph to those who use it. What are these features? What is required in a radiograph in addition to an adequate demonstration of the part examined?

Very simply the answer is *identification*. Any radiograph whatsoever should have included on it, preferably in indelible form, the following information.

(1) The subject's name and/or record number. If the name alone is used, the surname is insufficient; initials or a first name should also appear.

(2) The date on which the radiograph was taken.

(3) A correct sign of the right or left side of the subject.

(4) If the film is one of a sequence, proper indication of its position in the series; for example, 'control exposure', 'post-micturition', '10-min. after injection' and so on.

To this it is sometimes thought desirable to add:

(5) the patient's date of birth.

The provision of this information is properly a charge on the radiographer, for clearly the person who takes the film is best able to relate it accurately to the part examined, the time or interval of the examination and the identity of the subject. Consequently errors are unlikely to occur if the radiographer in practice and at the time of the film's exposure can record on it its correct identification.

This is not possible with the marking systems in use in many departments. Nonetheless, the theoretical responsibility remains and the radiographer who will not in fact actually mark the films as they are taken has an indisputable duty to ensure that whoever does mark them has accurate legible data from which to work. One scribbled label accompanying 3 or

4 cassettes into the darkroom is not an adequate discharge of this responsibility. It constitutes an open invitation to error, particularly when another group of cassettes similarly treated arrives simultaneously on the darkroom bench.

To facilitate the proper identification of films a number of systems and devices are generally available.

OPAQUE LETTERS AND LEGENDS

These permit the radiograph to be marked by means of the X-ray exposure itself. The letters or numerals may be themselves radio-opaque; that is they may be separate lead characters and used to make up any appropriate signal, or they may be painted in lead on Perspex plaques available either individually or already composed into useful legends; for example 'erect', 'supine'. Alternatively the letters or figures may be radioparent on an opaque base, that is, they are incised on a metal square or strip and thus provide dark characters on a clear ground. Some examples of these varieties are shown in Fig. 14.1.

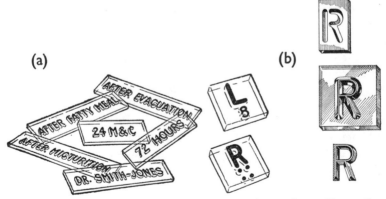

Fig. 14.1. (a) Radio-opaque legends and letters for use in marking radiographs. These are engraved on a Perspex base and filled with a radio-opaque material. The small character seen under the L and the group of dots under the R are to identify the radiographer. *By courtesy of Cuthbert Andrews.*

(b) Markers for radiographs.
      Upper: The letter is incised in a thin piece of metal.
      Centre: The letter is lead, mounted in a Perspex plaque.
      Lower: Single lead character.
By courtesy of Watson and Sons (Electro-Medical) Ltd.

In the case of individual characters it is usual to provide two or three small metal frames in which the letters or numerals can be contained. These frames or holders may be suitable for clipping to the edge of a cassette held vertically and for lying flat on the surface of a cassette or direct-exposure film.

Prepared legends of the kind described and the letters R and L for anatomical recognition are useful when correctly employed. They should be fastened to the cassette with adhesive tape before making the X-ray exposure, attention being given to the following points.

(1) The character or legend should not be placed in a position where it may obscure a feature of diagnostic importance.

(2) If the irradiated field is limited by a cone or collimator to an area appreciably smaller than the dimensions of the cassette, it is useless to place a radiographic marker close to the borders of the latter as it will receive no X-ray exposure and will consequently fail to appear on the film.

It is appreciated that these two considerations tend to be mutually opposed. In order to avoid the possibility of obscuring some significant area of the radiograph it is sensible to place these markers at one edge of the cassette. As a general rule this is correct procedure.

In order to avoid the circumstances described in (2) above, it is theoretically possible to give the area of the cassette which contains the marker a separate X-ray exposure if cover is first provided for the original radiographic field. However, this would appear scarcely a practical course in a busy department. It requires extra time in the use of the unit and, even though appropriate adjustment of factors should be made to give just a slight 'flash' exposure, the system decreases the life expectancy of the X-ray tube.

A better practice no doubt is to use smaller characters for marking the film and to place these with care. Fig. 14.2 shows a typical anatomical marker such as is used by many radiographers.

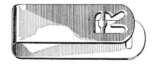

FIG. 14.2. Anatomical marker suitable for placing over the edge of a cassette to record on the film either the R or the L. It can be used in either vertical or horizontal positions. *By courtesy of Watson and Sons (Electro-Medical) Ltd.*

The clip form is generally convenient, particularly when films are taken with the cassette vertically placed. The letters are ½ in. by ⅜ in. and the dimensions of the clip such that on most cassettes the R or L appears within a couple of inches of the film's edge.

However, for say an occipitomental view of the nasal sinuses taken with a localizing cone on an 8 × 10 in. cassette, this type of marker is unreliable. It is sometimes visible, for example if the film is badly centred in relation to the patient or from the effects of secondary radiation, but in many cases the letter is not easy to read or is not apparent. Plate 14.1, following p. 206, shows how a smaller single character may be used to better advantage in these circumstances. Its dimensions are 0·8 in. by 0·4 in. Thought must be given to its position in order to avoid over-shadowing of important structures; indeed it is true that any marking system needs to be used intelligently.

Anterior Projections

The marking of any film for which the anterior aspect of the patient faced the cassette may require special attention. It is usual to present radiographs for report in the correct anatomical position; that is, the subject's left is on the observer's right, and conversely. This means that in the case of posteroanterior or anterior oblique projections the observer must read the film from the aspect which faced *away* from the X-ray tube during the exposure. If opaque legends of the type described are positioned on the cassette so that they are legible to the radiographer from the tube aspect—and this after all is the natural tendency—then they will not be readable by whoever must report on them, unless the film is first removed from the illuminator and the legend examined from the other side. To avoid this the radiographer should remember to reverse letters and numerals before fastening them to the cassette for any anterior projection.

Markers of the kind shown in Fig. 14.2 are generally available as A.P. or P.A. in type. In the latter the R and L are cut out as a mirror image and are intended to be used for anterior projections in order to avoid the difficulty described above. However, it is well to remember that there are certain disadvantages in having both types in circulation in the department.

So long as only one kind is available there can never be any doubt of the tube aspect of a film and sometimes certainty on this point is needed and indeed of crucial importance. As shown in Fig. 14.2, the tube aspect is bound to be that one from which the R and L is normally readable. In many departments it is felt that certainty of this kind outweighs the slight disadvantage of viewing the letter as a mirror image on anterior projections. The minor difficulty in vision is certainly not of a nature to create confusion between the right and left sides. It must be admitted that in any case the availability of both types of marker does not necessarily ensure their correct use and so entirely preclude the necessity of reading the letter in reverse from time to time. A radiographer in a hurry may fail to observe the type of marker employed, or having second thoughts of the plan of technique—perhaps in the case of a patient who has multiple injuries—may easily forget to alter the marker to match it. In these circumstances the observer may be in considerable doubt over the correct film aspect and the determination of the right and left sides.

PERFORATING DEVICES

Films, and indeed other records, may be perforated with letters or figures as a means of identification. Machines for doing this are available. A simple pliers type may be used for 1 to 3 letters. More elaborate presses cover a larger range of letters and may be suitable for including the date and the hospital's name.

Compared with other marking systems this method appears not very useful. Obviously most applicable when a large number of radiographs has to be marked with the same legend (such as the date or the hospital's identity), the necessity to change letters frequently makes these perforating devices quite unsuitable for names, even in a department which might not be considered very busy. They are most likely to be used on the processed film and the possibility of error in a patient's identity is thus a further disadvantage.

Rather more handy and reliable is a machine which perforates a lead strip which can be taped by the radiographer to the cassette before exposure. Letters are selected by turning a handle to the required character and pressing it down. The machine will cut the strip on completing the desired word. In this way not only the patient's name or number can be composed but other useful data, such as 'left', 'right', 'prone'. Strips of the latter kind can be used many times before they are discarded.

ACTINIC MARKERS

The use of individual, opaque or other characters to build the patient's name and possibly the date as well and thus record these on his radiograph is a procedure often too time-consuming in many X-ray departments. In some specialized examinations it may be an applicable method.

For example, such an arrangement might be placed in the exposure area of a rapid film or cassette changer and the information would then be automatically recorded on all films in that patient's series. In this type of case the time required to compose the name and position it suitably on the apparatus is very small in relation to the demands of the whole procedure. Not only does this ratio make the system worthwhile but time is likely to be saved at a later stage if the large batches of films which are often associated with the use of such changers are already correctly identified when they leave the unit.

There is the possibility of marking radiographs by a method which requires no specialized accessories of any kind. In view of other considerations however its simplicity does not constitute a recommendation for it. It involves the procedure first of writing on the films in the darkroom with an ordinary lead pencil and subsequently, when the radiograph is processed and dry, of transcribing this information in white ink or with a coloured 'Chinagraph' or 'Stabilo' pencil. These media are more easily recognizable than are ordinarily pencilled characters, though not necessarily much more durable. No doubt the disadvantages of the system are obvious.

(1) It does not provide permanent identification.

(2) While simple, it is also wasteful of time. The same information must be written on each film twice altogether and indeed in a busy department the sorting of radiographs and the transcribing process may occupy one person for several hours a day. This factor makes it totally unsuitable for automatic systems of processing.

(3) It does not provide necessarily a clear legend, though some may find advantageous the facility of being able to read this by incident as opposed to transmitted light.

(4) The system offers greater likelihood of error since it usually increases the number of people concerned with the marking of any one radiograph.

In view of these considerations systems of radiographic identification most commonly employed at the present time depend on the application of one or another form of actinic marker. This apparatus implies the use of some form of actinic radiation as the means of reproducing on the radiograph a written or printed legend. The radiation may be light or it may be X rays, depending on the equipment concerned, but in the latter

case it should be noted that the radiation source is not the diagnostic
X-ray tube nor is the exposure made simultaneously with the original
radiographic one.

All actinic markers possess in general those advantages which are the
converse of the points noted above; that is, if properly used, each—
(1) provides permanent identification;
(2) is economical of time;
(3) shows information neatly and uniformly;
(4) reduces the likelihood of error.

Actinic markers require some part of the film, usually a rectangular
strip along one edge, to be protected from X rays during the normal
radiographic exposure. This is in order to have in an established position
on every film an area of unchanged silver halide suitable for receiving
the exposure from the marker. Methods of accomplishing this will be
considered in a later section.

Photographic Markers

Photographic markers are those in which light is the operative actinic
radiation. A typical example is shown in Plate 14.2, following p. 206,
and is similar in principle to a photographer's printing box. If desired
it can be sunk in the top of the darkroom bench so that the top of the
marker is at a continuous level with the working surface.

The details to be recorded, that is the patient's name and number, the
date and other significant information, are first written or preferably
typed on a thin sheet of paper, small enough to occupy the window of the
box (about 2·5 × 0·8 in.) and thin enough to be translucent to light. The
model shown in Plate 14.2 has a magnetic bar which holds the titling
paper in position over the window and the window itself is illuminated
by a safelamp within. These are clearly useful refinements which give the
operator greater certainty and thus save time on the procedure.

The undeveloped radiograph is placed on the marker between the
guides so that the protected area of the emulsion lies over the window.
The spring pressure pad is then pressed down and this automatically
illuminates suitable lamps within the box. The light from these reaches
the film through the slip of translucent paper, thus recording on the emulsion any information it contains; the legend will appear white on a dark
ground.

In principle the device is admirably simple. In practice certain other
features are desirable if the marker is to be fully efficient. These are concerned with the production of a consistent density of background in order

to obtain on every radiograph a level of contrast which permits the legend to be easily read by the transmitted light of a standard X-ray illuminator. Variation of this background density obviously will occur with—
(a) variation of the light intensity due to fluctuations in the electrical supply;
(b) variations in emulsion speed of the film to be marked;
(c) variations in processing.
These effects may be such as to make the legend virtually unreadable because the ground is either too faint or too dark.

In order to eliminate the possibility of variations occurring under (a) above, good photographic markers of this simple type should operate from the discharge of a condenser, the condenser itself being fed from a stabilized supply provided by a neon valve within the unit. A few seconds are required to charge the condenser prior to every operation but this interval normally occurs in the usual procedure of unloading cassettes and is not noticed by the technician.

Most photographic markers incorporate a control which is adjustable to meet any alteration in film speed. Non-screen emulsions require exposure to an increased intensity of light and usually there is a specific setting on the marker for these. Equally the trial introduction in any given department of a screen-type film faster than that habitually employed could create difficulties if the marker had no means of reducing the light intensity, nor indeed would it be suitable for supply to a wide range of users. In some cases the potentiometer which provides this flexibility is freely available to the operator. In others it is intended for adjustment by the manufacturer's technician or engineer, either at the time of installation or on any subsequent request.

Variations in processing are not the responsibility of those who manufacture actinic film markers and of course do not normally occur in those departments where automatic systems are employed. However, one type of marker includes in the legend what is called a density reference. This is a small rectangle which will not alter in tone so long as processing is consistent. Its function is detective rather than prophylactic; it does not prevent the occurrence of these density variations but may reveal their source when they are noticed to be present.

The legibility of the information depends both on the background density and the difference between this and the lettering. Ideally, then, the latter should be recorded on the film as an area of no density at all. To this end it is important that the original writing or typing should be adequately black. The use of a ball-point pen is preferable to pencil. An ordinary sheet of carbon paper placed so that its active surface is in contact with the *back* of the titling paper can be used to enhance the opacity of the characters to transmitted light. A black fibre tip pen is helpful, too.

In another photographic marker of this kind the required information is written on a special carbon stencil with an empty ball-point pen, preferably upon a hard surface. On the radiograph the legend then appears black on a white ground, since the carbon is opaque to light except where its surface is incised by the style. It is a matter of opinion which form is easier to read.

Photographic markers of the kind so far described operate on a direct printing system, similar to the making of contact prints from any photographic negative. Another type uses a more elaborate method; it photographs, rather than photographically prints the information given.

An opaque card is used instead of a thin sheet of paper and this is placed against a guide, face downwards, on the window of the marker, with the undeveloped radiograph not on top of it but beside it. The card is illuminated from below, as opposed to transilluminated, and its image projected through 180 deg. on to the film. This is done, as shown in Fig.

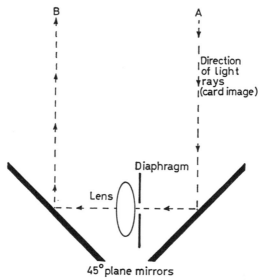

Fig. 14.3. Sketch to illustrate the operation of a photographic marker. The image from a card situated at A is transferred to a radiograph placed alongside the card at B. Control of exposure is obtained by varying the aperture of the diaphragm; this varies the amount of light passing through the lens.

14.3 by means of two aluminized mirrors each of which reflects the light through 90 deg. Between the two mirrors is a lens and a diaphragm.

Essentially this marker operates as a camera and perhaps an advantage of the principle is that the photographed image may be smaller than the original card; an area 3·5 in. × 1·12 in. is copied as a rectangle 2·4 in. × 0·8 in. This allows the original to be written more boldly or to have greater content relative to a direct printing device producing a legend of equivalent size.

Like the first one, this marker copies the data in white characters on a black ground. It is operated by a foot switch, has a safelamp illuminating the working area and an exposure control for different speeds of emulsion. This control—and we may note again its analogy with the mechanisms of a camera (Chapter XVI)—takes the form of variation of the diaphragm aperture and not directly of the exposure's duration which is fixed at 0·1 sec. for filament lamps and 0·001 sec. for flash tubes. The diaphragm is mechanically coupled to an illuminated scale which is at a level of brightness safe for reading in the darkroom. Inevitably this unit is quite a large piece of apparatus; indeed it requires in the darkroom as much space as a small table. It is illustrated in Plate 14.3, following p. 206.

Radiographic Markers

Radiographic markers are those in which the identification is recorded on each film by means of X rays. This is an efficient system which copies data neatly and clearly in black on a white ground. However, the apparatus required is more elaborate and consequently appreciably more expensive than any photographic marker. It consists of (1) the marking unit, (2) a machine for indenting the marker plates, (3) suitable metal plates on which the patient's name and other information will be embossed.

THE MARKING UNIT

The external appearance of the unit is shown in Plate 14.4, following p. 206.

It is about 3 ft. high and approximately a foot square, and is fully sealed against radiation leakage. A normal 13 amp., 220 volt A.C. mains supply is suitable for the operation of the X-ray tube which is similar to that found in clinical use in dental units. It has a focus of 0·8 mm and passes a current of 7 mA at a tension of 50 kVp.

To use it the operator fits the appropriate marker plates into a holder on the top panel of the unit, places the cassette face downwards against locating stops in relation to the window and then closes the lid. The latter action triggers the circuit supplying the X-ray tube which can be energized only by this means. The unit includes a timer which gives a choice of 4 pre-set exposure-intervals in order to provide for differences in the speed of non-screen and screen film and of various film-screen combinations.

THE EMBOSSING MACHINE

This is a modified standard addressing machine which will indent a metal plate with letters and figures as the user selects them. It may be operated by hand or electrically if the volume of work justifies the higher expense.

On the simpler type of unit, characters are selected by changing the position of a pointer on a marked dial; then operation of a hand lever embosses the letter on a blank plate placed in the holder of the machine. Forward movement of the plate carriage is obtained by depression of a button switch.

In the electric apparatus the embossing dies are located on a type drum which can rotate in either direction. The unit has the keyboard of a conventional typewriter and on slight depression of the appropriate key the selected character is automatically moved to the embossing position by rotation of the drum along the shortest route. The embossing action is automatic, as also is the subsequent movement of the plate holder into position for the next letter. In the event of a 'typing' error it is fortunately possible to back-space the carriage and alter the character without ill-effect. This apparatus is highly specialized, appreciably faster than a hand-operated machine and of course more expensive. It also occupies a fair amount of space. As it can cope with standard addressing work it might be used in a large hospital to serve other departments than radiology and this would make it a more economic proposition.

THE MARKING PLATES

These are of steel, coated with lead. They measure 3·5 in. × 0·94 in. Once a plate has been prepared with the patient's name and number it can be used indefinitely for any number of examinations at subsequent attendances. The date is usually recorded on a separate plate made out each day and this can include the hospital's name if desired. Transient information relating to a particular radiograph in a series, for example '10 min. I.V.P.', is better printed on the film by means of the prepared legends already described, in order to allow the name plate to remain valid for all X-ray examinations. Being robust, the marker plates are easy to handle and to file in small drawers.

A radiographic marker has the advantage that no darkroom is required for its operation. Consequently it is possible to place such a marker in every X-ray room or in a position in corridor or hallway where it may conveniently serve more than one room. Only one indenting machine is required for any number of markers. The plate can be embossed at some central point and can accompany the patient to the X-ray room clipped to his request form with any other documents normal to the department's record-keeping system. Immediately on conclusion of the examination it is the radiographer's responsibility to mark the films before the cassettes leave the room or its vicinity. Clearly this system almost excludes the possibility of errors in identification.

Photographic markers can be used under similar control by the radiographer if space in the X-ray room is given to the construction of a light-tight cubicle in which cassettes can be unloaded, the films marked and afterwards dispatched to the processing room in groups in some suitable container. In addition to the avoidance of error in identification, the system has peripheral advantages. These are as follows.

(1) Decentralized and therefore more practical responsibility for the condition of intensifying screens.

(2) Reduced wear of cassettes.

(3) Improved exposure selection which must result from associating with a particular X-ray unit only a restricted group of film-screen combinations.

Masking the Identification Area

The employment of any kind of actinic marker necessitates the provision on every film of a clear area which does not receive radiation during the radiographic exposure. This is achieved by the use of a thin lead mask which is mounted in relation to the front intensifying screen in the same position on every cassette. It corresponds in size to the window of the actinic marker and is situated where it is unlikely to obscure any radiographic detail of value, often for example in the top or lower right corner.

It is commonly advised that the film be protected from any fluorescence of the back screen as well, by means of either a twin lead strip or opaque adhesive tape. However, the practice is certainly not essential.

It is feasible to mount the principal lead strip on the front of the cassette. This gives clear indication to the user of its position; necessary

24

information if the identification is to appear always in the same position on the radiograph and not reversed top to bottom so that the lettering appears upside down to the observer.

However, better than external mounting of the strip is to place it within the cassette as it is then protected from the wear and tear of daily handling. The outside of the cassette can easily be marked in another way to show the situation of the mask, for example by the use of a coloured label or tape which is readily replaceable when worn. If the lead strip is placed within the cassette it is important that an appropriate portion of the front intensifying screen be cut away to receive it. Should it be fastened simply *on* and not *flush* with the screen surface, thin though the mask is, it will impair the contact of the screens and spoil radiographic definition.

Excision of a suitable area from the front intensifying screen—and from the back one as well if two lead masks are to be employed—can be undertaken with a sharp knife or perhaps a scalpel. It is not very easy work and needs care. The use of a template to locate the strip accurately is a great help. Without such an aid, lack of precision in measurements may result in the protected area failing to register with the aperture of the marker. At best this gives the radiograph an untidy appearance and at worst it may result in the loss of information.

The statement is sometimes made that the use of a lead mask is unnecessary. The rationale of this is that in the exposure of screen film very little activation of the emulsion occurs from the action of X rays; nearly all of it is effected by light. Significant protection of the film can be obtained simply by masking it from the fluorescence of both intensifying screens, usually by means of opaque plastic tape. This undoubtedly simplifies preparation of the cassettes but is bound to diminish the contrast and thus the legibility of the printed legend ultimately obtained. However, it may not be unacceptable. At present some manufacturers of intensifying screens will supply their products with a lead mask already in place on each of the paired screens. The position of the masks is specified by the customer at the time of ordering and their dimensions are appropriate for use with the majority of commercially available actinic markers.

Non-screen film must be effectively masked against X radiation. In this case a lead strip is placed directly on the appropriate edge of the film by the radiographer before making the exposure. Some exposure holders have a lead blocker already in position.

Anterior Projections

Reference was made in an earlier section to the mirror-imaging of printed information which occurs when an observer views anterior projections from their correct anatomical aspect. This is true of actinic markers as of others.

The effect can be avoided in most equipment if the titling paper or plate is reversed right to left in the window of the unit before marking posteroanterior or anterior oblique projections. This is not applicable to a marker of the kind described on pp. 316–317 which operates by reflected as opposed to transmitted light. In any case it may well be preferred to identify radiographs always by the same procedure, particularly if this operation is performed in the darkroom by technical rather than radiographic staff. Errors are less likely and a firm indication of the film's tube aspect is always present.

IDENTIFICATION OF DENTAL FILMS

The presentation of dental films requires special notice since these should not be marked directly with pencil or by any other means. For convenience of handling they are usually prepared for diagnosis by mounting the series relevant to the examination of a particular patient on a cut-out card or a translucent plastic sheet. The films should be arranged anatomically in accordance with the dental formula given below, with which no doubt the student is already familiar.

$$
\begin{array}{c}
\text{Upper} \\
R \quad \dfrac{8-1 \quad | \quad 1-8}{8-1 \quad | \quad 1-8} \quad L \\
\text{Lower}
\end{array}
$$

When the radiographs are placed in this way the observer is looking at the dental images as he would look at the teeth themselves, that is from their outer or buccal aspect. This aspect is also the tube aspect of each film.

Dental films are stamped with a circular embossment in one corner. This is convex on the surface which faces the X-ray tube during the exposure and consequently these radiographs should be fixed in their mount so that the 'pip' is towards the operator. It is usual when making dental X-ray examinations to insert the film in the mouth so that the embossed corner is coronal in direction rather than apical; and as each is taken to place it on the appropriate clip of the developing hanger in the correct anatomical position with the embossed projection facing the radiographer. This order should be maintained in the darkroom during processing.

If this technique is observed subsequent preparation of the films is a simple process of transferring each to a similar situation on the mount. However, if they should have become disordered it is not difficult to identify the upper and lower jaws if it is remembered that in respect of the lower jaw:

(1) the bone trabeculae make a horizontal pattern;

(2) usually the shadow of the mandibular canal can be seen;

(3) the molars have two roots.

In radiographs of the upper jaw the following evidence may be sought:

(1) air-filled cavities, due to the nasal translucency in the central incisor region and the maxillary antrum in relation to the distal teeth;

(2) triple roots to the molars.

Dental Mounts

These are frequently of the slide-in type similar in principle to some photographic mounts. Films can be slipped into position behind apertures of an appropriate size in a rigid card. These cards are available in a number of formats which hold from 1 to 14 dental films arranged in the main horizontally; some of the apertures may have the long axis vertical to conform with common radiographic practice in examining upper incisor and canine teeth with films so placed. Space is available on the mount for completion with the patient's name, the date and perhaps other details such as his hospital number and the name of the referring consultant.

Another type of mount is a plain, thin sheet of cellulose acetate, one surface being matt and the reverse aspect glossy. Held up to any source of light, for example even the window of a dental surgery, it transmits a diffuse regular illumination such as would a piece of ground glass. These sheets are available in sizes suitable for containing either one or two dental films or a number sufficient for examination of the whole mouth. Alternatively the material can be purchased in greater area—25 × 28 in.— and cut as the user requires.

Radiographs can be fixed in position on this mount by means of an ordinary manuscript stapler. However, this method is not ideal since it may be difficult to put the staples where none will obscure radiographic detail. A better device is a special dental mount cutter.

This little machine has a cutting head under which the cellulose acetate sheet is placed. On depression of the operating lever, four semi-circular incisions are made. These are appropriately spaced so that the corners of a standard sized dental film can be inserted through them and the film thus maintained in any desired position on the front of the mount; the pages of a photographic album are often similarly ordered to accept a standard size of print. The cutting head can be rotated to allow the format of the radiograph to be either vertical or horizontal. The patient's name and other details can be written easily with a lead or 'Stabilo' pencil or a ball-point pen on the matt surface of the mount.

PREPARATION OF STEREORADIOGRAPHS

Radiographs which are taken as a stereoscopic pair present special problems of identification, mounting and viewing, particularly as there is no standard practice in regard to their marking and there are current several methods of viewing these films.

The theory and technique of stereoradiography are not properly within the scope of this book but a simple re-statement of principle may be useful to the student at this point. Our normal, three-dimensional vision depends on the fact that the retina of each eye has a slightly different viewpoint of any object at which we look. In stereoradiography a pair of radiographs is taken. These are identical to each other in all features —and this must include factors of speed and processing—except that between the two exposures the X-ray tube is moved under conditions which make its focal spot correspond in turn to each eye of an observer looking directly at the patient. These films are then viewed simultaneously in the following way.

(a) The right eye looks only at the radiograph taken when the tube was shifted in a direction which is defined as the right.

(b) The left eye looks only at the radiograph taken when the tube was shifted in a direction which is defined as the left.

The two images become fused in a single impression which appears to the observer to be three-dimensional. He has an awareness of depth and 'reality' in the appearances recorded, which enables him to differentiate the levels of structures otherwise superimposed on a plain radiograph. Stereoradiographs are necessarily viewed under particular conditions, often by means of special equipment. In their correct presentation for radiological report we must consider first how properly each of the pair of films is to be identified, and secondly how they should be mounted and viewed together.

Marking Stereoradiographs

In addition to the customary identification of the patient, a stereo-radiograph preferably should carry two markers. One of these must indicate the anatomical right and left while the other refers to the right or left shift of the X-ray tube: this specifies equally the eye with which the film is meant to be viewed; it is erroneous to believe that the designation is equated with the patient's right and left. All confusion will be avoided if the second of these markers in fact is a complete legend and states 'R stereo' or 'L stereo'.

Where such legends are not available, the radiographer may adhere to the convention that the first letter on the radiograph is anatomical in reference and the second visual. Thus, a left shoulder taken with a right shift of the tube should carry the letters LR in the upper right corner; the film which resulted from the left shift would be marked LL in the same place.

If only one marker is available it can be used to perform both functions. That is to say, the letter R is used for the right tube shift and placed on the right of the patient; it is then changed for the letter L which is put on the patient's left during the exposure from the left shift of the tube. This is satisfactory when the examination relates to the trunk and head, but should it be of a limb the system must result in one of the pair of films being unmarked. The left tube shift cannot be indicated when a right limb is examined nor can the image be anatomically signed, and vice versa for the other side.

However, it may be felt that the absence of a marker is less confusing than the appearance on some of these films of both L and R, particularly to an observer who is not trained in radiology and perhaps is unaware that a stereoradiographic study has been made. A preference for either of these practices can be well justified and students may meet different methods current in individual departments.

Identification without Markers

While we may properly require stereoradiographs to be marked by the radiographer at the time of exposure, the circumstance is neither impossible nor altogether unknown that such a pair of films may require identification at a later stage, because markers have been omitted, or are not visible, or appear to have been incorrectly used.

To make such indentification the only essential is to have firm evidence of the tube aspect of the films concerned. When this is obtainable, the processed dry radiographs should be held to some light source with their tube aspect facing away from the examiner; they are placed one in front of the other so that their edges register. It will be seen that the images are not coincident but are laterally out of alignment. The film on which the image is further to the left is that taken with a left shift of the tube and intended for viewing by the left eye. Conversely the image which has moved to the right indicates the right stereoshift and should be viewed by the right eye. It is to be emphasized that for this determination to be correct the tube aspect of each radiograph should be turned away from the investigator.

Viewing Stereoradiographs

In order to have perception of depth, various methods are available for viewing stereographs. However, before considering these, some attention should be given to the direction from which the films are viewed and the significance of this on the impression received.

In the process of ordinary photography the details which appear in an image can only be those that are on the same side of the subject as the camera. From a stereoscopic pair of photographs we can obtain one view only: that is, a front view if the camera was in front of the subject.

However, this is not true of radiography. The ability of an X-ray beam to penetrate matter results, as we know, in recording on the film all layers of the subject. Detail in a radiographic image is composed of structures both near to and further away from the X-ray tube. Thus, in an anteroposterior projection taken stereographically we have the choice of ultimately viewing the subject either from the front or from the back.

If we look at the anteroposterior projection from the front, that is from the same point of view as the X-ray tube, we describe the effect as *orthoscopic*. If we look at such a radiograph from the back, that is in a direction counter to that of the X-ray beam, we call the image *pseudoscopic*. There is nothing complicated about this procedure. The reversal of direction is obtained, as would be expected, simply by turning over each of the films and looking at them from the other side.

We may take, for example, the anteroposterior projection of the sacroiliac joints made stereoradiographically. If we look at this pair of films as though we were occupying the position of the X-ray tube the pubic symphysis will appear nearer to us than the sacrum. If we reverse the aspect of the radiographs which faces us, so that we are now examining them from somewhere underneath the X-ray table, the patient's sacrum seems closer than the region of the symphysis.

In summary we can say that an orthoscopic image is obtained from the same direction as the exposure was made; while a pseudoscopic image represents a viewpoint counter to the direction of exposure.

Similarly to other radiographs, it is usual to view stereoradiographic films from the anatomical aspect. This means that anteroposterior projections will be examined orthoscopically and posteroanterior projections as a rule pseudoscopically. However, the ability to obtain both viewpoints from a single projection can be useful. Confirmation of the depth of a lesion which continues to be a little doubtful may sometimes be obtained if further observation is made from the aspect not employed before.

In stereoradiography, transposition of the subject, as in a mirror image, will occur if the film intended for viewing by the right eye in fact is seen by the left eye, and vice versa. This will make an orthoscopic image of the right limb appear as a pseudoscopic image of the left limb and is clearly rather a dangerous occurrence, particularly in relation to the head and trunk. It is caused either initially by incorrect marking of the stereoradiographic pair or later by mounting them on the wrong sides of the viewing apparatus.

Films which become reversed in aspect as well as being interchanged in position as regards right and left are probably more dangerous still. They remain in their proper presentation—orthoscopic or pseudoscopic as the case may be—but are again a mirror image in appearance, the right side of the patient seeming to be his left.

Stereoradiographs may be viewed by any of three methods.

(1) With a mirror stereoscope.

(2) With a binocular stereoscope.

(3) With direct vision.

THE MIRROR STEREOSCOPE

This, more often called the Wheatstone stereoscope, is quite an efficient piece of apparatus but rather cumbersome. Probably few departments are still using it, in view of the greater handiness of binoculars. Because of the infrequency with which it is met, a detailed description of the instrument will not be given.

The Wheatstone stereoscope has two full-sized X-ray illuminators which face each other at a distance of 50 to 60 inches. The distance between them can be varied at the will of the operator. At the midpoint between the illuminators a pair of mirrors is arranged in a V, each mirror being at 45 deg. to one of the illuminators. The user of the instrument stands facing the apex of the V, his nose being placed close against it. His right eye receives via the right mirror the image of a radiograph placed on the right illuminator: the left eye similarly receives the image of the film on the left. The observer can adjust the two to his sight until they superimpose and if he has the faculty of stereoscopic vision he will then see a single three-dimensional image. This arrangement is shown diagrammatically in Fig. 14.4.

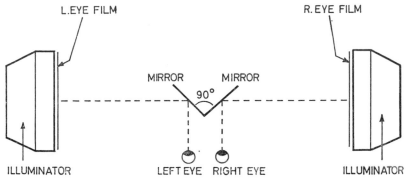

FIG. 14.4. Diagram to illustrate the design and operation of the Wheatstone stereoscope. *By courtesy of Kodak Ltd.*

In using the Wheatstone stereoscope the radiograph obtained with the right shift of the tube should be placed in the right hand illuminator and the left stereoradiograph similarly put on the left illuminator. However, it must be remembered that their images are to be viewed in a mirror and to avoid anatomical reversal of the subject the normal viewing aspect of each radiograph must be turned *away* from the observer and face the illuminator.

THE BINOCULAR STEREOSCOPE

Stereoscopic binoculars are easier to use than the Wheatstone stereoscope and may be thought also to give better results. They have the advantage of size: a pair of binoculars can be kept in a desk drawer as opposed to occupying a considerable quantity of wall space in the reporting room. If several pairs are available, more than one person at a time can look at stereoradiographs and this is clearly of benefit in consultation and teaching.

Stereobinoculars are similar in appearance to opera glasses. The films to be viewed are placed side by side on conventional illuminators, the right stereoradiograph being on the observer's right and the left one on his left. Prisms in the binoculars reflect and also refract the light, the latter phenomenon assisting in the convergence of the images. However, again it must be remembered that it is a reflection of the radiographs which is seen and if anatomical transposition is to be avoided their normal viewing aspect must face away from the observer.

DIRECT VISION

With guidance and practice many people can 'see' stereoradiographs in three dimensions without the aid of special viewing equipment and without incurring any sensations of strain. For those who can master it this is a quick and economical method and further has the advantage that the films can be read in any place where no more than conventional X-ray illuminators are available.

The radiographs to be examined should be placed side by side on the viewing area, their edges touching. The right stereoradiograph is put on the observer's left: he will look at it with his right eye. The left stereoradiograph is put on the observer's right: he will look at it with his left eye. Since no optical instruments are involved, other than the eyes, the normal viewing aspect of the radiographs should be presented to the observer.

He will begin the manoeuvre by standing at some convenient distance away from the illuminator and looking first at his own forefinger which is extended in front of him at arm's length and in the midline between the radiographs. He should not at this stage focus his eyes on his finger but should stare into the distance. A dual image will be apparent, and after a little time a third image which is smaller than the others and at a nearer distance.

When this is seen the observer should attempt to superimpose the images by converging his lines of sight; patients in the orthoptic department are familiar with this type of exercise, and in those who have had to practise it the ability seems to remain within easy recall. When he is successful in perceiving only the one, slightly reduced image the observer should remove his finger and keep his gaze on the radiographs, on which he should now focus. There should be no difficulty in seeing a single image of these and in obtaining the impression of depth.

Fig. 14.5 illustrates the positioning of the radiographs, the convergence of the observer's lines of sight and the production of the stereoscopic image in a plane within the shaded parallelogram.

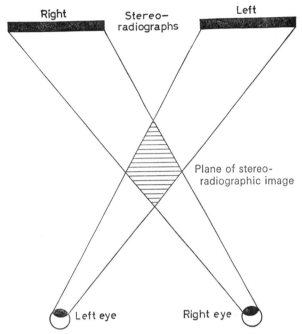

FIG. 14.5. Method of viewing stereoradiographs with unaided sight.

USE OF TRIMMERS

Films which have been processed in tension hangers show mutilation of their corners by the hanger clips. Channel hangers which are not kept scrupulously clean are prone to marr the edges of a film, particularly if drying is undertaken at too high a temperature and melting of the emulsion occurs. Even in automatic processing some systems involve perforation of one border of the film, although these marks are usually scarcely noticeable.

To remove this type of imperfection, film trimmers of one sort or another have long been occupants of the X-ray department and associated with the preparation of radiographs for report. At one time guillotines of the type employed for photographic prints were habitually used to trim the edges of processed radiographs. They often made the film more presentable in another way too, since careful application of the guillotine could result in marked improvement in the appearance of some radiographs which had been badly centred.

However, channel hangers are no longer in such general use and X-ray departments become always busier. At the present time film trimming—if it is done at all—is usually of the corners only. This not only is a tidying process but facilitates handling of the film when removing it from its envelope or inserting it. Furthermore the envelope itself is spared recurrent trauma from sharp or rough corners.

Corner cutters may be manually or electrically operated. In the latter case, insertion of the film under a guide plate brings its edge against a micro-switch. This triggers the circuit energizing an electromagnet and causes a semi-circular blade to move sharply upwards in a shearing action across the corner of the film. The severed portion falls into the base of the cutter, thus releasing the switch to its open-circuit position and allowing the blade of the cutter to become again disengaged.

A cutter which is electromagnetically operated in this way is about 3 times faster than the manual type, although also noisier. If many films have to be trimmed it avoids strain on the hand as well as requiring less time for the work. Both types of cutter have a deep cavity in the base which can be opened and emptied when full of film chips; the larger capacity of the electric cutter has some advantage in this respect.

The corners of most sheet film are already very slightly rounded by the manufacturers. In view of this and because film which has a polyester base is too tough a subject for the blades of most cutters, very few departments now continue to trim their radiographs.

DOCUMENTARY PREPARATION

In preparing radiographs for diagnosis, if the first necessity is correct identification the second is that the films should be properly documented: that is, they should be accompanied by their envelope, the patient's request form, radiological history and any previous radiographs. Record-keeping systems vary to some extent between departments and it is not within the scope of this book to describe them fully nor attempt their evaluation. Students in the course of training no doubt have the opportunity of becoming thoroughly familiar with the practice in their own hospitals and of appreciating how valuable a really efficient system is. Frequently adhesive coloured labels or printed numbers may be put on radiographs and their envelopes so that in the reporting room those of a particular examination can readily be related to others of a specific date. Colour coding of this kind can be adapted to the indexing of pathology or to the indication of other information which any centre may find desirable.

VIEWING CONDITIONS

It has been said, perhaps with some truth, that while thousands of pounds are often spent on highly refined apparatus in order to produce radiographs of impeccable quality, even perhaps at some particular instant in a rapid physiological phase, these same radiographs may ultimately come for diagnosis on viewing equipment which is not up-to-date and sometimes is quite inadequate.

Diagnosis. In this simple word we have the sole purpose of the whole complex exercise. We should remember that the effectiveness of any medical radiograph in the last analysis is never more than a subjective impression created in the mind of an observer. However delicate and precise is radiographic detail, it may as well not exist if he who is to read it cannot perceive it. In this sense no radiograph can be better than the conditions under which it is seen. Attention given to these conditions is a real contribution to radiographic quality. Perhaps their importance is sometimes overlooked in planning financial outlays for radiological departments.

The relationship between the perception of detail in a radiograph and the conditions of viewing is studied elsewhere in this book (Chapter XII). At this point it may be useful to consider the criteria by which we would judge these conditions and these can be very simply stated. In a good X-ray illuminator the following features are needed.

(1) The light should be even in intensity over the whole viewing surface.

(2) It should be as 'white' as possible.

(3) The source of light should not heat the radiograph even if this remains over it for a considerable period of time.

(4) The facility of varying the brightness of the illumination should be available.

Most reputable illuminators at the present time provide a diffuse regular lighting of a suitable standard. For radiographs of medical subjects the light source is most likely to be two 18 inch, 15 watt fluorescent tubes. Another type of cold cathode tube is available. This has a total length of 10 feet and runs up and down to cover the full area of the illuminator and form a continuous grid of light. It is described as having an operating life of more than 10,000 hours which would appear to make it an economic proposition although it is initially expensive. In both cases a reflecting surface, for instance white enamel, is placed behind the light source.

Some types of illuminator may be powered by a group of four or six standard pearl lamps of 40 to 60 watts. These do not show the tendency to flicker which may sometimes be associated with lighting from a fluorescent tube, nor is there any delay in the appearance of the illumination when the unit is first switched on. However, they are probably less satisfactory than fluorescent tubes. Lamp bulbs inevitably become hot in use and the viewing box requires adequate ventilation and perhaps has to be larger if it is to remain cool. Further, the tone of the light tends to be warmer; it has not the blue-white 'daylight' quality provided by some fluorescent tubes which is especially suitable for viewing the radiographic image.

Fluorescent tubes of course can vary in the 'colour' of white light produced. This point should be borne in mind when replacing them, particularly if they are not obtained from the original suppliers of the illuminator but are requisitioned from the electrician's stores in the hospital. In a single illuminator one tube should be the twin of the other, and, where a number of illuminators are banked together on a wall or desk to make a large viewing area, all must match. A disconcerting difference of appearance results when two radiographs of a series are mounted adjacently in lighting of dissimilar quality. This is particularly prone to mislead should a strict comparison have to be made, for example to assess the progress of a lesion in the chest or between a pair taken of the mastoid regions.

To compensate for inequalities which may be due to ageing of the tubes, incorrect replacement or even to the presence of strong cross lighting, a 'light trimmer' device is available on certain viewing units which are composed from 2, 3 or 4 individual panels. This gadget provides for matching both intensity of light and its colour value.

In the appreciation of detail in underexposed or overexposed areas of a radiograph the usefulness of varying the brightness of illumination has been described in Chapter XII. This may be done in three ways.

(1) A variable switch on the illuminator may alter the intensity of light over the whole viewing area. This has the advantage that some positions generally are arranged to give lower than 'normal' brightness. These assist visualization of a radiograph which may suffer from some degree of underexposure, for example a study of the chest made on the ward with a portable unit.

(2) A spot-light operated by a hold-on switch may be mounted in the viewer and provide a localized illumination of high intensity. In certain viewers which are intended mainly for industry and are otherwise powered by two parallel rows of conventional hot filament bulbs, this may take the form of a Photoflood lamp situated in the centre of the field. Adjustable masks can be closed down to the area of extreme brightness in order to avoid dazzle. Sometimes the film may be moved about on a counterbalanced carriage in order to bring any area of the radiograph over the central lamp. Alternatively the spot-light may be outside the main field of illumination; it is sometimes found for example on the right hand side of the front frame of the viewer.

(3) An entirely separate source of high intensity illumination may be used in conjunction with illuminators which do not themselves provide for any variation. This may be a thoroughly organized piece of apparatus with a built-in variable iris diaphragm to alter the diameter of the field from about 10 cms down to less than half a millimetre or nil. On the other hand a much simpler arrangement often gives adequate service, for example an Anglepoise lamp or even a plain unshaded pearl bulb.

In a radiological reporting room a number of illuminators are often grouped together on a wall to form an area where a series of radiographs may be examined and more easily compared without the recurrent need to change their position which a single illuminator entails. In operating theatres a smaller row is quite often used in a similar way and in this case the illuminators are usually mounted so that the front panel is flush with the wall surface. The seal may be water-tight to facilitate hosing of the wall, and even gas-tight and the switches spark-proof as a precaution against risks of explosion from inflammable anaesthetic vapours.

It is important when a number of illuminated panels are arranged like this that independent switching for each of them should be provided; otherwise if only one or two films are being examined there will be considerable dazzle from the unused areas. This is likely to impoverish radiographic quality.

The fronts of X-ray illuminators are necessarily of a ground glass or 'pearl' character. They may be either glass itself or Perspex. Because of the ease with which it acquires a static electric charge Perspex is not suitable for illuminators used in the operating theatre. In the X-ray department it is of course hardier than glass but more difficult to keep free of dust. A fluid designed to prevent the formation of static electricity is available for cleaning this type of panel. All illuminators should be regularly cleaned if they are not to lose efficiency.

Specialized Illuminators

In the course of various types of specialized radiographic experience the student is likely to encounter X-ray illuminators which have certain different features to make them suitable for particular work. There are small ones, for example, which are intended for the examination of a dental series; or we may contrast the needs of miniature chest radiographs with the lengths of 14 inch roll film used in certain serial changers for angiography.

Again, a demonstration or conference room may require a viewing unit working on the paternoster system, and perhaps motor driven, on which a very large number of radiographs can be mounted prior to their use in illustrating a lecture.

In sorting rooms, or whenever measurements must be made or lines drawn on a radiograph, for example in procedures designed to localize a foreign body, it is of some advantage to have an illuminated panel horizontally placed and flush with a working surface.

It will be appreciated by the student that the specially adapted features of any of these are quite apart from the fundamental design of all good viewing equipment. In this chapter our discussion has been mainly directed towards an understanding of these essential principles.

CHAPTER XV

Optical Principles of Photography

Even the most sophisticated cameras are merely refined applications of the same simple working principles. Some understanding of these principles is important to the radiographer since the X-ray tube and generator may be linked to a camera; for example in the units employed for mass miniature radiography of the chest or the equipment designed for cinefluorography. In these cases the radiograph is a photograph in the generally accepted sense of being an image recorded on a film through the agency of a camera.

THE NATURE OF LIGHT

From earlier studies in the course of training it may be assumed that the student radiographer has rather better than a nodding acquaintance with current theories of the nature of light. It will be remembered that many facts about the behaviour of light can be explained satisfactorily only by a combination of ideas. These are:
(1) that light consists of discrete amounts (quanta) of energy;
(2) that light is a series of wave forms.

Familiarity in detail with these concepts may not be important to the actual practice of photography. However it is worth noting that the quantum theory is the one taken into account when explaining the effects on a photographic emulsion when it is struck by light. On the other hand, the wave theory helps understanding of the different colours present in 'white' light and of the ways in which light can be deviated by a medium through which it passes.

By definition *optics* is the science of light, the study of its behaviour and of phenomena associated with it. More particularly we are concerned here with photographic optics. A large part of this deals with the formation of an image by a lens and is related to the geometrical aspect of light. Important to our understanding of the geometry of light is the assumption that its propagation is rectilinear when traversing a homogeneous transparent medium; that is, that in air at a uniform temperature, in a vacuum, or in clear glass of uniform density, it travels in straight lines. We can think of these straight lines as representing light rays and this concept is helpful when we try to explain what happens to light when it falls on a lens or a mirror.

The fact that light is propagated in a rectilinear manner need not be accepted by the student as an act of crude faith. It can be shown by a number of experiments. A very simple one may be performed with a card of convenient size in which a square aperture is cut. If this card is held between a light source and a plane surface the 'pattern' of light obtained on the latter demonstrates that the light has travelled in straight lines. This experiment and its result are depicted diagrammatically in Fig. 15.1. For the sake of simplicity in illustration the light rays are here

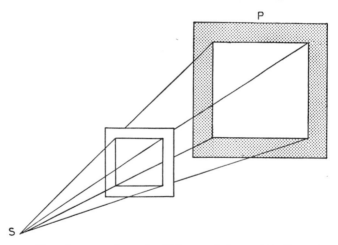

Fig. 15.1. Experiment to show that light travels in straight lines. A card, from which a central aperture of convenient size has been cut, is held between a light source S and a plane surface at P. A lighted area of similar shape, surrounded by the shadow of the card, is seen.

shown as emanating from a point source. In practice of course this is not possible: although the clear sun gives a good approximation to a point source and casts sharp shadows any source of light must have finite dimensions, but this does not affect the performance of the experiment nor the validity of the result obtained. Student radiographers perhaps will recognize that this experiment is repeated daily in the X-ray department whenever a light beam diaphragm is operated.

THE FORMATION OF IMAGES

When light falls on an object three main effects may occur, to a greater or lesser degree.

(1) It may be absorbed.

(2) It may be reflected; that is, it will reappear on the same side of the object as it originated.

(3) It may be transmitted; that is, it will pass through the object or material in question. In the context of photographic optics the last two are of immediate significance; particularly of course the transmission of light through glass since it is upon the characteristics of this that the ability of a lens to form images depends.

Refraction

When a ray of light is transmitted through one medium into another of different density—for example from air into water or glass—its direction is generally altered. This is not true of the *normal* ray, that is for a beam at right angles to the receiving surface. In all other cases the beam appears to bend as it passes from one medium into the other ciprocal relation'. The distances concerned in this case are those from many practical instances occurring in everyday life, for example the apparent distortion of a stick thrust at an angle into clear water. The effect is illustrated diagramatically in Fig. 15.2. In a general statement

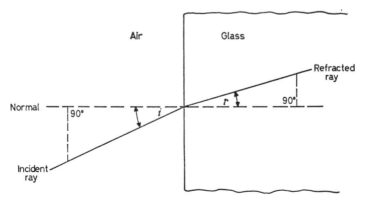

FIG. 15.2. Refraction of a ray of light passing from a rare medium (usually air) into a denser one such as glass. The ray of light is bent nearer to the normal (a line at right-angles to the surface on which it is incident); the angle *r* is smaller than the angle *i*. *By courtesy of Ilford Ltd.*

we may say that light passing obliquely from a rare into a denser medium is bent *towards* the normal: rays are reflected *away* from the normal when their passage is from a dense into a rarer medium.

There is, naturally, a mathematical expression for the amount of refraction which occurs in any particular instance. This is given by the equation:

$$\frac{\text{Sin } r}{\text{Sin } i} = n$$

where *i* is the angle of the incident ray with the normal, *r* the angle of the refracted ray and *n* a factor known as the refractive index of the material concerned. In photographic optics the significant material of course is glass.

When refraction is studied in more detail by means of light passing through a glass block which has parallel sides it is found that the oblique beam is refracted twice. As we would expect, on entering the glass it is bent towards the normal at the point of incidence: on leaving, the deviation of the ray is away from the normal. This state of affairs is depicted in Fig. 15.3.

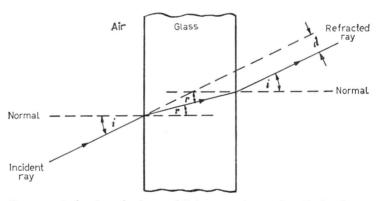

Fig. 15.3. Refraction of a beam of light traversing a glass block. The ray is deviated twice. A lateral shift in its passage is produced, equivalent to the distance *d* in the diagram. *By courtesy of Ilford Ltd.*

It will be noticed that the effect of the second part of the process is to balance the first. This means that though it has been shifted laterally by its passage through the glass, the light leaves the block in the same direction as it entered.

A somewhat different result is obtained when the experiment is applied not to a rectangular block of glass but to a triangular prism. Here the refracting surfaces of the glass are not parallel but at an angle to each other. In these circumstances the light is bent as before on entering the glass and bent again on leaving it but in the same direction, that is towards the base of the prism. This is illustrated in Fig. 15.4. It will be seen that the effect of the prism is to provide a means of changing the direction of a beam of light.

When two identical prisms are placed base to base, as shown in Fig. 15.5 their combined action results in rays from a point source being brought together again at another point some distance from the prism.

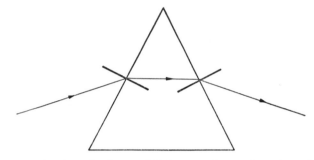

FIG. 15.4. Refraction of a beam of light traversing a triangular prism. In this case the direction of the beam is changed. *From The Science of Photography (H. Baines) by courtesy of The Fountain Press.*

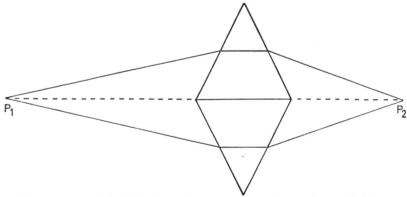

FIG. 15.5. Two identical triangular prisms placed base to base will bring light rays from a point source (P_1) together again at another point (P_2) some distance beyond the prisms.

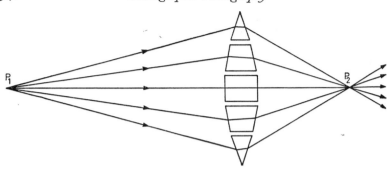

Fig. 15.6. A simple converging lens shown as a number of prisms. From a source P_1 light rays are refracted by the lens, resulting in their focus at a point P_2. *By courtesy of Ilford Ltd.*

This is the way in which a simple converging lens operates. It can be considered as a series of prisms (Fig. 15.6). Any light reaching such a system may conveniently be considered as having emanated from a large number of point sources covering the surface of the object, each such point being similarly imaged. It can be depicted here only two dimensionally.

Dispersion

White light consists of a mixture of lights of many different wavelengths, these differences being perceived by the eye as differences in colour. The term dispersion refers to the separation of a beam of white light into its different coloured components by a prism and can be produced in this way because the refractive index is a constant for any given material only if the light concerned is monochromatic (i.e. of one wavelength). Where several wavelengths are present in a beam, as in white light, it is found that long wavelengths are refracted less than short. It is this difference in refraction which results in the analysis or dispersion of the beam into the various colours which compose it.

This is a significant effect in photographic optics since it implies that a lens constructed of one type of glass only cannot bring different colours of light to a common focus. However, this difficulty is not insurmountable. Different types of glass have different refractive indices and different dispersive powers and so a compound lens can be constructed from two or more simple lenses in different glasses so selected that dispersion tends to be cancelled while focusing power is retained.

Reflection

When a surface reflects light it may do so in two ways which are described as being either direct or diffuse.

DIRECT REFLECTION

This is the type of reflection which occurs in a mirror. The light is not scattered but redirected along a definite line on the same side of the reflecting surface as its origin. The effect is illustrated in Fig. 15.7 which shows that the angle of the incident ray with the normal is equal to the angle of the reflected ray.

This kind of reflection is sometimes termed *specular reflection*.

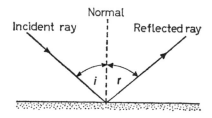

FIG. 15.7. Direct or specular reflection, such as occurs in a mirror. The angle *r* is equal to the angle *i*. *By courtesy of Ilford Ltd.*

DIFFUSE REFLECTION

This form of reflection occurs from a rough or matt material and is due to the myriad tiny irregularities of such a surface. Light striking it is reflected by these at many different angles to the main plane of the substance. The term *scattered reflection* is sometimes used of this.

It is of course by diffusely reflected light that we 'see'. The details of an object from which *all* light is directly reflected cannot be perceived. We do not see the surface of a mirror unless there is dust on it to create irregularities and thus reflect some of the light diffusely. Some substances exhibit both direct and diffuse reflection: in addition to the dusty mirror we have examples in varnished or polished wood, a playing card or similar surfaces.

TOTAL INTERNAL REFLECTION

This is a type of reflection which occurs in certain specialized circumstances. It has been said that light passing from a dense to a rarer medium is refracted away from the normal. This means that as the angle of incidence increases the direction of the refracted ray moves nearer the boundary plane between the two media in the manner illustrated in Fig. 15.8. Ultimately, for a certain angle of incident ray, the line of the refracted ray will be the boundary line between the media. When this is so the angle of incidence is termed the *critical angle*. When the angle of the incident ray is greater than the critical value then total internal reflection occurs.

For glass the critical angle is of the order of 40 to 42 deg.; it depends on the refractive index of the glass concerned. The significant point at present is that light striking the boundary at 45 deg. will be totally reflected in the manner shown in Fig. 15.8. Figure 15.9 illustrates the employment of this property of glass in a right-angled prism such as is used in some document copying cameras; the reflection rectifies the lateral inversion caused by the lens and thus gives right-way-round copies.

IMAGE FORMATION BY A MIRROR

The image of an object which is obtained in looking into a plane mirror is a *virtual image*. No light from the object actually passes

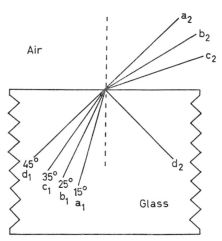

FIG. 15.8. Total internal reflection. In the figure, a number of rays of light a_1, b_1, c_1, d_1, are passing from a block of glass into air. They are at different angles of incidence. As this angle increases, the direction of the refracted rays a_2, b_2, c_2, becomes nearer to the boundary between glass and air and eventually passes it. This has happened in the case of the ray d_1, which is internally reflected along the line d_2.

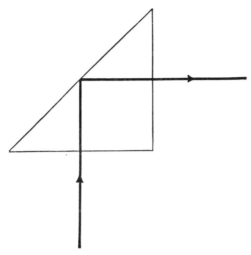

FIG. 15.9. Total internal reflection by a right-angled prism.

through the mirror: the image gives the impression that it is beyond the glass but it can be observed only from the same side as the object originating it. Virtual images are produced by divergent beams and cannot be projected on to a screen.

However, not all mirrors reflect a virtual image. In contra-distinction to this term, the image formed by a *concave* mirror is called *real*. Real images are produced by convergent beams of light and they can be projected on to a screen: their formation is an important aspect of mirror optics, since a suitable mirror system may replace a conventional lens in some circumstances. A relevant example of this is found in some equipment used for fluorography (photography of the fluorescent screen).

The experiences of everyday life make familiar to us all the fact that a mirror image, whether virtual or real, is laterally reversed, right appearing as left.

IMAGE FORMATION BY A PINHOLE

When light passes through a small aperture an image is formed beyond the aperture. The classic demonstration of this is to hold a card, perforated at its centre by a pinhole, between a candle and a light screen in the manner shown in Fig. 15.10. The rectilinear propagation of light

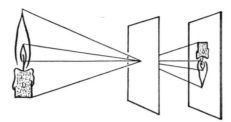

FIG. 15.10. Image formation by a pinhole camera. *From The Science of Photography (H. Baines) by courtesy of The Fountain Press.*

in all directions results in the inversion of the image; the lines in the diagram represent some of the image-forming rays.

A pinhole is a simple way of forming an image and a camera employing this inexpensive principle can be used to obtain photographs. However, it has practical limitations which prevent it from being a very serviceable device. The sharpness of the image produced is related to the size of the pinhole, assuming a given distance between the pinhole and the screen. A relatively large hole admits more light and results in a brighter image but it becomes ever more poorly defined. If the size of the aperture is reduced, initially a sharper image results but eventually diffraction from the edges of the pinhole begins to impair definition. There is an optimum size of pinhole which gives an image of maximum sharpness. Even assuming a hole of this ideal size, the definition obtained with a pinhole camera is never really good, nor are short exposures possible owing to the very limited brightness of the image. These disadvantages are scarcely offset by the good points of such a camera —cheapness, lack of optical distortion and a splendid simplicity in operation.

IMAGE FORMATION BY A LENS

A lens is a system of one or more pieces of glass which causes regular convergence or divergence of light rays passing through it. A lens which consists of only one piece of glass is described as *simple*. Except for those found in the most elementary cameras, photographic lenses are of the *compound* (or *complex*) type: they consist of several components, each of which may consist of a number of pieces of glass cemented together. At present the action of a simple lens will be considered, to facilitate understanding of the subject.

Fig. 15.6 shows a simple converging lens as a number of prisms. Light rays radiating from a point source P₁ are refracted and—providing that the angles of the prisms are appropriate—are brought together again at a point P₂ to form a sharp, bright image: they are described as coming to a *focus*.

Simple lenses may be either *positive* or *negative*. Positive lenses converge light to a point on the side of the lens remote from the source. Negative lenses diverge light: the image is formed on the same side of the lens as the object originating it and—like the image reflected by a plane mirror—is a virtual image. Fig. 15.11 illustrates the formation of a virtual image by a negative lens.

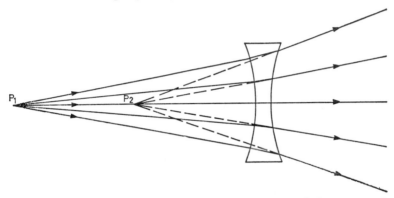

a plane mirror, it is a virtual image; it cannot be projected. *By courtesy of* P₁ is on the same side of the lens as the object. Like the image reflected by a plane mirror, it is a virtual image; it cannot be projected. *By courtesy of Ilford Ltd.*

Simple lenses are not necessarily all the same shape. A number of them are listed below and Fig. 15.12 illustrates their cross-sectional appearances. As a simple principle we may remember that *positive*, converging or convex simple lenses are thicker at the centre than at their edges, while *negative*, diverging or concave lenses are thinner at the middle than at the periphery.

DOUBLE-CONVEX. This is perhaps the 'typical' lens. It has two convex surfaces.

PLANO-CONVEX. One surface is plane and the other convex.

DOUBLE-CONCAVE. Two surfaces are concave.

PLANO-CONCAVE. Comparable with the plano-convex, this lens has one plane and one concave surface.

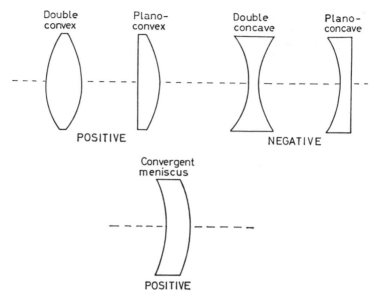

FIG. 15.12. Types of simple lenses.

MENISCUS. This lens has two curved surfaces, the centres of both curves being on the same side of the lens: more simply, we can say that it is crescent-shaped. Meniscus lenses may be of either positive or negative type. They are often used in inexpensive 'snapshot' cameras.

Lens Axis

This term refers to the line which contains the centres of the curved surfaces of a lens. In Fig. 15.12 it is represented in each case by the dotted line.

Camera lenses, while they may contain both negative and positive components, must in their overall effect be of the positive type: otherwise the image could not be recorded on a film placed in the camera behind the lens. For this reason, and for readier understanding, it seems sensible in discussing further the principles of image formation to concentrate our attention on the behaviour of a thin, simple, positive lens.

Focal Length

When light from a point on a very distant object, such as the sun, reaches a lens the rays may be regarded as being parallel; the object is said to be at *infinity* in respect of the lens. The plane on which the image of a distant object is formed is termed the *focal plane* and its intersection with the axis of the lens determines the *principal focal point*. More simply we can say that the principal focal point is the focus for parallel light. The distance again from the principal focus to the lens is the *focal length* of the lens. Fig. 15.13 illustrates these features.

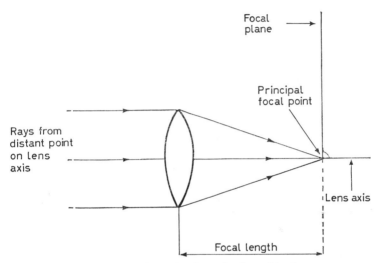

FIG. 15.13. Image formation by a simple positive lens.

Rays which emanate from points on the object above the lens axis come to a focus in the focal plane *below* the lens axis; that is, the image is inverted by the lens just as was the image formed by a pinhole.

The focal length of a lens is extremely significant in determining its suitability for any particular purpose, since it has a marked influence on the scale of reproduction of the image, and the angle of view (that is, the amount of the subject included on the film); it is also an important factor in the relative brightness of the image.

SCALE OF REPRODUCTION

For a given object-to-lens distance the height of the image is related to the focal length of the lens in the manner shown in Fig. 15.14. The longer the focal length the greater is the image size. The ratio relating the size of the image to that of the object in reality is the same as the ratio between two distances which we shall consider shortly; those between the image and the lens and the object and the lens.

In considering a lens of certain focal length, we find that the image of an object is diminished if the object is remote from the lens, magnified if it is nearer to the lens than two focal lengths, and reproduced in its natural dimensions if the distance between it and the lens is exactly twice the focal length. However, when the object-to-lens distance is less than the focal length, the light rays transmitted by the lens are divergent. Consequently they form a virtual image, not a real one. This condition obtains when a positive lens is used as a simple magnifying glass.

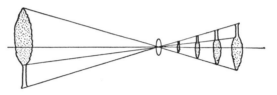

FIG. 15.14. Variation of image size with the focal length of the lens. The greater the focal length, the larger is the size of the image for a given object-lens distance. *From the Science of Photography (H. Baines) by courtesy of The Fountain Press.*

We may notice as a feature of negative lenses that the image is always diminished; for this reason the term *reducing* lenses is sometimes applied to these.

Summarizing this we can state that for an object at some given distance the ratio of reproduction is governed by the focal length of the lens: and that for a lens of any given focal length the ratio of reproduction is governed by the distance between it and an object.

CONJUGATE DISTANCES

The term 'conjugate' here is perhaps rather intimidating to the student of photography who is not also a scholar in Latin. It implies things which work in close association with each other, meaning in a literal sense 'yoked together' and in a mathematical sense 'joined by a reciprocal relation'. The distances concerned in this case are those from an object to the lens (*the object conjugate distance*) and from the image to the lens (*the image conjugate distance*): for a lens of any stated focal length these distances are closely related to each other. They are linked by an expression termed the *lens equation*.

Conventional symbols for the statement of this are to let u represent the object conjugate, v the image conjugate and f the focal length of the lens: the lens equation can then be written as follows:

$$\frac{1}{u} + \frac{1}{v} = \frac{1}{f}$$

This formula and others derived from it can be employed in practical photography in calculations to obtain, for example working distances, whether using a camera or an enlarger. It is doubtful whether knowledge of this expression is ever put to any useful purpose in an X-ray department.

Where the object conjugate is relatively great (more than ten times the focal length of the lens) the image conjugate can be taken for practical purposes as equal to the focal length of the lens. Thus, in most 'ordinary' photography the conjugate distances are not of direct significance. However, in special circumstances the fundamental facts expressed in the lens equation become relevant.

We may refer, for example, to the photography of some small object (clinical photography perhaps of a tooth or isolated skin lesion) which is to be shown in its natural size. In these circumstances u becomes equal to v and we can write the lens equation as

$$\frac{1}{u} + \frac{1}{u} = \frac{1}{f}$$

or
$$\frac{2}{u} = \frac{1}{f}$$

or
$$u = 2f$$

This means that the distance at which the object should be photographed is twice the focal length of the lens. The position is shown less mathematically in Fig. 15.15 and it can be seen how in these circum-

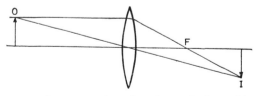

Fig. 15.15. Geometric construction of an image I of an object O, photographed at a distance of twice the focal length of the lens. In these circumstances the image is the same size as the original. *From The Science of Photography* (H. Baines) *by courtesy of The Fountain Press.*

stances the image recedes from the principal focus by a distance equal to the focal length of the lens. This means that the intensity of light at the image plane is only one quarter of what it was at the principal focus since the distance has been doubled and the same quantity of light must now illumine an area four times greater; the image will be commensurately reduced in brightness. Allowance for the diminished brilliance of the image must be made when photographing objects very near to the camera. During more conventional photography the distance of the subject from the camera does not affect the illumination of the image, since the image conjugate can be assumed virtually equal to the focal length of the lens.

Relative Aperture (F-numbers)

The brightness of an image formed by a lens must depend upon two factors:

(a) the amount of light transmitted by the lens;
(b) the area over which the light has to extend.

Assuming the lens has perfect transparency, (a) is proportional to its size, or more accurately to its area: this is proportional to the square of the lens diameter. (b) is the area of the image and this becomes greater as focal length is greater, increasing with the square of focal length.

It will be seen that these two factors work in opposite ways to each other: a lens having a large diameter produces a bright image; a lens of long focal length implies an image of diminished brilliance. From this we can say that image brightness is proportional to:

$$\left(\frac{\text{lens diameter}}{\text{focal length}}\right)^2$$

However in this particular form the expression would be awkward to handle. Almost always the diameter of a lens is smaller than its focal length and consequently the function becomes a fraction. To avoid such an arithmetical inconvenience we invert the formula and consider the ratio of focal length to lens diameter. This function $\frac{\text{focal length}}{\text{lens diameter}}$ is called the *relative aperture* or f-number of the lens. It is written usually as a small f followed by an oblique stroke and a numerical value: thus $f/8$. In Europe the relative aperture of a lens often is expressed simply as a ratio: thus $1 : 8$. Both forms of statement mean the same thing.

We need to remember that as we have inverted our original expression f-numbers increase as image brightness becomes less. A lens of $f/8$ is one which has a diameter one-eighth of its focal length. The student should have little difficulty in remembering this if it is observed that the oblique stroke indicates 'divided by': for example, we may write one quarter with equal intelligibility as 1/4. The f/8 lens might have a diameter of 5 mm and a focal length of 40 mm; or it might have a diameter of 1 inch and a focal length of 8 inches. In either case an image of similar brightness results—theoretically we can say that these lenses have comparable speed. However, the image produced by the second is much larger than the first.

The f-number is a generally accepted and useful statement of the speed of a lens. One having a relative aperture of f/2·8 is 'faster' than another of f/5·6 because it admits more light. However other factors can be significant, since it is the amount of light *transmitted* by the lens which really is the relevant quantity. Our original statement assumed a lens of perfect transparency, capable of transmitting 100 per cent of the light received. In practice there are likely always to be some losses due to absorption and reflection, especially if the lens is compound in type and has several components. A complex lens may in fact lose up to 50 per cent of incident light.

This discrepancy between the geometrical measure of a lens' relative aperture and its actual transmitting ability can be handled in two ways. Light loss due to surface reflection can be much reduced by *blooming* of the lens. In this process each glass-air surface of the lens is coated with a thin layer of some material having a refractive index intermediate between that of the glass and air. Certain fluorides are suitable for this, being of appropriate refractive index and capable of forming a uniform hard layer which will adhere well to glass. In this way reflection from each surface of a lens can be very much reduced. Bloomed lenses usually have a blue or purple appearance. As they are only thinly coated they should be given careful protection, in order to avoid having to clean them often. When cleaning these lenses proper materials should be used, for example a lens tissue together with much caution.

In addition to treatment which diminishes light losses, a lens may be individually calibrated by photometric means which take into account its transmission as well as its geometry. This has introduced a system of T-numbers which represent a measure of the amount of light passed by a lens in relation to the transmission of a perfectly transparent lens. A T-8 lens is one which passes as much light as the theoretically ideal f/8 lens: its relative aperture in fact will be of the order of f/6·3. This concept of T-numbers is of value mainly for exacting work where there is no margin for error in exposure selection and it is important to know accurately the practical speed of a lens, for example in cinematography.

The subject of f-numbers and exposure will be given further consideration in the next chapter.

Depth of Focus

It is convenient to consider image formation in terms of light rays emanating from a point or a number of points on the object studied. It is assumed that the lens is capable of rendering such a point as a point on the image. In practice however perfect resolution is unattainable. Even with sharpest focusing a point on the object appears in the focal plane as a small circle of light to which is given the name—perhaps inappropriately—of the *circle of least confusion*.

It might appear from this that it is impossible in any circumstances to obtain an image which looks completely sharp. This would be so were it not for the fact that the human eye is satisfied with something less than pinpoint definition. There is a limit to the smallness of detail which the eye can perceive: when this limit is reached the image appears sharp because the eye cannot appreciate any further increase in sharpness. We can say that it will accept as a true point a circle of confusion of which the diameter is no greater than a thousandth part of its distance from the eye.

From this it is evident that the permissible diameter of the circle of confusion will vary depending on whether we are considering—for example—a negative or contact print which will be examined in the hand, or an entry in a photographic exhibition which will be hung on a wall and viewed from a position several feet away.

However, at a distance of not less than ten inches—this being considered the minimum normal viewing distance—the average correctly functioning human eye will accept as perfectly sharp a circle 1/100 inch in diameter. The circles of confusion may be less than or equal to this maximum without affecting the appearance of the image to an observer under general conditions. Obviously this implies some latitude of focus. Fig. 15.16 illustrates how points immediately in front of and immediately behind the plane of sharpest focus appear sharp because the circle of confusion is within the limits above defined. The distance between these front and rear boundaries constitutes *depth of focus*.

In order to clarify a principle, the foregoing discussion has been based on a situation referring to a photographic negative from which contact prints are to be made. Where enlargement is envisaged, the permissible diameter of the circle of confusion in the negative must be reduced in proportion to the expected degree of enlargement; for example, if we intend to enlarge a 35 mm negative by 5, the permissible diameter of the circle of confusion becomes only 1/500 inch.

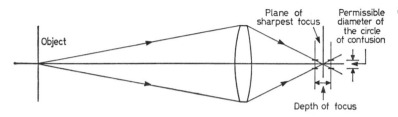

FIG. 15.16. Depth of focus. *By courtesy of Ilford Ltd.*

From a practical point of view depth of focus means the distance through which the recording film may be moved without the image of a flat object becoming appreciably unsharp. It is related to the f-number and the focal length of the lens. Depth of focus increases with larger f-numbers (i.e. smaller relative aperture) and in normal circumstances with greater focal length. This characteristic of the lens is not of any direct practical significance to the average photographer but it is of course important to the manufacturer since it indicates tolerance levels for the positioning of the sensitive material in the camera in relation to the lens. In most miniature cameras depth of focus may be very restricted because they commonly possess lenses of wide relative aperture and short focal length: this is one of the features which require such cameras to be precision built. The student should notice that depth of focus is not synonymous with depth of field: this will be considered in the next chapter.

ABERRATIONS OF LENSES

Lenses are not perfect instruments. They do not in all circumstances form a completely faithful image of the physical aspects of an object. The defects which they may display are termed *lens aberrations*. A simple lens will exhibit a number of aberrations but photographs can be success-fully taken with it in an inexpensive camera because its relative aperture is kept small. Aberrations as a rule become more intrusive in their effect as aperture increases and that is why the 'fast' lenses of sophisticated cameras must be highly complex structures. Different kinds of glass are combined and radii of curvature accurately computed in order to correct errors of reproduction inherent in a simple lens.

Lens aberrations fall into three main categories.

(1) Chromatic errors.

(2) Spherical errors.

(3) Diffraction errors.

The first group are due to the fact already stated that the refractive index of glass varies with the wavelengths of the incident radiation. Not all wavelengths are brought to a focus at the same point and white light, as we know, consists of a variety of wavelengths. The second group are due to the spherical shape which the lens requires if it is to be manufactured economically and with precision. The third group arise from the diffraction of a beam of light, or similar radiation, which occurs when it passes through a narrow aperture: the student perhaps will remember the use of this phenomenon in the analysis of X-ray spectra and that it is explicable in terms of the assumption that light is a series of waves. Diffractive errors become more pronounced at smaller relative apertures and less pronounced the shorter is the wavelength of the incident light.

An exhaustive study of lens defects is unnecessary in this book. However, the main features of certain aberrations are described in the remainder of this chapter, with an indication of how they may be remedied or minimized. Even after correction most lenses retain residual tendencies to these errors which may become apparent under critical conditions.

Chromatic Aberrations

As described in the section relating to dispersion, shorter wavelengths are refracted by a simple lens more sharply than long and consequently the focus for blue light is nearer to the lens than the focus for red light. The image is said to suffer from chromatic aberration and will appear to lack definition in all parts of the lens field.

Chromatic aberration can be reduced if the lens is constructed of two types of glass in the way described in the earlier section on dispersion. A positive element of crown glass is cemented to a negative element of flint glass. These two types of glass have different refractive indices. A lens constructed in this way is called an achromatic lens, or more briefly an *achromat*.

A special form of chromatic aberration results in the appearance of little fringes of colour at the edges of the image. This is called *transverse colour aberration* and is due to the formation of a small spectrum at points away from the lens axis. It is seriously significant only in colour work of high precision and can be remedied in manufacture by 'symmetrical' construction of the lens. This implied originally that the lens was made up of a pair of components symmetrically arranged. The principle is illustrated in Fig. 15.17(a). In modern terminology such a lens has two separated components but their arrangement may not be exactly symmetrical. The term is to be contrasted with *triplet lenses* in which three separated components are concerned. Such a lens is illustrated diagrammatically in Fig. 15.17(b). Most good camera lenses at the present time are based on one or other of these forms of construction.

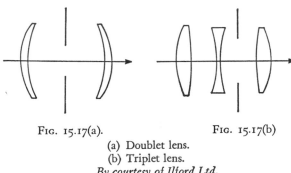

Fig. 15.17(a).   Fig. 15.17(b)
(a) Doublet lens.
(b) Triplet lens.
By courtesy of Ilford Ltd.

It may be noted that lens errors, such as lateral colour, which are not present in the centre of the field are sometimes termed *oblique*, in distinction to direct errors which affect all parts of the image.

Spherical Aberration

This again results in unsharpness of the image and is due to peripheral rays coming to a focus nearer the lens than do those passing centrally. It can be reduced to a minimum in a simple double-convex lens if the radius of curvature of the posterior surface of the lens is approximately six times that of the front surface. In a compound lens spherical aberration may be corrected by combining a suitable positive with a suitable negative element in which the spherical aberration is equal in magnitude but opposite in sign.

Coma is a special type of spherical aberration affecting rays which strike the lens obliquely. It can be reduced by the use again of symmetrical construction of two elements, each having equal and opposite errors.

Curvilinear Distortion

Unlike other aberrations, the presence of curvilinear distortion affects the shape of the image but not its sharpness. Furthermore, curvilinear distortion is not diminished by reduction in aperture. It causes the image of a square object to appear with its sides bowed either outwards (*barrel distortion*) or inwards (*pin-cushion distortion*). The effects are illustrated in Fig. 15.18.

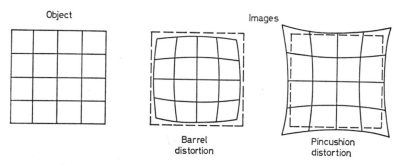

FIG. 15.18. Curvilinear distortion. *By courtesy of Ilford Ltd.*

Curvilinear distortion is an oblique error and is due essentially to an alteration in scale of the edges of an image. If the scale is too small at the edges we see barrel distortion; if it is too large, pin-cushion distortion results. The type of deformity which may occur in a particular camera depends on the position of the limiting diaphragm (see Chapter xvi): placed in front of a simple lens it produces the barrel effect; behind the lens it causes the pin-cushion deformity. The error can be corrected by constructing the lens of two separated elements and placing the diaphragm between them: in this way its position behind one and in front of the other has a self-cancelling action on the two defects.

Curvature of Field

Not to be confused with curvilinear distortion, this is a defect which causes the plane of sharpest focus to be not flat but saucer shaped. The effect is illustrated in Fig. 15.19.

In practice this means that an image sharp at the centre is unsharp at the edges and vice versa. In the case of a simple positive lens a suitable meniscus shape will flatten the field to some extent.

In some instruments a curved focal plane cannot be avoided and arrangements may be made to bend the film slightly to follow the field.

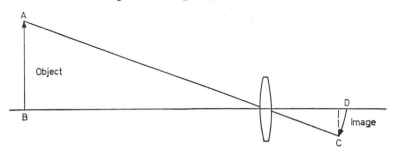

FIG. 15.19. Curvature of field. *By courtesy of Ilford Ltd.*

This is true of the mirror focusing system employed in the 'Odelca' 70 or 100 mm cameras for photofluorography. Students who have seen this apparatus operated or are in practice familiar with its use will perhaps have noted the convex platten which holds the film in place.

Astigmatism

This is another oblique aberration. Broadly speaking we can say that a lens which exhibits astigmatism fails to render horizontal and vertical lines sharp at one time. This is not a fully accurate statement, since it is strictly applicable only to lines which respectively are radial and tangential to the lens axis: however, it certainly expresses the effect on the observer's eye and is an acceptable conclusion for general purposes.

Astigmatism is an important defect and is associated with curvature of the field. Early attempts to correct astigmatism in a lens tended to increase the curvature of the focal plane: a flat field was obtained only with the introduction of astigmatism. However, progress in the manufacture of optical glasses has made this no longer true; glass can be produced which has a low refractive index combined with high dispersion and vice versa. The correction of astigmatism is now effected by means of a particular relationship between dispersive power and refractive index in the glasses of a compound lens. Flatness of the field is maintained. Such a lens is described as an *anastigmat* or an anastigmatic lens.

CHAPTER XVI

The Camera

In this chapter will be considered the practical application in a camera of the optical principles previously discussed. Any camera has certain necessary attributes, though the degree of refinement which they exhibit may vary considerably, as also will the cost of the camera in proportion. The essentials are stated below.

(1) The camera must not admit any extraneous light.

(2) It must have a lens at one end and at the other a means of supporting a light-sensitive material in some suitable frame at right angles to the lens.

(3) The lens must be focused or capable of being focused in the image plane occupied by the film.

(4) It must generally be possible to 'aim' the camera by the use of a view-finder. In radiographic practice the 'view-finder' may be quite different from the devices usually signified by the term: for example during modern cinematography of the fluorescent X-ray image the 'view' taken is seen and selected through observation of the image intensifier or the television monitor screen.

(5) There must be a means of controlling both the amount of light admitted by the lens and the duration of its passage.

It is convenient to consider (5) first. Two features of the camera take part in this: they are the *diaphragm* and the *shutter*.

THE DIAPHRAGM

Camera lenses are not always employed at their full aperture. One of the reasons for this is an effect known as *vignetting*. This occurs when the edges of the various components of a lens cut off oblique light rays and no compound lens is wholly free from it at full aperture. We have considered in the previous chapter features of a lens which affect definition at the field edges, namely the oblique category of lens aberrations. Here then are two reasons at least which make desirable in a camera some method of restricting the aperture of the lens, so that whenever possible we use only its central part rather than it periphery.

This is achieved by means of an *iris diaphragm* or—in a very simple camera—by means of a *stop*, that is, a metal plate which has a number of circular apertures and is capable of being moved to bring each into an appropriate position in front of the lens. This process of decreasing the effective aperture of the lens, whether by means of a diaphragm or a stop, is known as *stopping down*.

The iris diaphragm, as its name must suggest, is analogous in operation to the way in which the human eye adapts itself to light. It consists of a number of light metal blades or leaves which are equally spaced round the lens in a circle and can overlap: this construction is shown in Fig. 16.1. Open, they form a virtually circular aperture centred on the axis of the lens.

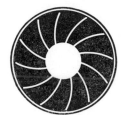 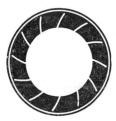

FIG. 16.1. An iris diaphragm.

The components are closed by rotation of a ring in the lens mount, the circle which they form becoming then decreased in diameter in a continuously variable fashion; the actual extent of the aperture is dependent on the degree of rotation of the ring. Where the lens is compound in type it is common practice to place the iris diaphragm between its components rather than in front of the total lens assembly.

Effective Aperture and Exposure

It has been said earlier (Chapter xv) that the brightness of the image formed by a lens, that is in a camera the intensity of light reaching the film, is proportional to the square of the lens diameter. Putting it another way we can say that the exposure-time required for a certain film density is inversely proportional to the square of the lens diameter. From this it follows that alteration of the diaphragm aperture in order to restrict the effective diameter of the lens necessarily affects exposure-time and consequently it is important to provide the operator with some means of knowing what the aperture is, or rather of attaching to it some definite value.

This can be done by means of the f-number. The derivation of this function has been discussed in the previous chapter and the student will recall that when the f-number is numerically low the lens aperture is wide: a small f-number requires less exposure-time relative to a higher one.

It is usual to calibrate the iris diaphragm by a series of f-numbers giving a diminishing succession of image brightnesses, such that each requires twice the exposure time of its immediate forerunner. As the amount of light passed by a lens is inversely proportional to the square of the f-number, the factor by which this series of numbers must increase is $\sqrt{2}$ (approximately 1·4). In the United Kingdom the standard series of f-numbers is:

f/1	f/8
f/1·4	f/11
f/2	f/16
f/2·8	f/22
f/4	f/32
f/5·6	

In Europe the figures are different although their relationship to each other is the same. They are:

f/1·1	f/9
f/1·6	f/12·5
f/2·3	f/18
f/3·2	f/25
f/4·5	f/36
f/6·3	

Moving the iris diaphragm from one number in these series to the next (thus requiring the exposure time to be either halved or doubled) is described as an alteration of 'one stop' or as a 'whole stop'. A change from one number to the next but one in the series is an alteration of 'two stops': it will require the exposure time to be quartered or quadrupled.

Most cameras have the lens diaphragm scaled in such a series of standard numbers. In practice, especially in colour transparency work where exposure is critical, photographers may employ variations of 'half a stop' or even 'one third of a stop', and for this reason some exposure meters or other types of exposure calculator are scaled to the nearest third of a stop. In this case a typical run of numbers would be:

f/2; f/2·2; f/2·5; f/2·8; f/3·2; f/3·5; f/4.

This form of calibration includes numbers from both the British and European series. In any particular camera the maximum aperture of the lens, which can usually be found engraved on the lens mount, is quite likely to lie between a pair of standard numbers, for example f3·5.

Depth of Field

It will be remembered that depth of focus in a camera (Chapter xv) referred to the latitude available in the plane in which the film is located. From the user's point of view a much more useful piece of information is the latitude available in the plane in which the object is located; that is, when the camera lens is focused on some point we need to know to what extent other points, situated behind and in front of the first, will appear equally sharp in the photograph. This is what is meant by the term *depth of field*.

In a way similar to the production of depth of focus, latitude is available in the object plane because of the eye's acceptance of a small circle, the circle of confusion, as a point. The geometry of its occurrence is depicted simply in Fig. 16.2.

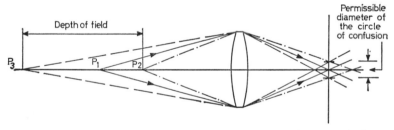

FIG. 16.2. Depth of field. The lens is focused on the point P_1. P_2 in front of this point and P_3 behind it appear acceptably sharp on the film because their images come within the permissible diameter of the circle of confusion. *By courtesy of Ilford Ltd.*

It may be noted that, unlike depth of focus, depth of field is not usually disposed equally about the plane of sharpest focus: for most subjects greater depth is available beyond the point on which the camera is focused thin in front of it.

Depth of field varies with certain factors.

(1) It is greater when the focal length of the lens is short relative to another.

(2) It is greater when the ratio of reproduction is small. This means that in close-up photography depth of field is reduced, though its disposal at

the same time becomes more symmetrical and is found to be virtually equal on either side of the plane of exact focus.

(3) It is greater as the f-number is higher.

The first two statements indicate that depth of field is much increased in a miniature camera compared with a large one and from (3) it will be apparent that the first and most flexible method of controlling depth of field in any particular instance is by means of the iris diaphragm. On stopping down the aperture greater depth is obtained.

Calculations which estimate the total depth of field in any particular case tend to be complicated and may prove inaccurate owing to the influence of factors which cannot be readily assessed: curvature of the field, for example, affects depth and a certain type of lens correction may alter its disposition in relation to the plane of sharpest focus. However, most photographers are more interested in knowing in general terms the limits of the field which will be sharp in the picture and many cameras have included on the lens mount a most useful scale for this purpose. Index marks correspond to each f-number of the diaphragm and indicate the nearest and furthest distances which are in acceptably sharp focus when the camera is focused on the distance denoted by some central indicator, usually an arrow or similar device.

THE SHUTTER

The shutter is the mechanism in the camera which controls the duration of the exposure. Like the lens the function of the shutter is intricate and sensitive. Its quality affects the efficiency, versatility and inevitably the price of the camera.

In the early history of photography the requirements of the camera shutter were not every exacting. Exposures of several seconds' duration could be satisfactorily achieved if the operator simply uncapped the lens by hand and then replaced the cover when he deemed the film to have received an adequate amount of exposure to the available light. At the present time the situation is very different from this.

The development of both faster sensitive materials and lenses of increased relative apertures has made it necessary to obtain exposure intervals of merely fractions of a second and of course these intervals must be accurately timed, in some cases down to one thousandth of a second. Efficiency of this order can be achieved only by a specifically designed, well functioning mechanism. The fundamental requirements of such a mechanism are:

(1) it should expose each part of the film equally;
(2) it should allow all the light passing through the lens at any selected aperture to strike the film for the full duration of the exposure;
(3) it should operate without vibration and without noise;
(4) it should be simple and rapid to set in motion.

In the history of photography a wide variety of shutters have been described and used. Detailed knowledge of them is not important to the student radiographer and for the present purpose we need consider only their two main categories, *lens shutters* and *focal plane shutters*.

Lens Shutter

These shutters are situated close to the lens. If the latter is simple in type the shutter may be either in front of, or behind it. However, in the case of a complex lens the usual position for the shutter is between the components. The student will remember that frequently the diaphragm also is placed here. This juxtaposition has advantages. The beam of light entering the camera is narrowest at the diaphragm and to permit and then occlude its presence the shutter's travel need be only minimal. Even illumination also is easier to obtain when the shutter is close to the diaphragm.

The simplest form of lens shutter is a thin metal plate with a slot in the centre. During exposure it is flicked across the lens from one position to another. In both its terminal positions the lens is covered, but the transit of the open slot permits light to enter the camera for a short period, usually about 1/40 second.

However, most lens shutters are of the iris diaphragm type: three or four interleaved blades uncover the lens by a rotary action, the moving force being provided by a spring. In some self-setting shutters this spring is compressed and released through a single movement of the exposure button. In others, which must be pre-set, a preliminary 'cocking' action of the exposure mechanism is required. In many modern cameras this is done when the film is wound on and this interlocking device prevents dual exposure of the film. The arrangement has advantages of considerable increase in speed and a finger-touch lightness of release. Consequently there is less likelihood of movement of the camera when the exposure is initiated.

Such shutters may provide for exposure intervals varying in duration from 1 second to 1/500 second. Very often their actual progression is arranged in a manner similar to the standard series of f-numbers, the value of each setting being halved and doubled by its immediate neighbours: thus, 1, 1/2, 1/4, 1/8, 1/15, 1/30, 1/60, 1/125, 1/250, 1/500. When this is so, a reciprocal relation can be maintained between shutter speed and lens aperture by means of a mechanical interlock between the controls of the shutter and the iris diaphragm. Alteration in the first automatically opens or closes the diaphragm in order to maintain a constant value of exposure received by the film. Many cameras in amateur use have such an 'exposure value' scale on the shutter and exposure meters or charts usually have calibration for it.

Focal Plane Shutters

The essential feature of this type of shutter is that it consists of a small blind which has across it a transverse slit and moves over the film, as close to the latter as possible. Its situation, theoretically at, and in practice very close to the focal plane, is responsible for the shutter's designation.

The speed of this type of shutter may be varied,
(a) by alteration in the tension of the spring which moves the blind,
(b) by adjustment in the width of the slit which traverses the film; in the latter case there may be either a number of slits of different dimensions or variable separation between a pair of blinds.

The outstanding advantage of the focal plane shutter is its potential speed. Exposures of the order of 1/1000 of a second are possible with it. However, it should be noted that a focal plane shutter cannot expose all parts of the image simultaneously. If the subject of the photograph is moving fast then the slit, as it traverses the film, may record on it a later phase of movement at some points relative to others. Distortion of the image inevitably results, although it will be sharp; for example, moving car wheels may appear oval.

Comparison of Shutters

It is sometimes said that focal plane shutters are more efficient than lens shutters. This is not really so. Technically the efficiency of a shutter is the ratio between the amount of light actually transmitted by it and the quantity which would have been transmitted had the shutter been fully open for the total time of the exposure. Inevitably some, perhaps small, but definite interval of time is needed before the shutter is fully open, and again time is needed for it completely to close. The bigger are these intervals the less efficient is the shutter.

In regard to the focal plane shutter, time is required for the slit to uncover the lens aperture, just as time is required for the blades of a diaphragm shutter to open. It is fair to say that the efficiency of a good

diaphragm shutter and of a focal plane shutter is about equal. In both cases efficiency is greater in two circumstances:
(a) when the lens is stopped down;
(b) when the time of exposure is long.
In relation to the first, this is because a smaller lens aperture is more quickly uncovered to its full extent. In the second case, as the time required to open the shutter fully remains virtually constant for all shutter speeds, it represents a smaller proportion of the whole interval of movement when the latter is long rather than short. Shutter efficiency is therefore relatively greater.

Each type of shutter has characteristics which may make it suitable for a particular category of work. The focal plane shutter offers the advantage of higher speeds. However, when the exposure interval is less than 1/50 second, it is less easy to synchronize with a flash light. In the case of a diaphragm shutter the most intense peak of the flash has to coincide with the moment when the shutter is fully open. However, a focal plane shutter requires the flashlamp to have a high *uniform* intensity over the whole period when the slot is moving across the film. The lamp must have constancy of output over a longer interval of time and is necessarily used at poor efficiency since its illumination is reaching only part of the film at any one moment.

In the case of any given camera it is rarely possible to choose the type of shutter employed, since the latter is usually a basic feature of the camera's design. However, the shutter available obviously is a very significant feature in selecting a camera for a particular purpose and indeed is hardly less important than the characteristics of the lens.

FOCUSING

Certain simple cameras are of the type known as *fixed focus*. This is because the lens has a small relative aperture, usually $f/11$ to $f/16$, and approximates to the condition of the pinhole camera. The latter has infinite depth of field and the image is sharp whatever may be the distance of the subject from the camera. Consequently no focusing adjustment is needed. However, with the typical fixed focus camera, for example the popular box type, the nearest distance at which sharp pictures can be obtained is 9–10 feet. In any more sophisticated camera which has a lens of larger relative aperture, the position of the focus, that is the point at which the image is sharp, depends on the distance of the subject from the camera; there must be provision for altering the distance between the lens and the film in order to maintain the latter in the plane of sharpest focus, or else a means of altering the focal length of the lens to achieve the same effect.

Focusing is performed in a number of ways depending on the type of camera concerned. A stand camera, of the type employed in photographic studios, may have a bellows extension which allows the camera front and the lens with it to move forward along rails; these are usually calibrated with a scale giving different object distances. In some cases the back of the camera may also be moved independently. Back focusing permits the object-to-lens distance to be kept constant and this is advantageous when working to a definite scale of reproduction, as for example in copying work.

In another method of camera extension, the lens is mounted on a rotating ring which gives it an axial forward or backward movement. The ring is calibrated with distances in the same way as the rails of a stand camera and this type of focusing mechanism no doubt is familiar to most people from personal experience. It is found on any miniature camera and others in general use.

Some folding cameras are focused by altering the focal length of the lens, rather than the lens-film relationship. The direct association of the conjugate distances with focal length has been discussed in Chapter xv. It will be seen from application of the lens equation that the lens-image distance can be kept constant if focal length is varied for varying object distances.

These cameras have the shutter placed between the components of a compound lens and the front component is capable of forward movement by means of mounting it on a coarse screw thread. Alteration in this way of the distance separating the two components alters the focal length of the whole assembly. It is an inexpensive method of focusing but is unsatisfactory at close distances owing to impairment of the lens' performance.

Aids to Focusing

Stand cameras—that is those mounted on a stand or tripod and not designed to be held in the hand—do not require either a view-finder or any device to assist focusing. Accurate focusing of the subject, as well as its composition, are carried out by direct vision on a ground glass screen at the rear of the camera. When the photographer is ready, the glass screen momentarily is held back by the fingers against spring tension. The cassette, carrying a sheet film of appropriate size, can then be inserted in its place and the dark-slide withdrawn ready for use.

This method of viewing and focusing has marked virtues of directness, accuracy and simplicity. However, it is slow of course and would be quite unsuitable for moving subjects. In the case of small hand cameras, reliance on the calibrated scale for most purposes is sufficiently accurate, though it is to be assumed that the photographer either can evaluate without error or is in a position to measure the distance from him of his subject. Owing to decreased depth of field, the exactness of this estimation becomes more important the closer the distance concerned.

To obviate mistakes in this category some cameras incorporate a rangefinder which is usually linked to the focusing mechanism. Essentially the range-finder consists of two small telescopes which are separated by a few inches but give images which can be seen in a single eye-piece. One of these can be swivelled to make its image coincident with its fellow's. The subject either appears as two separate whole images or is seen in two discrete halves. In either case, when alignment is secured in the range-finder, if the latter is coupled to the focusing mechanism, the lens is then correctly focused on the subject. This device offers obvious advantages of speed in operation.

The *reflex* camera adapts the direct viewing and focusing system of larger cameras. In this case the ground glass screen forms the top of the camera and the image is visualized on it by means of a plane mirror placed at 45 deg. to the lens axis. The principle of the camera is illustrated in Fig. 16.3.

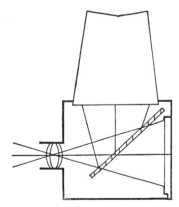

Fig. 16.3. A reflex camera. *From The Science of Photography (H. Baines) by courtesy of The Fountain Press.*

Focusing adjustments can be made and the subject viewed until the moment of exposure. Release of the shutter first moves the mirror upwards so that the image is lost on the screen and falls now on the film, correctly focused since the latter and the screen are equidistant from the lens.

To avoid the time lag required by the movement of the mirror and to enable the photographer continuously to view his subject, some reflex cameras employ a twin lens system. The upper lens is used for focusing and the lower—which is mechanically coupled to it—projects the image on the film. The main disadvantage of the device is that the image viewed on the screen is not identical with the one photographed, since the two lenses are not on the same level. The difference in viewpoint between the lenses produces an alteration in the apparent relative positions of near and distant objects. This phenomenon is known as *parallax* and the error can be significant when the subject is close to the camera. For example, in the case of a portrait it may result in failure to include on the film the upper part of the sitter's head.

THE LENS

The lens no doubt is the most important feature of any camera and to a large extent determines its suitability for a particular type of work. The optics of image formation by a lens and some aspects of lens performance have constituted a large part of the previous chapter. It is unnecessary to discuss these facts further, nor is detailed knowledge of the construction and use of different lenses required by the student radiographer. However, in this section are listed some varieties of lens, together with a little comment on their characteristics. It may be noted as an attractive feature of high quality miniature cameras that a ready interchange of lenses is possible. Thus the one instrument may be made suitable for a wide variety of work by the selection of the appropriate lens.

'Normal Focus' Lens

This term is applied to a lens of which the focal length is equal to the diagonal of the film it is intended to cover. It gives an angle of view about equal to that of the human eye when it is wandering inattentively without movement of the head. Such a lens is likely to be used at a reasonable distance from the subject, neither very close to it nor remote from it, and thus gives the appearance of a normal perspective. The angle of view provided by a lens is determined by the focal length and itself determines the amount of the subject which will be included in the film.

Wide Angle Lens

This type of lens is capable of covering a film which has a diagonal longer than the focal length of the lens. Such lenses usually embrace a field of about 75 deg., though some have been successfully constructed to include angles of as much as 180 deg. Because they are often used in confined spaces and close to important objects, they tend to give a steep, exaggerated perspective and are sometimes employed to make deliberate, though possibly false emphasis of some feature of a subject: for example, a small room can appear majestic and spacious by the use of such a lens.

Wide angle lenses are valuable for work in confined conditions where the camera-subject distance is limited, though they must be used with care if the unpleasant effects of distortion at the edges of the field are to be avoided. Their relative aperture is generally small, for example f/16.

Long Focus Lens

This lens is designed to cover a film having a diagonal markedly shorter than the focal length of the lens. It gives a concentrated narrow angle of view and is useful when a large image must be obtained of a subject which the photographer is unable to approach closely; for example it could be of value for photography in the operating theatre. A *telephoto* lens is a long focus lens of special construction which enables the camera body, i.e. the distance from the lens to the film, to be much shorter than the focal length of the lens would normally necessitate.

Varifocal Lens

This lens is probably better known as a *zoom* lens. It is often used to direct attention in cinematography or television since the camera appears to move in close to the subject. The principle of its operation is that the focal length of the lens is altered by varying the separation between its components. During this process the lens is kept focused and the f-number constant either by mechanical coupling of the controls or through a system of optical compensation. In some varifocal lenses so great an alteration in focal length is possible that the effect produced varies over the complete range of wide angle to telephoto.

CAMERAS USED FOR RADIOGRAPHY

The cameras encountered in X-ray departments in the line of duty are few and well defined in type. They are all used for photography of a fluorescent image. This is often the image observed on an intensifier during fluoroscopy and in this case the photography may include both single shots and cine recordings. Dynamic physiological processes can be studied by means of cine equipment: for example, the movement of blood through the heart or of the urinary tract during micturition. On the other hand, single shot photographs may be taken of the specially utilized fluorescent screen found in equipment for mass miniature radiography of the chest.

In all these applications, that part of the apparatus which contains the film and permits this to receive the image of the lighted screen under controlled conditions of exposure either recognizably *is* a camera, or is functioning in the capacity of one.

Cine Cameras

Cineradiography is not a new idea. In the 1930's certain leading radiologists, both in Europe and the United Kingdom, were impressed with its potentialities in physiological research, and apparatus was devised and used to record a moving image produced by X rays and subsequently to project and study it. A sinister aspect of cineradiography has been the relatively high dose of radiation which it must entail for the patient and this was certainly one consideration which discouraged its clinical application for a number of years.

However, at the present time the extended use of intensifying systems has made generally obtainable a much brighter fluoroscopic image. Concurrently with this development, the march of photographic science has been towards faster emulsions at acceptable levels of grain and contrast. As a result of these trends, and the availability of X-ray equipment offering increasingly high output, cineradiography in the armamentary of the clinical radiologist has become a practical proposition.

There is to be noticed here a distinction in terms. Cineradiography strictly is the direct cinematography of the radiographic image; that is, the film receives some or all of its exposure from X rays. The student is advised, however, to become familiar with the word *cinefluorography* for this is the procedure commonly practised at the present time. It implies recording on a continuous film, moving at a minimum speed of 16 frames per sec., the light image presented by a fluoroscopic screen.

Films recorded at speeds slower than 16 frames per sec. are often described and shown as cine films but more accurately should be called serial radiographs. The eye's persistency of vision is such that it will accept as continuous a succession of images which replace each other at the rate of 16 or more per sec. Below this figure the lag is too great for the eye successfully to merge each image into the next. Serial radiographs projected at a rate faster than that at which they were exposed result in acceleration of the movement and—if the motion was rapid—in an appearance of jerkiness.

Cinefluorography may be photography of the conventional fluorescent screen but it is much more likely that the light reaching the film will be from a system which has greatly intensified the brightness of the original image. It is not within the purpose of this book to explain or evaluate any particular method of image intensification. No doubt the student will be familiar with at least one type of intensifier from parallel studies in the M.S.R. course and perhaps from practical experience of the clinical application of such apparatus. At the present time all these units offer the possibility of a camera's insertion into the system: it may be photographing the intensified image directly or it may be coupled to a television monitor which is receiving the image.

THE TYPE OF CAMERA

Cameras used for this work have been 16 mm and 35 mm and there is a considerable field of opinion and discussion on the qualities of the results obtained. In some cases the smaller lens may be faster than that obtainable for 35 mm film and the reduction in radiation dosage which this implies is a valid argument for its use.

However, 35 mm film offers approximately four times the recording area of 16 mm and particularly when a fine grain emulsion is combined with slow, fine grain processing an image of superior detail undoubtedly is obtained. It would be very easy to improve the quality of the cinefluorographic record if no attention need be paid either to the radiation received by the subject or to the severity of the load imposed on the X-ray tube and generator. The lens-film-developer combination above described undoubtedly results in the highest quality image, though only at increased cost in radiation and electrical factors.

In adopting procedure for cinefluorography the operator must make such practical selection from the apparatus and materials available as will appear to him to produce an image of good diagnostic quality, free from grain and of satisfactory contrast, which at the same time does not require an impermissible level of radiation input. For example, it has been stated that each of the following alternatives carries comparable radiation dosage.

(1) f/2·3 lens; 35 mm film of intermediate speed; X-ray developer.
(2) f/0·95 lens; fine grain 16 mm film; slow, fine grain developer.

However, the contrast of the image obtained by (2) is bound to be lower and detail may be lost on projection. Quite apart from photographic factors, the detail of the image is further affected by the siting of the camera within the fluorographic system. When the picture is taken from a television monitor, as opposed to the intensifier itself, it may be expected that resolution will be poorer.

It is clear that the optimum balance of so many variables is not easily obtained and that the selection of an appropriate lens-film-developer combination requires both experience and nicety of judgement in the chooser.

THE SHUTTER

The shutter mechanism of cine cameras operates on a different principle from those employed for still photography. It takes the form of a disc which continuously rotates when the camera is in action. The disc has a cut out or open sector which will allow light to reach the film and a solid or closed sector which will cover the film during that interval of time when the latter is being moved forward, ready for exposure of the next 'frame'. The rotation of the disc is synchronized with the film movement. Camera speed can be controlled to suit different subjects and effects. For example motion can appear to be accelerated if the film is exposed at a slower speed (small number of frames per second) than that at which it is subsequently projected. Conversely, rapid movement can be slowed and in consequence more readily analysed if it is filmed at a high number of frames per second and projected at the conventional rate of 24 f.p.s.

The matter of filming speeds may appear a little confusing to the student. Sixteen frames per second was used originally for silent cinematography because it is the minimum speed which will give a smooth appearance of movement. Later when sound was introduced, a rate of 24 f.p.s. was adopted because this allowed more space for better sound quality. Television uses a framing speed of 25 f.p.s.

In many commercially available cine cameras the shutter-open time is 180 deg.: this means that the pull-down of the film occurs during half a revolution of the rotating disc and exposure occurs during the next half turn. Thus, if the camera is driven at 25 f.p.s. the film is exposed for half of 1/25th (i.e. 1/50th) of a second. Increasing the number of frames per second, as might be required for a rapidly moving subject, necessarily decreases the actual interval of exposure. In terms of cinefluorography this would mean the use of higher milliamperages to obtain adequate density of the film and associated with it would be implications of heavier tube loading and increased patient dosage.

Because of these factors some cameras have been designed specifically for cinefluorography, with improvement of the ratio between the shutter-open period and the film pull-down. The latter is accelerated and the shutter has a 270 deg. clear sector: that is, it is closed for only a quarter and open for three quarters of the period of one revolution. At 25 f.p.s. this would result in an exposure interval of approximately 1/30 second, with consequent lightening of the tube load and reduced patient dosage. A typical 35 mm camera planned for cinefluorography has a lens aperture of f/0·75, a 270 deg. shutter and a speed variable from 0 to 50 frames per second. This is an instrument capable of a very satisfactory performance.

The use of the phrase 'slow' or 'fast' shutter should be noted. A 90 deg. shutter is faster than one of 270 deg. because it is bound to give a shorter interval of exposure.

It may be observed that a camera synchronized with half-wave rectified 50-cycle mains supplied to an X-ray tube and driven at 25 f.p.s. would not require a shutter at all, provided the film movement were timed to occur during the suppressed half cycle and the fluorescent screen had no appreciable afterglow. This arrangement was in fact used during earlier cinefluorographic work.

A currently more important aspect of correct phase relationship occurs when the camera is photographing the image presented on a television monitor. Here it is essential that the camera be driven at a speed which is a multiple of the frequency with which the picture appears on the monitor and is in correct phase relationship with it. If the phasing is wrong, an unexposed bar will appear on each frame of the film, due to the fact that the shutter was open during a blank interval on the television screen, Synchronization and phasing of the camera can be achieved if it is driven by a phased synchronous motor operating from the same mains supply as the television system, but the limitations imposed by the phasing may preclude cinematography at high speeds.

Video Tape Recording

Systems of image storage which have become available seem to indicate that cinefluorography in the future will be done without a conventional camera. The conversion of the fluorescent image to an electronic signal is now an established technique. It is possible to transfer the latter to a magnetic tape in a process similar to sound recording. The video tape can be 'played back' on a T.V. monitor or on any number of monitors. No special projection equipment is needed. The system has been in use for commercial television, particularly in America, for some time. A sound commentary can be either included on the tape at the time of the original recording or added to it later.

Video tape for cinefluorography offers certain advantages. Briefly these are as follows.

(1) No processing is required. The recorded examination can be viewed at once. This feature would be particularly valuable during procedures such as angio-cardiography.

(2) The system entails a smaller radiation dose for the subject than does an equivalent record on film. This is because the tube factors chosen for fluoroscopy—of the order perhaps of 0.5 to 2 mA at 80 to 115 kVp—require no alteration for video tape. Even the fastest film used with a wide aperture lens is bound to need more 'exposure' than this and tube milliamperages five or six times greater may be noted in the course of filming.

(3) Video tape can be used again and again if the image is first erased. The tape is expensive but each reel provides virtually two hours' running time. The image is satisfactory for retention as a permanent record if desired and sections of particular interest in a reel can be cut and made into short loops, similarly to conventional film.

(4) The contrast and brightness of the taped image are very flexible since they can be varied through the appropriate controls of the viewing monitor to suit the taste of an individual observer at any time. A processed film certainly cannot offer this kind of freedom.

Video tape has replaced cine film in many applications and seems likely to continue to do so. Its projection—like that of cine film—can be slowed to facilitate analysis of rapid movement. However, in this respect it is perhaps the less satisfactory recording agent. Its slow motion is not so smooth as in the case of a film which can be exposed at high speeds and projected at much lower speeds without the introduction of perceptible jerkiness. In respect of video tape the fact that we are looking at a slow succession of individual frames tends to be intrusive and a total appreciation of the movement studied becomes more difficult to obtain. For this reason cinefluorography of the cardiac image on film —particularly if the patient is a child—retains its supporters, although video tape may often be used in these circumstances as the ideal means of making a preliminary survey.

Still Camera Units

MASS MINIATURE RADIOGRAPHY

The use of a miniature camera and 35 mm roll film to record a single image of the fluorescent screen has been long established as a means of rapidly and inexpensively submitting a large number of people to X-ray examination of the chest. These cameras had a lens aperture of f/1·5 and a focal length of 50 mm.

However, to a very large extent the 35 mm camera in this context has been replaced by 70 mm and 100 mm systems. These units will be considered in more detail in the next chapter but it may be noticed that they do not include a recognizable camera of any conventional type.

The image of the fluorescent screen is obtained not through a lens but by means of a concave focusing mirror (the Bouwers concentric mirror system). The mirror system is considerably faster than the refractive lens previously in use for this work: for example, the 'Odelca' 100 mm camera has a relative aperture of f/0·65 (focal length 213 mm) and the 70 mm camera has a relative aperture of f/0·63 (focal length 160 mm). This represents a difference of about two 'stops'; that is, the mirror system provides a speed approximately four times greater than that of the refractive lens. The reduction in radiation dosage and the facility of using a larger film in single cut sheets, with equivalent or improved radiographic detail, both offer obvious radiological advantages and sufficiently explain the present ascendancy of these camera units.

Recording the Intensified Image

Several types of equipment are available for single shot photography of the appearance on the image intensifier. As in the case of the cine camera, these units may record the image either off an associated television monitor or directly from the anode phosphor of the intensifier tube. Each system has its own advantages and disadvantages and the choice between them is largely a matter of the personal opinions of the user.

From the T.V. Monitor

The advantages of recording the image produced by an intensifier system and visualized on a television monitor are several fold.

(1) The monitor and its associated camera need not be in the same room as the X-ray apparatus and could be, for example, directly in the processing room.

(2) The system is therefore space- and weight-saving in the X-ray room.

(3) No increase in the X-ray tube current is needed for filming and therefore the exposure can be made more quickly: there is no delay while tube filament circuits are boosted and the anode brought up to speed.

(4) The density of the film can be flexibly adjusted by means of the brightness and contrast controls on the television monitor.

(5) The operator can readily see what is being recorded.

(6) A lower dosage to the patient is implicit in (3).

However, there are certain indisputable *disadvantages* in making a film record in this way.

(1) The image inevitably loses some sharpness and brightness in the television system.

(2) The T.V. monitor is notoriously the least stable part of the intensifier system. This is not to say that it is mechanically or electrically unsound and subject to frequent breakdown; but it *is* subject to voltage variations. These variations are noticeable when the light reaching the television pick-up tube is poor—as it always is in the case of the conversion of an X-ray beam compared with the light levels of, for example, a television studio. The voltage fluctuations on the monitor in turn produce variations in film blackening which impair radiographic quality.

(3) The line-scanning process on which all television relay depends may result in a visible pattern of lines upon the film.

In the case of poor quality equipment the above features would certainly outweigh the good points earlier listed. Nevertheless, considerable advances have been made in the photography of the monitor image. Components can be carefully selected and circuits stabilized to ensure that the output of the cathode ray tube—and consequently light levels and degrees of film blackening—remain constant. The cathode ray tube itself is specially made. It is described as being a 4 in. × 6 in. tube which gives a circular field 3 1/4 in. (90 mm) in diameter. It has a fine line scan (625 double interlaced lines per frame) and an optically flat face for better definition over the whole field.

With this television monitor a variety of cameras can be used; for example, 35 mm or 16 mm cine cameras are suitable. If single shot photography is intended, the use of 100 mm cut film (4 in. × 4 in.) is particularly appropriate in view of its 1 to 1 ratio with the field of the cathode ray tube.

A separator cassette similar to those described in the next chapter (p. 394) is associated with a box camera which has a simple lens, no focusing mount and a shutter operating (by means of a relay) at 1/25 sec. When the exposure is completed a wedge with a guillotine action pushes the exposed film from its leading position in the supply magazine into the receiving magazine and the cassette is immediately ready for the next exposure. The simplicity of the camera's optical system means that very little light is lost between the cathode ray tube and the film and this offers obvious advantages in increased efficiency.

If the T.V. monitor and camera were situated in the darkroom it is not beyond the bounds of possibility for the receiving cassette to feed films directly into an automatic processor designed for 100 mm film (see p. 407). This is a high degree of automation indeed.

Another type of camera which has been—and is being—used for recording the monitor image is the Polaroid-Land camera described in Chapter 1. This offers a means of obtaining a dry print within a few seconds which, if so desired, may be immediately enclosed in the patient's notes.

FROM THE INTENSIFIER TUBE

From the viewpoint of picture quality the best method of photographing the appearances of the fluorescent screen undoubtedly is to record the image directly from the anode of the intensifier tube—assuming that the intensification system includes such a tube. The image on the anode phosphor is at its sharpest and brightest and so logically this is the position from which it should be photographed. Furthermore, the image is necessarily free of the scanning lines and 'noise' inherent in television systems. (*Noise* is the term used in electronics for the intrusion on a television signal produced by extraneous variations in current through any of a number of components; it is inevitably present in some degree, although in good equipment it is minimal.)

However, there are *disadvantages* associated with the method.

(1) The camera must be attached to the image intensifier, thus adding to the bulk and weight of the equipment which the radiologist must handle during fluoroscopy. The camera could add 30–40 lbs. extra load.

(2) Before each exposure, fluoroscopic values of X-ray tube current must be boosted to a level suitable for radiography and the anode of the X-ray tube accelerated to full speed. This means a minimum interval between exposures of 1–2 secs. which in practice may be a few seconds longer depending on the mechanism employed for moving the film into a position ready for exposure. However, in some cases the filming procedure can be made more rapid by maintaining the exposure handswitch in the 'prepare' position so that the tube anode does not slacken its speed.

(3) There is inherently a bigger radiation dose to the patient owing to the increase in exposure factors for radiography.

Direct photography of the image on the output phosphor of the intensifier tube depends upon a mirror of the light-splitting type. This is a partially silvered mirror which reflects some portion of a beam of light and permits another portion to pass through it. In the equipment the light from the image intensifier tube passes through a tandem arrangement of back to back lenses with the beam-splitting mirror operating between them.

For photography of the fluorescent image the mirror is automatically moved into a position from which it allows most of the light to reach the camera—and thus the film—while only a small portion reaches the T.V. system and the observer. A student who has seen this kind of equipment in operation will have noticed how faint the television picture becomes during filming. This is because only about 10 per cent of the light from the image intensifier is reaching the television pick-up tube and operating the monitor.

During fluoroscopy of course the beam-splitting mirror is in a position which favours the observer at the expense of the camera. The change-over of the mirror from fluoroscopy to photography occurs during the 'prepare' period for the X-ray generator. It is one more reason why this cannot be so rapid a method of photography as filming of the television monitor.

Photography from the output phosphor of an image intensifier tube is equally possible as a cine record or in single shots. A single-shot camera may utilize 100 mm cut film in interchangeable supply and take-up magazines of the kind described in the next chapter (p. 394). This camera has a shutter which is situated in the optical system (see p. 363) and automatically opens on the 'prepare' position of the handswitch.

Another camera which is available employs perforated 70 mm roll film. It is associated with a 9/5 in. image intensifier and has a 9 in.

(210 mm) lens pre-focused on infinity with a fixed aperture of f/4·5. It projects a circle 63 mm in diameter. This camera does not have a shutter. It is versatile, as it will take not only single shots but exposures at the rate of 3 or 6 frames per second which would be suitable for recording movements of a slow character.

The choice between 70 mm and 100 mm film is very much a matter of personal opinion and experience. Processing aspects of both films are discussed in Chapter xviii. The 70 mm film is rather more difficult to view as it requires magnification and when cut into short lengths shows a tendency to curl. Its smaller format seems in some instances to give a brighter image of better detail, but this is an appearance rather than a positive reality. On balance, the 100 mm is probably the more popular format generally speaking: the films are easier to handle and the camera itself less bulky.

CHAPTER XVII

Fluorography: Equipment

The photography of the fluorescent image has received some attention in the previous chapter, specifically in relation to certain types of camera which may be employed for it. It is necessary now to consider in greater detail what is implied in some aspects of this procedure and what features are significant in X-ray units designed for the work.

A patient interposed between a source of X rays and a fluorescent screen with which he is in contact will produce on the screen an image of approximately life-size; in fact it is magnified to some extent owing to the comparatively short anode-screen distance generally employed. When this image is photographed by means of either a lens or an optical system which may replace such a lens then it becomes reduced in scale and the result is described as a miniature radiograph.

By far the commonest, though not the only application of this principle has been in making X-ray examinations of the chest among large groups of the populace, and few terms in radiographic practice can be more familiar to the general public than the name *mass miniature radiography*. This nomenclature has largely been replaced in technical references by expressions more accurately descriptive of the procedure; *fluorography, photo-fluorography* or *radio-photography* may all be encountered by the student.

The principal advantages of the system no doubt are well known. The miniature is very much cheaper than a full-size 14 × 17 in. radiograph and since the film is mechanically advanced or changed in the camera examinations can be performed in a rapid sequence. When such units undertake large surveys it is usual to have two operators, one of whom remains at the control table, while the other is responsible for radiographic positioning and centring. Other members of the team document and marshal the patients prior to examination and ensure their free outflow on its completion. In this way the time required for the radiography of each subject is very short, of the order of a few seconds, and in practice the pace of the system is probably set by the clerical staff who have to complete the patients' identification cards.

THE CAMERA UNIT

The basic arrangement of all fluorographic units is sketched in Fig. 17.1. It is seen that the camera, whatever its type, is placed at the end of a light-tight tunnel which connects it to the fluorescent screen. The image reaching the camera is a light image only, owing to the sheet of clear lead glass which covers the fluorescent surface of the screen. Between the patient and the screen is situated a secondary radiation grid (not shown in the diagram). By means of a side-arm or some equivalent arrangement the X-ray tube is linked to the screen and is centred upon it, as also is the camera through the light-tight tunnel; all three therefore move together as a single unit and centring in respect of the patient can be readily executed through a single control lever. This moves the whole assembly up or down upon its supporting columns, the mechanism being usually power-assisted in view of the weight of the equipment. A typical unit for fluorography is depicted in Plate 17.1, following p. 206.

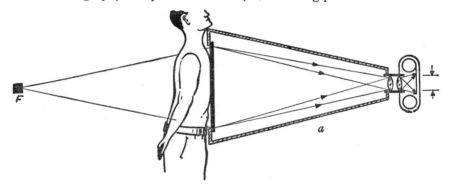

Fig. 17.1. Outline sketch of essential equipment for fluorography; an X-ray source and a fluorescent screen connected by a light-tight tunnel to a camera. The image on the screen is recorded by the camera on a miniature film. *By courtesy of The Centrex Publishing Company (Philips Technical Library)*.

In summary we can say that fluorography requires the following equipment.
(1) An H.T. generator and X-ray tube.
(2) A fluorescent screen.
(3) A camera, by which is meant an optical instrument to form the image and a suitable film holder to allow it to be recorded on a sensitive emulsion.

THE CAMERA

It has already been mentioned that the first cameras used for mass radiography were 35 mm and employed a coated refractive lens of a conventional type. This was centred and focused on the fluorescent screen by means of an optical device which was reputedly accurate to within one thousandth of an inch. In theory once this determination had been made during installation of the unit, the lens by virtue of the camera's rigid construction remained indefinitely in correct relationship to the fluorescent screen. In practice of course its setting would be examined at intervals.

The camera incorporated two cassettes; one contained unexposed film, while the other received the exposed portion of the roll. Each had a capacity of 25 metres of film, this being sufficient for some 720 35 mm radiographs. At any time, as a daylight operation, the exposed film cassette could be removed and an empty spare cassette recoupled to the remainder of the roll. This facility of course is necessary in using roll film if any particular series of radiographs are to remain together as a discrete group and not run into others which may follow them on the reel but are not related to them by any significant factors of occasion or subject.

The exposed film cassette incorporated a guillotine for shearing the film and could not be removed from the camera until this had operated. The unexposed film cassette possessed a recording device which indicated the amount of film remaining on the reel. Electrically interlocking contacts in the camera prevented any exposure being made if the film were not correctly inserted, had failed to advance at the termination of exposure, or had become exhausted. Some of these features—easy removal of the film, recording devices and electrical interlocks—continue to be found in the more advanced equipment in use at the present time.

The Bouwers Concentric Mirror System

Advances in mirror optics have led to the development of fluorographic equipment in which an optical system replaces the refractive lens in the camera. Allusion has been made in the previous chapter to the practical aspects of the mirror system. Briefly they are:

(1) simpler construction;
(2) wider relative aperture, with even illumination from the centre to the periphery of the field;

(3) a focal length approximately 3 to 4 times greater, resulting in a larger radiographic image and improved appreciation of detail.

In any radiograph which must be enlarged for viewing, by either a magnifying glass or a projector, clarity of detail may be lost owing to the perceptible graininess which occurs on magnification to a high power. Because of this possibility emulsions for fluorography should be of fine grain. They are consequently slower than other X-ray emulsions and this is a reason why the procedure requires more radiant energy than full-scale radiography of a comparable subject.

No reasonable assessment can be made of a 35 mm radiograph unless it is enlarged considerably. The mirror cameras now in use yield pictures which are 70 mm or 100 mm square. The larger of these seldom require magnification and radiological reports are commonly made simply from direct vision of the radiograph. For the smaller film projection up to full size or the use of a magnifying glass are no doubt advantageous, but in any event less magnification is required than for a 35 mm film.

Mirror optical systems used in fluorography depend on a spherical mirror; this is a curved mirror of which the reflecting surface is defined as part of the surface of a sphere. This is shown in Fig. 17.2. As might be

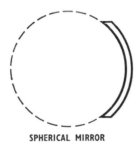

SPHERICAL MIRROR

Fig. 17.2. Diagram of a spherical mirror. The reflecting surface is part of the surface of a sphere. *By courtesy of Kodak Ltd.*

anticipated the image formed by such a mirror is subject to spherical aberration (Chapter xv). In the Bouwers concentric mirror system, now widely employed, this is corrected by means of a low power lens which has a spherical error opposite to that of the mirror; the two elements possess a common centre of curvature and the general scheme is depicted diagrammatically in Fig. 17.3a. In Fig. 17.3b a cone lens has been added for improvement of the system's resolving power. It should be noted that the focal plane is curved. (Chapter xv; curvature of field.)

28

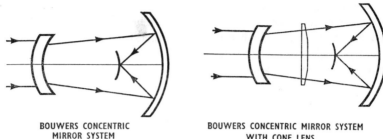

BOUWERS CONCENTRIC
MIRROR SYSTEM

BOUWERS CONCENTRIC MIRROR SYSTEM
WITH CONE LENS

a

b

FIG. 17.3. (a) The Bouwers concentric mirror system used for fluorography in place of a refractive lens. Light from the fluorescent screen (depicted as parallel arrowed lines) passes through a correcting lens; this lens eliminates spherical distortion produced by the mirror. The mirror reflects and converges the light on a convex focal plane.

(b) The Bouwers concentric mirror system with the addition of a cone lens to improve resolution. *By courtesy of Kodak Ltd.*

With this arrangement definition over the whole area of the field and the resolution obtained are so good that on high powered magnification the fine structure of the secondary radiation grid can be seen to be recorded on the film. The thickness of the lead elements is 0·07 mm.

The complete arrangement of the camera unit is shown in its fundamentals in Fig. 17.4. It will be appreciated from this and from the illustration appearing in Plate 17.1 that the spherical mirror is of a size comparable with the fluorescent screen. A large mirror increases the speed of the apparatus.

Summarizing these points we can say that in the majority of fluorographic units at present in use the camera is of the mirror type and that its optical system consists of:

(1) a spherical concave mirror;
(2) a meniscus correcting lens;
(3) a cone lens.

EXPOSURE CONTROL

A camera used for fluorography of course does not require a shutter. Exposure is effected in the X-ray generating system and its duration controlled usually by a photo-electric timer.

The full operation of this type of radiographic timer is not within the intended scope of this book and no doubt the student will study its detail

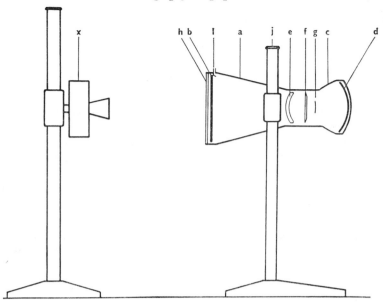

FIG. 17.4. Schematic arrangement of camera unit for fluorography. *By courtesy of Kodak Ltd.*

a ... c	The camera tunnel.
b	Fluorescent screen.
d	Concentric mirror.
e	Correcting lens.
f	Cone lens.
g	Film at focal plane.
h	Secondary radiation grid.
i	Card-holder for film identification.
j	Camera stand.
x	X-ray tube.

in another connection. In resumé we may say that the essential difference between this timer and others used in radiographic practice is that the photo-timer does not mark a specific physical period but terminates exposure when the film has received a pre-determined energy which will give it on development a certain density. If the subject is thin and a high tube tension is selected, then the actual time of exposure will be short. If converse conditions obtain, then the interval is bound to be longer—how much longer can only be appreciated by observation of the milliampere-seconds meter and the requisite mental arithmetic, since the radiographer receives no direct indication of the *time* of exposure. With this type of apparatus the exposure interval cannot be pre-set but can be only recorded.

The photo-electric cell on which the fluorographic photo-timer depends receives part of the light from each apical area of the lungs. It is this quantity which determines the duration of the exposure. Within certain obvious limits of over- and under-exposure, there is a considerable range of individual opinion on the densities which constitute a well exposed radiograph of the chest. To allow for variations in the criteria of the examining radiologist or chest physician, or for a change in film speed, a density control is incorporated in the photo-timer. An adjustable knob can be set to any chosen position in a scale numbered perhaps from 0 to 10: these figures are arbitrary, unrelated to any form of densitometric calibration, and there only for convenience.

This selector knob is easily accessible but once its position has been decided it should not be subjected to frequent alteration by the operator. To use the density control to increase the exposure obtained for an obese patient is to make nonsense of the photo-timer's principle and purpose. Equally incorrect is the assumption that the presence of photo-electric timing will produce a satisfactory radiograph in any circumstance. The operator has still to make a proper selection of tube kilovoltage and in doing this the presence of the grid, the relatively slower response of the film and the limitations of the optical system should be remembered. Tube tensions appropriate to fluorography usually are above those in general employment for direct radiography of the chest. A well established practice, though one perhaps not very commonly employed, is to relate their determination to the anteroposterior diameter of the thorax and a known satisfactory exposure for a 'normal' or average subject.

A timer called the Iontomat also is in use for the automatic control of fluorographic and indeed other radiographic exposures. The principle is the same as that just described but a distinguishing feature of its operation is that the radio-sensitive element is not a photo-electric cell but an ionization chamber. It should be noted that this is passing current in proportion to the quantity of X rays incident upon it, whereas the photo-electric cell responds to light. However the foregoing discussion on exposure control is equally applicable to either device.

FILM IDENTIFICATION

Proper film identification is an important part of all radiographic procedures. It has been said that an undated radiograph is without value; even more obvious is the necessity to attach to each film the correct

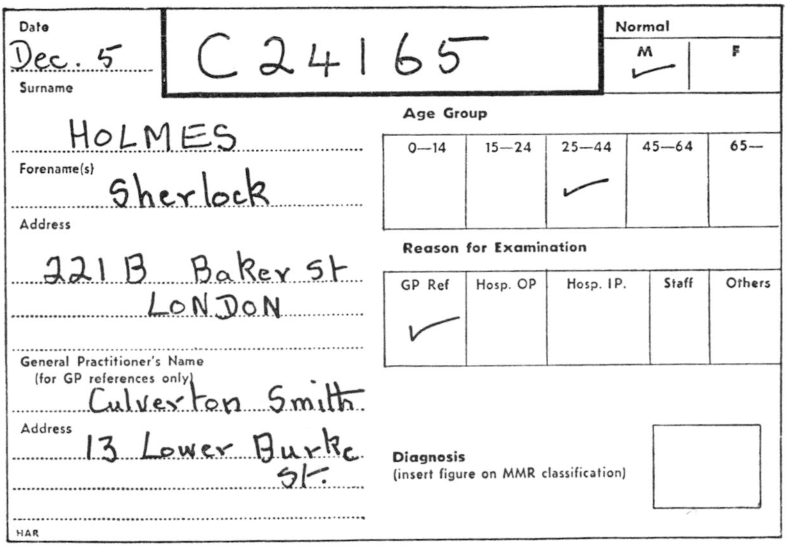

Date		Normal	
Dec. 5 $C \ 2 \ 4 \ 1 \ 6 \ 5$		M ✓	F
Surname			

	Age Group				
HOLMES	0—14	15—24	25—44	45—64	65—
Forename(s) Sherlock			✓		

Address	Reason for Examination				
221 B Baker St. LoNDoN	GP Ref	Hosp. OP	Hosp. IP.	Staff	Others
	✓				

General Practitioner's Name
(for GP references only) Culverton Smith.

Address 13 Lower Burke St.

Diagnosis
(insert figure on MMR classification)

HAR

FIG. 17.5. Identification card for use with a fluorographic unit. Only details printed in the upper central frame are recorded on the fluorogram.

patient's name or record number. In the case of a miniature radiograph the latter may be more practicable. The length and nature of a name cannot be foreseen and the legend preferably should appear large enough for reading without the aid of a magnifier; figures also have the advantage in mass surveys that they can be serially printed in advance on an appropriate number of cards. However, from the operative aspect of providing fluorographic units with an automatic means of film identification it is immaterial whether a name or a number is recorded.

The method adopted is photographic; that is selected details from a record card are photographed by the camera at the same time as the fluorescent image—in fact under automatic control it occurs immediately on completion of the X-ray exposure. For this purpose the patient's card must be placed in front of the camera in a suitable relationship to the fluorescent screen and illuminated for an appropriate interval. In the older 35 mm units the card was fed into a slot at the top of the camera tunnel. In the 'Odelca' 100 mm and 70 mm units, a card tray is provided below the fluorescent screen and can be pulled forwards by means of a handle to permit the card's inspection. Plate 17.2, following p. 206 shows the card-holder in the open position.

The card is a standard size, in Europe 7 × 3 ¼ in. (187·3 × 82·6 mm) and in the United Kingdom 6 × 4 in., but only a limited area, 90 × 20 mm, is actually recorded on the film. This rectangle, known as the *identity frame*, may occupy the top left or right hand corner or the top middle portion of the card, as shown in Fig. 17.5. Its position is indicated on the card by a heavy black line. Though different sizes of cards may be employed through the provision of an appropriate card holder, the dimensions of the identity frame are fixed: within it should be written or printed prominently the patient's number or name.

In use, as each patient presents with his card it is placed in the tray and the latter pushed into the closed position for exposure. Illumination of the card is provided by a small fluorescent tube within the holder and in order to obtain a constant density from the card's exposure, irrespective of film speed, the operation of this light is usually through the discharge of a suitable condenser in the feed unit. In certain equipment a control knob may be provided to adjust the card's exposure to the correct density and a monitor lamp to indicate that the card has received exposure.

The legend, whether number or name, appears on the radiograph in a central position along its lower border, that is in the subphrenic area of the chest where it is easy to read and unlikely to obscure any feature of diagnostic significance.

The camera unit incorporates a number of important electrical inter-locks to ensure that it is impossible to take a radiograph which is not positively related to the person examined. The function of these means that:

(1) no film is transported from the magazine to its correct position in the focal plane unless there is a card ready for exposure in the holder;
(2) no subsequent exposure can be made until the card is changed.

It is evident that in this equipment considerable thought in design and executant skill have been devoted to the end that film identification shall be a fool-proof procedure. However, sad experience must add the observation that it is possible to obtain a radiographic exposure from the unit if the card either is inserted upside down, or back to front, or is incomplete. In this unhappy circumstance of course no legend can appear on the radiograph to which it relates.

It is common practice to date the radiograph simultaneously with its exposure. In distinction to the previous procedure this is not done photographically. The X-ray tube itself, in making the radiographic exposure, records on the fluorescent screen and thus on the film the image of a group of perforated metal figures suitably arranged in a small frame. This can be fixed in any convenient area on the front of the unit; for example it should not obscure any significant feature if it is placed in an upper corner or immediately below the chin rest. It is of course necessary for the operator to remember to change the appropriate numerals at the beginning of each day.

FILM FORMATS

The photographic characteristics required in emulsions used for fluorography will be considered in the next chapter. Our present concern is with the size of film necessary and its suitability for various purposes.

Fluorographic units currently in use employ film in a number of formats. The following dimensions are available:

(a) 3 m × 70 mm roll film, each reel being sufficient for 40 exposures;

(b) 100 ft. (30 metres) × 70 mm roll film which is sufficient for 450 exposures;

(c) 100 mm × 100 mm in single sheets;

(d) 70 mm × 70 mm in single sheets.

The last in fact is little used in present practice.

The category of film employed will depend upon the type of work which the fluorographic unit is to handle. The larger film offers the sound radiological advantage of easier visibility of detail, so that any subsequent recall of subjects for a full-scale radiograph should be minimal. However, there are other considerations.

Where the unit is demountable and has to be assembled at different sites of operation, or where its installation is within the confines of a touring caravan or truck, the smaller size and weight of the 70 mm apparatus may prove decisive factors in its choice. It further represents a possible saving of film costs, though this is comparatively slight.

When the number of candidates for examination is very large, of the order of several hundred, roll film—as opposed to cut film—is speedier to handle. This is particularly true of its processing: the advantage offered in the actual rate at which examinations can be made is relatively small.

A helpful feature of cut film is that when circumstances make it desirable a single radiograph can be exposed, removed and processed at once to meet an individual need. Of equal benefit is the facility of being able to compare side by side a number of radiographs of the same patient taken over a period of time.

The 100 mm cut film is undoubtedly the one of choice for an installation handling a small variable number of candidates in the range 0 to 50. This is group radiography rather than mass radiography and 100 mm camera units are frequently found in hospital where they may undertake the examination of all out-patients' chests, those of members of staff and perhaps other selected groups such as patients referred by their general practitioners and contacts with cases of pulmonary tubercle.

Because of the higher radiation input which fluorography requires and to avoid the possibility of incurring further dosage from subsequent examination on a large film, it is not usual to survey on these camera units either pregnant women or anyone occupationally exposed to ionizing radiation. Both the dose factor and the unpredictable, and usually longer intervals of exposure inherent in the operation of the photo-timer make children also—up to the age of about 14 years—unfavourable subjects for examination by this method.

FILM CASSETTES AND MAGAZINES

The type of magazine which the camera unit incorporates is dictated by the size of film which it will employ. Several cassettes are available. It is well to note in regard to the loading of those associated with a system of mirror optics that the sensitized surface of the film (fluorographic emulsions are coated on one side of the base only) should face *away* from the X-ray tube: that is, this aspect will be then towards the reflecting surface of the mirror. If error occurs it will be with cut film, since the pack can be as easily placed with the emulsions facing the wrong aspect of the cassette as the correct way round. The mistake will not be discovered until the films are processed and this may not be until fifty examinations have been made.

Single Film Cassette

It is possible that the student will see references to a single film cassette in manufacturers' leaflets but it is not in contemporary use to any extent. It is available for supply with the 70 mm camera and allows a single 70 mm × 70 mm sheet to be exposed for test purposes. This could be to make a check of exposure or perhaps in order to examine a single subject. The facility appears to be so little needed, however, that the student is unlikely to meet this cassette in the course of any practical experience with 70 mm units.

The most interesting feature of this cassette is the curved pressure plate which holds the film within a frame for exposure in a slight arc, corresponding to that of the focal plane. This convex plate is necessary because of the camera's curvature of field (Chapter xv). It is precision made and should be handled carefully to avoid any risk of abrasion, since this type of damage may result in a localized loss of definition in the radiographic image. Such unsharpness arises because indentations and prominences on the surface of the plate may interfere with the film's critical alignment with the focal plane.

Because of the curvature of field, this convex platten is a feature of all the cassettes used in fluorographic mirror cameras but in the others to be described it is less accessible and for that reason perhaps less likely to come to harm from careless handling. However, it should be noticed by the student as an important part of the unit.

Serial Cassette

This cassette is depicted in Plate 17.3, following p. 206. It has an interchangeable magazine which will accept 70 mm film in lengths of 3 metres. The magazines can be changed in daylight and a spare one is provided with the cassette. A darkroom of course is necessary in order to load the magazine with fresh film. Since each roll permits 40 exposures the number of examinations which can be made at one time is a little restricted, unless a suitable darkroom or a sufficient number of already loaded magazines are available.

The operation of the serial cassette is manual, by means of the large turning handle, a new 'frame' of the film being thus wound into position for exposure. An electrical interlock is included to prevent subsequent exposures should the operator inadvertently omit this, or should the film fail to wind forwards correctly. The number of completed exposures is indicated by a counter and each magazine contains sufficient for 40 examinations.

The serial cassette is not in wide use, no doubt owing to its small capacity and the need for manual operation.

The M.C.S. Cassette

The letters here stand for *mass chest survey*. The appearance of the cassette is shown in Plate 17.4, following p. 206 and it is mounted on the side of the camera in the position seen in Plate 17.5, following p. 206.

It can be appreciated from Plate 17.4 that the M.C.S. cassette has two large magazines, incorporating a feed spool and a take-up spool, each capable of accepting 100 feet (30 metres) of 70 mm film. This cassette is designed for the examination of large numbers and is employed in many mass radiography units.

The film is wound forwards automatically in the cassette, each frame being numerically recorded by a numbering device. This has numerals 9999 to 0 and can be set by hand to any required number within this range. It can usefully be employed to indicate to the operator the number of exposures still available on the reel, each full reel being sufficient for 450 examinations. The take-up magazine incorporates a cutter to shear the film. This permits the removal of the magazine and its contents at any time. Thus processing can be undertaken after any number of exposures, up to that of the complete reel, has been made. To decrease fatigue in a reporting session it might be helpful, for example, to cut the film after every 75 examinations so that interpretation could be made in blocks of reasonable length. However, while this is a practicable procedure for a camera operating at base, it would complicate the operation of a unit on tour.

A further refinement of this cassette is a device which enables any particular frame, or perhaps a number of frames, to be identified—even by touch in the darkroom if necessary. This is hand-operated and essentially is a punch which nicks the edge of the film at the selected frame. It could be useful as a means of rapidly identifying in a roll a radiograph requiring early report or special selection for any other reasons of survey.

Apart from the insertion of the roll of film in the supply magazine, loading of the M.C.S. cassette is a daylight operation. The cassette is actually a T-shaped structure, the part visible outside the camera being the cross arm of the letter. The leg of the T projects into the camera to the focal plane. It is in fact a double leg: at the terminus of one limb is a frame and at the terminus of the other a convex platten which will hold the film against the frame when it is ready for exposure. Explanation of the loading procedure will be easier to follow if reference is made to Fig. 17.6.

A large control knob on the front of the cassette, which can be seen in Plate 17.4, is unlocked by a clockwise twist and pulled towards the operator. This action withdraws the platten on a guide rod from the camera into the body of the cassette. The pressure frame remains in position. The free end of the reel of film in the supply magazine (on the right in Plate 17.4) is drawn straight through the cassette into the take-up magazine (on the left in Plate 17.4) by means of a simple guide. This is composed of two thin strips of metal fastened together at one end and

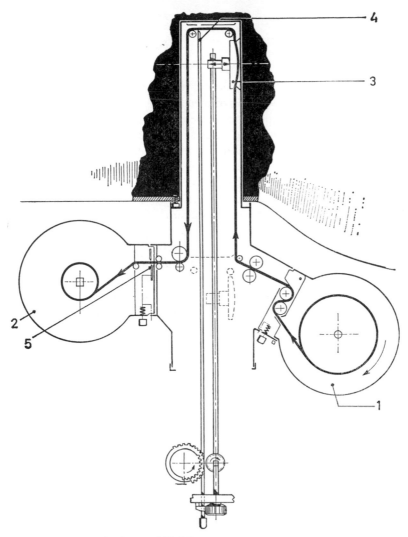

FIG. 17.6. Internal scheme of M.C.S. cassette.

(1) Supply magazine with feed spool.

(2) Take-up magazine with spool.

(3) Platten in position in the focal plane; the convexity of the film as it is held by the platten against the pressure frame should be noted.

(4) Identification device which can be operated to nick the edge of the film at any selected point, and facilitate its selection on the roll. The cutter is withdrawn during loading of the cassette.

(5) Guillotine to shear the film and permit removal of the take-up magazine at any time.

The dotted outline seen between the magazines indicates the position of the platten during the loading process. The leading end of the film is thus free to pass through the cassette, as indicated by the broken horizontal line. *By courtesy of N.V. Optische Industrie de Oude Delft.*

designed to pass easily through slots at the front of the cassette. The film is then fitted between the leaves of metal and is held by them. When the guide is drawn back through the cassette the film necessarily follows it. It can then be released from the guide and fed into the take-up magazine.

With the film now engaged in the magazine, the central rod, which has the platten at its other extremity, is pushed back into the camera by means of the control knob. It carries ahead of it a loop of film which thus passes between the platten and the pressure frame. When the control knob is locked again the operation of a cam behind the platten moves the latter into contact with the frame and thus holds the film in correspondence with the convexity of the focal plane. To facilitate movement of the film through the camera, four nylon runners are fitted at the end of the guide rod just beyond the pressure plate.

During the loading operation the loop of film between the two magazines necessarily is exposed to daylight, as indeed must be any 'trailer' in a roll film camera. However, the total loss is very small: it represents the sum of 7 frames.

Like the serial cassette the M.C.S. cassette has interlocks which prevent incorrect operation. If the film becomes torn or the magazine is exhausted, no further X-ray exposure can be obtained from the unit. The camera can be heard to wind indefinitely until it is switched off. On completion of the normal radiographic exposure, a monitor lamp situated at the base of the camera in the interlock unit visually signals that exposure of the record card has been made.

The Roller Separator Cassettes

Whereas the serial cassette and the M.C.S. cassette were for 70 mm roll film, the separator cassette is for cut film.

In clinical practice at the present time virtually all the camera units employing cut film are of the 100 mm type. For this reason the separator cassettes to be described are those for 100 mm × 100 mm film: the student is unlikely to meet any but these in the course of experience. A separator cassette includes:

(1) a supply magazine into which sheets of unexposed film are loaded in the darkroom and from which they are automatically fed to the focal plane in the camera;

(2) a take-up magazine into which each film automatically passes on completion of the exposure.

A system of dark-slides, which either must be closed by hand or in later units may be self-operated, makes it possible to withdraw either magazine as a daylight operation without risk of fogging films, whether these are in the withdrawn magazine or in the other.

Plate 17.6, following p. 206 shows the supply magazine being withdrawn from the separator cassette on the top of the camera, and in Plate 17.7, following p. 206 can be seen in detail the take-up magazine beneath and the action of its removal. The general illustration of a 100 mm unit which appears in Plate 17.8, following p. 206 shows the relationships of the magazines and the separator to the whole camera assembly. They may be compared with the position of the roll film cassette shown in Plate 17.5.

Separator cassettes in use at present are usually of the variety known as a roller separator cassette.

This cassette offers fast transport of film: it is said that the actual rate at which a sheet of film moves through the camera is of the order of 30 m.p.h.

The roller separator cassette can be operated in any reasonable position, that is with vertical (top to bottom) transport or with horizontal or even oblique film transport. As can be seen from Plate 17.8, in units employed for chest fluorography the transport is vertical and in a downwards direction. Plate 17.9, following p. 206 shows a 100 mm camera unit being used for angiography and here the supine position of the patient necessitates placing the cassette parallel to the floor and consequently a horizontal transport of the films. However, users are not encouraged to adopt a position of the camera which would require vertical transport upwards. In view of the force of gravity one can understand why. Even if no practical difficulties occurred, the sequences of films through the unit would be bound to lose speed.

In the roller separator cassette the cycle of events is as follows.

(1) In the static condition unexposed films in the supply magazine are held forward by a spring plate, the first in the batch being positioned above a pair of film guides.

(2) On preparing the exposure switch, these guides which are situated at the lower corners of the film move a few millimetres medially. They slightly curve the film and separate it from its fellows in the magazine.

(3) A hook engages the edge of the film which is thus freed and slides it to the first of a set of rollers.

(4) The rollers bring the film to the focal plane where, as in other cassettes, it is curved by a pressure plate to conform to the field's convexity.

(5) At this point the camera is ready for exposure; the operator receives

a visual signal that is so in the form of a green light on the monitor unit.

(6) After exposure the pressure plate withdraws and the film is gripped by the next set of rollers which direct it into the take-up magazine. A guide within the magazine ensures that, as each film enters, it is stacked in correct order in the container.

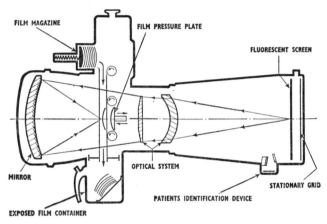

FIG. 17.7. Diagram of fluorographic unit employing 100 mm cut film and the roller separator cassette. *By courtesy of Watson and Sons (Electro-Medical) Ltd.*

Fig. 17.7 which schematically illustrates a 100 mm camera unit shows the main features of the separator cassette and should assist the reader's understanding of the mechanism. However, descriptions of a mechanical operation must tend to be meaningless and difficult to remember unless they can be linked with some working reality. Students are well advised to take any opportunity to see one of these units in use and to review the above account in association with visual observation.

Two types of roller separator cassette are available for use with 100 mm cameras. The *standard cassette*, indicated as the R.S.S. cassette, is used for single exposures, as in radiography of the chest for large groups. The *rapid cassette*, indicated by the letters R.R.S., is similar in operation but is associated with a programme selector of a kind similar to those of other film changers. It can be used for filming fast physiological sequences; for example, the unit is applicable to the techniques of angio-cardiography.

The programme selector permits a series of 40 films to be taken in eight groups of five. A numbering device in the card-holder of the unit advances one numeral every time a film arrives in the pressure frame for exposure. Each radiograph therefore is photographically marked not only with the patient's name but with a number indicating its place in the series.

On the programming panel, exposure frequencies can be pre-selected by means of a separate control knob for each of the eight film groups. The maximum rate is 6 exposures per second but other possibilities are any whole number up to 6.

It should be noted that the rapid roller separator cassette does not possess any electrical interlock. However two red lamps provide a warning signal in the event of the following erroneous conditions:

(1) the supply magazine is empty, or absent, or incorrectly fitted to the separator;

(2) the take-up magazine is not fitted;

(3) there is no patient's card in the card-holder.

If a suitable camera can be available it is not only a helpful but an entertaining exercise to observe the operation of a separator. This can be easily done if the supply magazine is removed and a spare sheet of film (100 mm × 100 mm) held lightly in the hand in the position normally occupied by the leader in the magazine. The contact for the safety monitor which the magazine usually holds open must be manually depressed before the roller separator will function.

Removal of the cover plates on the sides of the camera will permit observation of the film's passage through the exposure gate. The take-up magazine must of course be empty or films in it will be irreparably fogged.

THE X-RAY GENERATOR

In clinics and hospital departments the fluorographic camera unit may be operated from any standard generator having an output of 100 mA at 95 kVp or higher. However, where the service is mobile it is necessary to give special attention to the X-ray generator. The whole equipment may be permanently mounted in a large van, or it may be transported and then unloaded and re-assembled in some suitable building. In either case, its general compactness is a significant feature: in the latter circumstance it is desirable that the apparatus can be unpacked from the truck and fitted together again without recourse to specialized tackle or a large number of personnel. Also important is the current consumption of the generator. It may have to operate efficiently from a mains supply of 15 amperes.

Because of these considerations an X-ray generator and appropriate controls have been designed specifically for mass radiography, with ready transportability, low input and ease of operation as cardinal features. The high tension transformer is housed in a cylindrical tank about 2½ feet high. The four rectifying valves occupy another tank of similar dimensions and both may be provided with carrying handles on either side.

Carrying handles can also be fitted to the control table. Its general appearance and compactness can be seen in Plate 17.10, following p. 206. A special feature to notice is the 'gear lever' type of exposure switch. The L-shaped gate provides two positive positions, the lever being moved down to 'prepare' and then laterally to effect exposure.

In the sloping top panel of the control table, in addition to the hand switch, are placed those instruments required during routine fluorography; line voltage compensator and meter, kilovoltage selector and milliampere-seconds meter. In the vertical panel below are circuit breakers and other radiographic controls which include a synchronous timer with a range of 0·05 to 1 second, a milliamperage selector for three values of tube current (50, 100 and 200 mA), and a switch which enables the photo-timer to be disconnected in order to take large films by direct radiography. Certain other controls which are easily accessible behind a panel are used mainly in setting up the apparatus in order to adapt it to varying conditions of mains supply; for example, a coarse voltage adjustment and another for mains resistance. Also included are spare fuses and switches.

The generator provides an output of 200 mA and 90 kVp and even at maximum load its current demand is less than 30 amperes on a 240 volt supply. All electrical connections associated with the unit are made by means of plugs and sockets, so that dismantling and re-assembly may readily be performed without tools.

The X-ray tube is of the rotating anode type with effective foci of 1 and 2 mm. It is linked to the camera by a side arm which inclines it caudally 5 deg. This can be noticed in Plates 17.1 and 17.5. The anode-screen distance is 36 inches, the tube aperture being appropriately limited by a diaphragm. This may be shaped to conform to the general contours of the lung fields. This feature can be seen in the diaphragm in use in Plate 17.8. In some instances the aperture may be adjustable to enable the lower part of the X-ray beam to be masked if the patient is small. Where the unit is permanently sited in a clinic or hospital the conventional light beam collimator can of course be fitted, but it is an unsuitable elaboration in apparatus which is to be frequently dismantled.

Though a desirable and even requisite feature of any X-ray installation, the use of adequate protective lead screens is particularly important in mass radiography units, which often will be operating in confined space; especially of course where the equipment is permanently mounted and examinations are performed in a van. In any case it would be impracticable to provide enough cable to allow the control stand to be other than relatively near the camera unit.

MONITORS AND INTERLOCKS

References have been made in this chapter to the provision of interlocks and monitoring devices on fluorographic equipment. The student is referred to the sections relating to the card-holder, to the serial and M.C.S. cassettes for 70 mm roll film and to the roller separator cassette for cut film. The purpose of these devices is to eliminate as far as possible operational errors due to human oversight and also to give warning of such faulty conditions as exhaustion of film in the supply magazine or circuit failure in the film marker.

There is available a self-contained safety monitor unit which is a standard accessory to the 100 mm camera unit employing the normal roller separator (R.S.S.) cassette. This unit can be wall-mounted near the camera in a position readily observable by the operator. It can be seen on the wall to the patient's left in Plate 17.8, following p. 206.

The monitor has a vertical row of four pilot lamps, the uppermost one being green and the others red. They operate as follows.

GREEN	This lights up when the film is in the pressure frame and the camera is ready for exposure.
RED Supply magazine	This is illumined when the supply magazine is empty or not in place.
RED Take-up magazine	This is illumined if the take-up magazine has not been fitted or the exposed film has failed to reach the magazine.

29

RED Card-holder

This signals if the card-holder is open or if the patient's card has not been changed between exposures.

No exposure can be obtained from the unit if (a) the green lamp is *not* alight and (b) any of the red lamps are alight.

The safety monitor may have associated with it another unit which is related to the card-holder and provides both a signal that the recording lamp has correctly lighted and a control to adjust the required density of the legend to variations in film speed. Reference to these features has been made in the section on film identification. The two units together provide a very comprehensive check on the functioning and operation of the camera.

In summary we can say that the purpose of an *interlock* is to prevent a radiographic exposure being made in the event of either incorrect performance by the operator or failure of some parts of the camera mechanism: and that the function of a *monitor* is to indicate by the illumination of a lamp the region where fault lies. These are important features of radiographic equipment which is to be used to make a large number of examinations in conditions which give neither time, space, nor even perhaps opportunity to retain subjects for any check on radiographic quality. In many instances processing in fact may not be undertaken at the camera's site of operation and films must be conveyed back to base for development and inspection.

APPLICATIONS OF FLUOROGRAPHY

Emphasis has been on the use of fluorographic camera units of the type described in this chapter for radiography of the chest and certainly it is in this field that they have major application at the present time. However, their possibilities in relation to other radiological procedures should not be overlooked. In Europe, notably in the Netherlands and in Germany, considerable attention has been given to the use of the 100 mm camera for examinations of the gastro-intestinal tract and even of the skeletal system. Use of the rapid roller separator (R.R.S.) cassette extends the applications of the unit to angiographic procedures and to bronchography and intravenous pyelography.

For these investigations of course the unit must be placed under the X-ray table. It is seen in this position in Plate 17.9, following p. 206. To make this a reasonable physical possibility the length of the camera tunnel has to be reduced and this is done by placing the mirror system at right angles to the fluorescent screen and using a 45 deg. plane mirror to reflect the fluoroscopic image into the focusing system. The arrangement is depicted diagrammatically in Fig. 17.8.

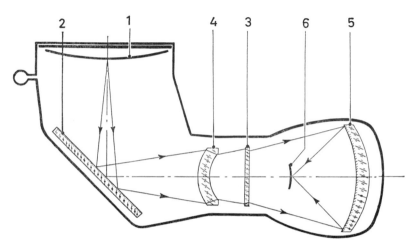

FIG. 17.8. Schematic arrangement of fluorographic camera unit for under-couch use. The mirror system is at 90 degrees to the fluorescent screen and a 45 degree plane mirror reflects the fluorescent image in the required direction.

    (1) The fluorescent screen.
    (2) 45 degree plane mirror.
    (3) and (4) Optical system.
    (5) Bouwers concentric mirror.
    (6) Film.
        By courtesy of Watson and Sons (Electro-Medical) Ltd.

In an earlier chapter (Chapter XVI, p. 375) are described some other possibilities in the photography of a fluorescent image, mainly associated with recording the appearances seen on an image intensifier.

It has been stated that if even 50 per cent of X-ray investigations could be made on miniature film a very substantial economy would occur in the present high costs of radiology. In view of this it seems likely that experiment with fluorography will continue.

CHAPTER XVIII

Fluorography: Photographic Aspects

Film emulsions employed in fluorography are unique in radiographic practice, inasmuch as no X-rays are incident upon them: it is light only which activates the silver halide layer. Furthermore, in comparison with the level of illumination available to the conventional photographer even on rather a dull day, the brightness of the fluoroscopic screen must be considered as poor. Inherent in the procedure of fluorography are certain photographic requirements which need particular consideration. These relate not only to the sensitive materials but to their processing and viewing.

THE FLUORESCENT SCREEN

The emission of light by a fluorescent screen under the action of X rays should now be familiar to the student. Personal observation, if nothing else, will have made it evident that this is not a white light and also that, compared with other forms of photographic lighting, it is not very intense. Before considering what type of film emulsion will be best suited to these conditions, we may usefully examine for a moment the characteristics of this luminous image.

It is important to recognize that fluorescent screens employed in radiography are of the following distinct categories.

(1) Intensifying screens used in direct contact with the film in order to increase the actinic radiation reaching it.

(2) Fluoroscopic screens giving an image for observation directly by the eye.

(3) Fluorographic screens from which the image is recorded by a camera placed at some appropriate distance.

The first have been considered in some detail in an earlier chapter (Chapter v). In regard to the second group, the over-riding consideration must be to obtain maximum brightness even if this necessarily is at the expense of some detail sharpness. Even when well adapted the human eye in darkness or in a low level of illumination is less sensitive to contrasts. In these conditions fine detail cannot be appreciated by an observer and it is a waste of time to concentrate on obtaining high resolution from a screen conventionally used for fluoroscopy, when this must be effected at the cost of decreased luminous emission. Fluoroscopic screens have a relatively thick coating of phosphor and a larger grain size: their intrinsic unsharpness may be as high as 1 mm but they are much brighter than would be an intensifying screen activated by the same energy.

The fluorescent material usually employed for fluoroscopic screens is zinc cadmium sulphide. Zinc sulphide fluoresces predominantly blue and cadmium sulphide predominantly orange. By suitable adjustment of the ratio of zinc to cadmium the light emitted by the combination can be made yellow-green in colour. It is to this region of the spectrum that the human eye has greatest sensitivity at low levels of illumination and this clearly is a significant point in making the available brightness of the screen most effectively useful.

In contra-distinction to those features which are desirable for fluoroscopy, we recognize the principle that an intensifying screen should possess ability to render detail in preference—within the limits of combined radiographic unsharpness—to a high level of luminosity.

Keeping in mind these two rather different desiderata, we can appreciate that a screen designed for fluorography should have some characteristics of each of the others. As the only actinic radiation incident on the film is the light from the screen, this should be as intense as possible if exposure-time is not to be impractically prolonged. Equally the production of radiographic detail is important if fluorographic studies are to be technically comparable with direct radiographs, particularly as in some cases they may be viewed enlarged. In order to decrease their intrinsic unsharpness, screens designed for fluorography are thinner than those intended for fluoroscopy and naturally the luminous emission is not so high.

Colour of Fluorescence

The colour of light emitted by the screen is important in relation to the spectral sensitivity of the film with which it is associated. At the present time screens used in fluorographic units are of two kinds, one fluorescing yellow-green and the other blue. The first is zinc cadmium sulphide and the other zinc sulphide activated by a small quantity of silver. They will be employed respectively with an orthochromatic or panchromatic emulsion or with one sensitive mainly to the blue band of the spectrum.

It may appear to the student rather confusing that two types of fluorographic screen are in general use: it would seem a fair conclusion that analysis must show one to be more effective than the other, when their spectral characteristics are irreconcilably different. However, there are points in favour of each.

The obvious advantage of the green-emitting screen is that it can be used with fast materials. The wider spectral sensitivity of orthochromatic and panchromatic emulsions implies a more rapid response and consequently a reduction in exposure-time can be made. This is a desirable end in nearly all radiological procedures and certainly is so in relation to examinations of the heart and lungs.

However, it must be remembered that neither of these types of film can be handled safely in the lighting ordinarily found in radiographic darkrooms. Orthochromatic emulsions require a dark red light. If they are fast they should not be exposed even to this for more than a few seconds. Panchromatic material should be manipulated in total darkness, though it may withstand *indirect* illumination from a deep green lamp for a very limited period of time: such lighting is permissible in order to observe the time during processing but not to facilitate handling of the film.

This means that in a general radiological department such materials have a high nuisance value. They are more troublesome to manipulate because of reduced visibility. Either another darkroom must be provided for their processing or additional appropriate lighting in the main darkroom, in which case technicians manipulating ordinary X-ray film at the same time must suffer the irritation of having the illumination unnecessarily reduced or totally withdrawn. Furthermore in standard X-ray developers these orthochromatic and panchromatic materials may require different processing periods and this in itself is a minor disadvantage as it offers increased likelihood of human error.

Consideration of these processing factors may determine the preference for the blue-emitting screen. In the United Kingdom some 100 mm cameras employ these, while 70 mm and the older 35 mm mass radiography units usually have green-emitting screens and use orthochromatic or panchromatic emulsions. A proportion of the 100 mm equipment no doubt is associated with general radiological departments in hospital and may not command exclusive processing facilities. Mass radiography concerns, on the other hand, tend to be self-contained and in this case it is manifestly easier to meet the needs of the faster film materials on which the majority of the work will be done. These differences may explain the continued co-existence of the two types of screen. In the U.S.A. there appears to be a greater preference for the blue-fluorescing variety, while in Europe generally opinion is in favour of the green-emitting fluorographic screen.

THE FILM MATERIAL

The standard formats of fluorographic film have been listed in the previous chapter. It is clearly important that the spectral sensitivity of the film should be linked to the spectral emission of the fluorographic screen and consequently the emulsions available for fluorography are of the kinds already suggested; that is either blue sensitive, orthochromatic or sometimes panchromatic.

In distinction to normal radiographic film which is directly influenced by radiation contrasts in the subject, fluorographic film can be affected only by the contrasts available in the screen image; these inevitably have a shorter range. Consequently fluorographic materials should have high contrast if changes in the luminosity of the screen are to be made readily apparent.

At the same time emulsion speed is of some importance, in view of both the limited brightness of the fluoroscopic image and the desirability of using short exposure intervals when examining intra-thoracic structures. Up to a point, the resolving power of the material is of slighter significance than its contrast and speed; the limits of resolution are unlikely to be with the grain size of the emulsion but rather will be found elsewhere, in the optical system or most probably in the structure of the fluorescent screen.

Since these emulsions are exposed not to penetrating radiation but to light which is meeting the sensitive surface from one aspect only, they are single coated. In the case of roll film the base is 0·13 mm in thickness and permanently grey-dyed as an anti-halation measure. The 100 mm cut film has a somewhat thicker base (0·2 mm) which is blue-tinted and has an anti-halation backing which clears during development.

PROCESSING EQUIPMENT AND PROCEDURE

The processing of most fluorographic films is best regarded as a photographic rather than a radiographic operation. This is said in order to emphasize that a more stringent procedure is required for these than for other X-ray materials. Cleanliness, unvarying attention to detail, and rapidity and economy of method are high qualities in any darkroom technician. Nevertheless it must be recognized that a radiograph may receive something less than this exacting standard of attention and frequently not be noticeably the worse for the carelessness. Fluorographic film is much more likely to show evidence of haphazard treatment in the darkroom.

A strong reason for this is that the negative is a miniature. With the exception of the 100 mm cut film, the fluorographic image must be viewed enlarged and this means that such imperfections as scratches, splashes or dust on the emulsion surface become unpleasantly prominent and may interfere with the observation of radiographic detail.

This is particularly true when the fluorographic record is a 16 mm or 35 mm cine film. Because of the troubles which may be encountered in handling efficiently in a radiographic darkroom considerable lengths of cine film, the practice of some X-ray departments is to have such fluorographic studies commercially processed. This can be done by institutes normally undertaking the work for the cinematic industry. It is without doubt true that this is the preferable procedure if the object is to obtain a 16 mm copy from a 35 mm original or to make any copies for demonstration or lecture purposes.

Opinion is varied on whether the 16 mm or 35 mm camera generally gives better results in fluorography but is undeniably a disadvantage of the latter that the equipment required for its projection is expensive and is unlikely to be generally available in lecture or conference rooms, even assuming that is so in the film's 'parent' hospital. This and considerations of wear and tear in projecting frequently a valuable negative make it virtually essential to have a 16 mm copy of any 35 mm film which is of clinical or other interest. It must be recognized that this kind of work requires special equipment and skill and is correctly that of professionals concerned with cinefilm production. While it lies outside the scope of radiographic photography some knowlege of its proper terminology may be useful to the radiographer who has to give instructions for such work to be done. These are briefly discussed at the end of this chapter.

However, in many cases the preference of the X-ray department may be to undertake the initial processing of its own cinefluorograms and certainly all other fluorographic studies are likely to be processed in their places of origin; we may include in this, films taken by a mobile mass radiography unit and brought home to their base for development. In processing any type of fluorographic material advantage should be taken of certain specialized equipment which is available and facilitates the production of satisfactory fluorograms, free from processing faults. This is discussed in greater detail in the sections which follow.

Cut Film

This film has dimensions 100 mm × 100 mm and in the United Kingdom is of the blue-sensitive category since the camera unit often has a blue-emitting screen. It is by a long way the easiest type of fluorographic material to process. The small, individual cut sheets are as familiar to handle as other X-ray films and the spectral characteristics of the emulsion such that the normal lighting of the radiographic darkroom (olive green or orange) is safe for its manipulation.

Plate 18.1, following p. 414 shows a hanger which holds nine 100 mm radiographs and is suitable for use in a conventional processing unit, having 2-, 3-, 5-, or 10-gallon tanks. The hangers are really the only specialized items of equipment required.

These films are developed in a standard Metol-hydroquinone X-ray developer for 5–9 minutes and in a standard Phenidone-hydroquinone X-ray developer for 4–8 minutes, depending on the degree of density and contrast desired.

Where the department employs automatic processing for its normal radiographic work or for roll film, this unit may be of a kind which cannot accept a film as small as 4 inches in either dimension, unless—like the roll film—it is provided with a leader. This is clearly impractical if many such films must be processed. The trend towards automation for X-ray processing generally has resulted in the production of a small automatic processor specifically for 100 mm radiographs. One of its practical virtues is that it occupies very little space, a helpful feature since it almost certainly cannot be the *only* processing equipment required in a department. The length of the processor is 4 ft. 9 in. (145 cms.); its height is 3 ft. 3 in. (103 cms.) and its breadth only 17 ½ in. (44 cms.).

This unit produces a dry finished radiograph in 8 minutes and will operate from a 13 amp. mains socket. It requires cold water at a conventional tap pressure and can therefore be connected directly to the normal water supply: the quantity required is between 3 and 6 litres per minutes or 80 gallons an hour. Other quite simple installation needs are a 1 ½ inch waste pipe and a 6 inch air duct capable of dissipating 1 kW of heat.

The working temperature of the developing and fixing baths is 79°–82°F (26°–28°C) and the films remain in each for about 2½ minutes. The speed of transport is adjustable, as also is the temperature. With the further possibility of altering the concentration of the developer or its type, processing is adaptable to varieties of film or to individual conceptions of what may constitute ideal image quality. Chemical replenishment is made by means of pumps.

Between the different sections of the unit the film is taken up by rollers which remove from it the liquid of the preceding bath. This makes rinsing of the film unnecessary between development and fixation and accelerates both washing and drying processes. The temperature of the washing water is 68°–77°F (20°–25°C). Apart from the rollers film transport is by means of a rotating spiral in the base of the unit. Depending upon the adjustment of the transport sequence, the unit has an output of 120–150 fluorograms per hour.

A notable feature of this unit is that it automatically unloads films from the magazine of the separator cassette as a daylight operation and consequently a darkroom is not necessarily required for its functioning. Under suitable conditions the unit could operate as a self-contained entity in the X-ray room itself.

However, limited darkroom facilities must be available for reloading the separator cassette. We may note again at this point that in carrying out this procedure the sheets of cut film should be placed in the magazine so that the emulsion surface will face away from the X-ray tube. It is good practice on removing the films from their wrapping either to drop them as far as possible singly into the magazine, or—more quickly—to separate them by running the ball of the thumb over the pack. Practised card-players have the right aptitude here. This is to assist the introduction of a thin layer of air between the films. In a damp atmosphere particularly, individual members of a box may tend to adhere to each other and if more than one is taken up by the camera mechanism normal operation of the unit is prevented. Should it occur it is not hard to determine and correct the fault, but it is better still to forestall its eventuality by the habitual exercise in the darkroom of this loading technique.

Roll Film

Darkroom manipulation of roll film is inevitably more difficult for two main reasons.

(1) The increased spectral sensitivity of the material.

(2) Radiographers or technicians with experience of a general radio-

logical department may find long lengths of roll film disconcerting to handle, especially at first. Both these considerations suggest that a separate darkroom for the processing of fluorographic materials is to be recommended but in hospital this may seldom be possible, particularly of course if such processing is only occasional.

In regard to (1), cine films, whether 16 mm or 35 mm, will certainly be panchromatic for reasons of speed. The safest procedure is to process these in total darkness, although *indirect* illumination from a very dark green filter is permissible for a brief period of time. This implies either the provision of separate safelamps or changing the filters on existing lamps in a general radiographic darkroom. In addition a lengthy period of visual accommodation is needed before such limited illumination can be of any practical assistance to the operator. It may well be not only prudent but quicker and easier to undertake processing without any light at all.

Roll film employed in the M.C.S. or serial cassettes of the Odelca mirror camera will be 70 mm and very probably a fast orthochromatic material. The use of a dark red illumination is possible but exposure of the film to this cannot safely exceed a few seconds. For the reasons already given the radiographer or technician who must process it in a general radiographic darkroom may well decide to do so without illumination.

In regard to the length of film involved, the M.C.S. 70 mm cassette contains 100 feet (30 metres) and the Arrieflex 35 mm cine camera has 200 feet (60 metres) on the full reel. It is obviously important to handle a roll of this kind with some respect or it may become unwound with a freedom which escapes the operator's control. Festoons of film on the darkroom floor will lead at best to abrased areas on the emulsion and at worst to actual tears of the base, either of which may render part of the film useless.

Roll film can be successfully processed in certain automatic systems of the roller type, provided that a leader of plain cut film is attached to the end of the strip. The two films should be spliced edge to edge with a piece of chrome tape on either side, in the manner shown in Fig. 18.1.

A 16 mm film will be narrower than the splicing tape and the latter's projecting portion should be cut away: the unwanted section is marked with a dotted line in the diagram.

If the roll film is kept over to one side of the automatic unit other radiographs can be processed simultaneously, provided that they are not so large as to overlap the smaller width of film. In a general department,

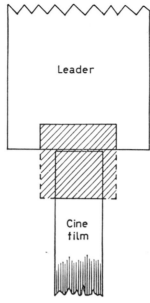

Fig. 18.1. Method of splicing a leader to cine film using chrome tape. The chrome tape is wider than the cine film, and the sections marked by a dotted boundary should be removed.

when assessing the through-put of film for replenishment purposes, the occasional cine film can be ignored, owing to both its narrowness and the thinness of the emulsion layer. However if a slow emulsion is being processed the period of time in the fixing solution may not be long enough, and a test piece should be processed first in order to check that fixing in fact is adequate. As cine film is subject to certain physical strains during projection, satisfactory hardening is also significant.

In those cases where automatic processing is not applicable, specialized units and devices are available and may be considered as essential items for roll film. Some of these are described below.

PROCESSING FRAME

This in effect is an ordinary developing hanger which can be immersed in a conventional processing tank. A typical example is illustrated in Plate 18.2, following p. 414 which shows a 70 mm film being wound into position, the frame being supported and rotated on a stand for the purpose. Some of these frames are of an adjustable nature and will accept film of different width from 35 mm to 70 mm. None are suitable for long lengths of film, the maximum capacity being usually 10 feet (3 metres).

In winding the film on to the frame care should be taken to make certain that the emulsion surface is on the outer aspect. If it is inside, some areas will be in contact with the sides of the frame and proper dispersal of the processing solutions over these areas will be prevented. Striations of unprocessed emulsion will mar the result.

In order to ensure that the position of the film is correct it may be wise to check in the darkroom the location of the emulsion surface. Fluorographic film is not necessarily wound on the spool in the same direction and an operator unfamiliar with it may be misled. For example, 3-metre rolls of 70 mm film which are supplied for the Odelca serial cassette are wound with the emulsion outwards; the same type of film on a spool containing 100 feet and intended for the Odelca M.C.S. cassette is wound with the emulsion on the inner aspect of each turn, and so is cine film.

If processing is undertaken in total darkness and the operator is in doubt, the only method of determining this point is by touch. Perhaps the best way of doing this is to rest a slightly damp finger on some unimportant portion, for instance the first inch or so of the roll. The emulsion surface will feel a little sticky in comparison with the reverse aspect.

SPIRAL PROCESSING OUTFITS

A number of spiral processors are available. These vary in elaboration, details of design and the size of film for which they are appropriate. However, in general they consist of similar components.

(1) A spirally grooved spool which is large enough in circumference to accept a suitable run of film, for example lengths of 24 or 100 feet.

(2) A loading device to facilitate winding the film on to this reel and rewinding it on to its original spool when necessary.

(3) A set of circular processing dishes or tanks, usually four, of a size to accommodate the reel.

(4) A lid to fit these dishes.

(5) A spin drier.

Plates 18.3 and 18.4, following p. 414, illustrate the Hansen unit which probably exemplifies the most refined of these systems.

The spool and loading unit. In this equipment the core of the spool is made up of three loose rings. The upper flange of the spool can be placed on the core so that all of these rings are between it and the opposite flange; or alternatively so that only one or two of the rings separate the two halves of the spool. This is illustrated in Fig. 18.2 and it can be seen that

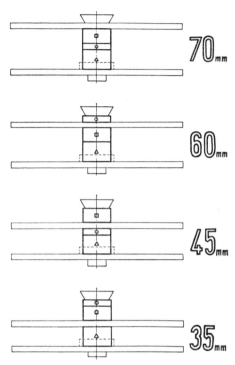

FIG. 18.2. Elevation diagram of the Hansen processing reel showing how the separate components of the centre section can be varied in position to alter the width available between the flanges of the reel. *By courtesy of N.V. Optische Industrie de Oude Delft.*

the device makes the reel adaptable to four different widths of film. Each of the flanges of the spool consists of a large number of toothed radii, the serrations of which are aligned with each other. The diameter of the reel is 11·5 in. (29·25 cms).

The spooling unit is motor controlled and on completion of processing can further be used for winding the film back on the small spool which it will hereafter occupy for projection in the case of a cinefluorogram. This facility is helpful in keeping considerable lengths of film under control, in performing the operation quickly and in ensuring that the film is wound at an even and acceptable tension.

In operation the processing spool is first adjusted for the size of the film concerned and is then placed on a turn-table, with which it engages and will synchronously rotate. The film guide is a metal channel, the sides of which are adjustable in separation to accommodate the different widths of film. A needle at the free end of the guide engages a spiral groove on the rotating turn-table and causes the guide to move outwards in an ever widening orbit.

In its starting position the guide is swung inwards as far as possible towards the core of the spool. The roll of film is placed on an adjacent spindle. A small right-angled fold is made at the free end of the film and it is then fed down the guide until it passes just beyond the extremity of the latter. By means of a variable control the motor is then started at a gentle speed. The synchronous rotation of the spool and movement of the guide will engage the film in the teeth of the former and feed it continuously on to the reel.

Successful engagement of the film with the reel can be detected aurally and by touch if a finger is kept lightly on the edges of the film at the entrance to the guide. Once the film is felt to move it need not be handled further by the operator at any stage in the ensuing procedure. The 'no touch' technique is common even to the simplest spiral processing outfits and offers obvious advantage in the avoidance of artefacts.

As soon as the spool has begun to accept the film, its speed of rotation can safely be increased by turning the regulator gently clockwise. Preferably it should be slowed down again towards the end of the run if the approach of this can be recognized in time; a finger placed lightly on the edge of the feeding spool after an interval will indicate the amount of film remaining and may help the operator to judge the moment at which to reduce speed.

When the whole film has been wound, the apparatus should be allowed to continue running slowly until the film guide has passed completely out of the reel and the needle is no longer engaged in the turn-table. This procedure avoids possible damage to the grooves of the turn-table which is of a plastic material and consequently no robust opponent for a steel needle. Attempts to disengage the needle in the dark, rather than let the guide disengage itself, may easily result in defacement of the grooves. The passage of the needle also helps to keep the channels free of dust or other fortuitous particles.

The reel of the Hansen processor will accept 100 feet (30 metres) of film. It is possible to put on the spool at one time a number of shorter lengths of film provided adequate spacing, that is two empty grooves, is maintained between them. The end of a film which is to be followed on the spool by another is less likely to touch the folded beginning portion of its successor if it is cut in a crescent shape.

Once in position, the film remains on the spool until processing and drying have been completed. The lid of the Hansen tanks has a central hole which can be aligned with another in the core of the spool. The lid is placed over the spool which is allowed to remain where it is on the turn-table of the apparatus. A knob provided for the purpose is then screwed through the lid into the core. This gives a means of agitating the film during development by manual rotation of this knob from time to time and also allows the whole assembly to be easily lifted from one tank to another during processing, without the necessity of actually touching the film itself at any time.

The processing tanks. The Hansen tanks are used for the following.

(1) Preliminary immersion in a wetting agent. This is not an essential procedure.

(2) Development; this tank is marked on the side by a white disc.

(3) Rinsing.

(4) Fixing.

(5) Washing.

If a wetting agent is employed the same tank can be used for this and for rinsing.

The significance of processing materials will be considered in a later section. However, we may notice that the quantity of solution required in each tank during the first four stages will depend on the width but not the length of the film being processed. It is obviously important to respect the manufacturer's instructions in this and to be sure before processing is begun that the quantity of solution which has been prepared is correct for the film concerned. Apart from the waste of materials it is not serious if too large a quantity is made up: but if too little is prepared only part of the spool may be covered by the solutions and thus along one or other edge of the film an unprocessed band will result.

In respect of fluorographic films which are in general use in the United Kingdom and for which the Hansen processor is suitable the quantity of solution required in each tank is:

35 mm   4 litres or 1·1 imperial gallons.
70 mm   7 litres or 1·9 imperial gallons.

The washing tank of this equipment differs from the others in possession of certain special features. The reel of film, from which the lid has now been separated, is placed in the wash tank in the usual way and over it can be fitted a perforated cylindrical bar, capable of being connected via suitable tubing to an ordinary water tap. The direction and

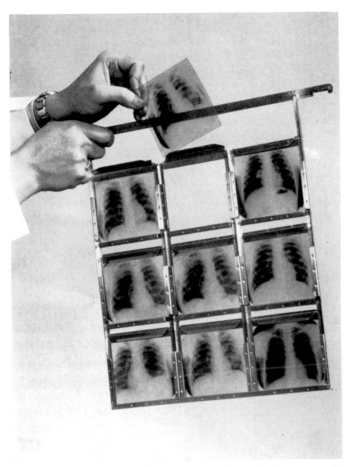

PLATE 18.1. Hanger for processing 100 mm radiographs by means of conventional manual unit. *By courtesy of Watson and Sons (Electro-Medical) Ltd.*

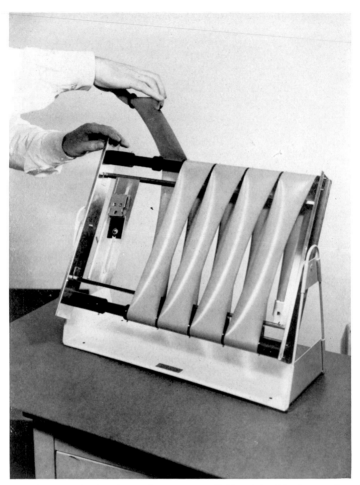

Plate 18.2. Developing frame for 70 mm roll film. The film is transferred from its spool by rotation of the frame between its supports; on removal from the stand, the frame can be immersed in a conventional tank. *By courtesy of Watson and Sons (Electro-Medical) Ltd.*

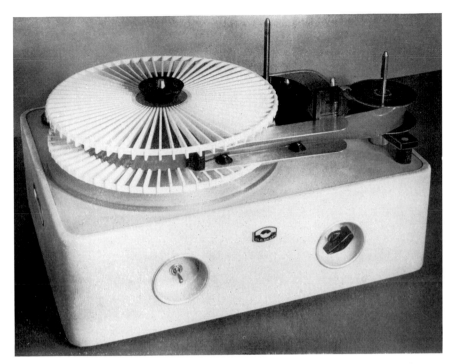

PLATE 18.3. Hansen processing reel and loader. The large serrated reel rotates on a turn-table in a clockwise direction taking film, fed via an adjustable guide, from the small spool seen in position on the right. The guide moves outwards in a widening circle by means of a needle engaged in the grooves of the turn-table. The toggle switch has on/off positions, and the rotary control to the right adjusts the speed of the processing reel. *By courtesy of N.V. Optische Industrie de Oude Delft.*

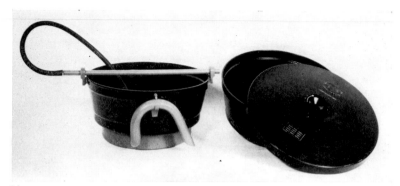

(a)

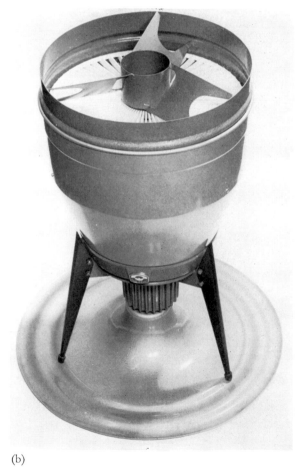

(b)

PLATE 18.4

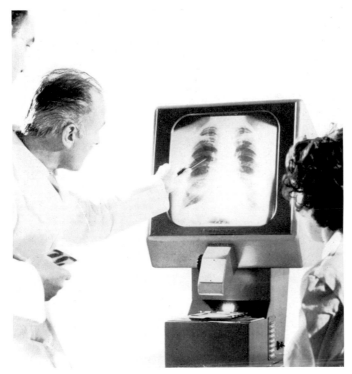

PLATE 18.5. Projector giving full-size enlargement of 100 mm cut film. *By courtesy of N.V. Optische Industrie de Oude Delft.*

PLATE 18.4. (Left) Hansen processing tanks (a) and spin drier (b). The processing tanks are a set of four; the illustration shows two of these, one of which is for washing. Water enters the washer from the top through perforations in the cross rod, which is connected to the water supply by the rubber tubing shown attached. Because of its curvature, the overflow pipe leading from the bottom does not operate until the tank is almost full. The lid of the other tanks and the processing reel can be screwed together by means of the central knob; subsequent rotation of this agitates the reel within each tank. For washing and drying, the lid is removed from the reel, which the illustration shows in position in the drier. Hot air, driven through the centre and slanted sections of the lid, causes the reel to rotate. *Drier by courtesy of Watson and Sons (Electro-Medical) Ltd.*

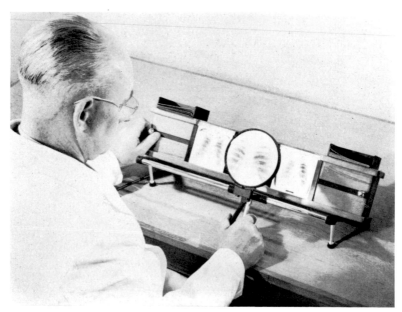

PLATE 18.6. Viewer for examination of 100 mm radiographs, either directly or with a magnifier. Up to 3 radiographs can be illuminated simultaneously; alternatively one or two thirds of the lighted area may be masked by slides at the side. *By courtesy of Watson and Sons (Electro-Medical) Ltd.*

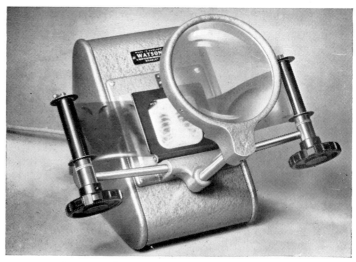

PLATE 18.7. Illuminator for 70 mm roll film. *By courtesy of Watson and Sons (Electro-Medical) Ltd.*

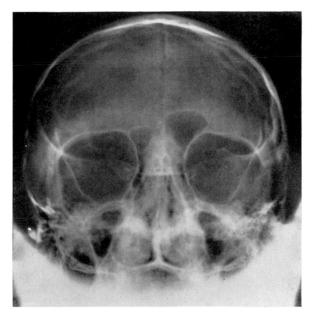

PLATE 19.1. (a) Radiograph prior to injection of contrast agent. This is Film
1 in the subtraction procedure.

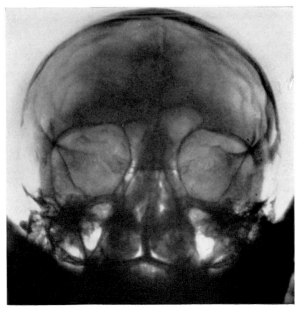

PLATE 19.1. (b) Positive image copy of Film 1. This is Film 11 in the subtraction procedure.

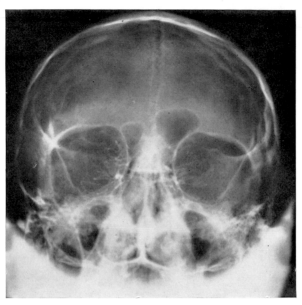

PLATE 19.1. (c) Radiograph made after the injection of contrast agent (cerebral angiogram). This is Film III in the subtraction procedure and is identical to Film I save for the presence of the contrast agent.

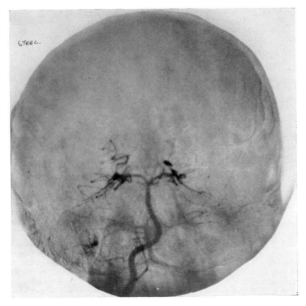

PLATE 19.1. (d) The subtracted image made by superimposing Film II and Film III and printing through them. This is Film IV in the subtraction procedure.

force of the jets from this cross bar are such as to cause the spool to rotate continuously. An overflow device allows the running water to be directed into some adjacent sink or drain.

This overflow pipe leaves near the bottom of the tank beneath a perforated false floor, situated about 2 inches above the base. However, since it then runs along the outside of the tank in an upward direction before taking a final downward passage, the pipe does not actually permit any water to escape until the tank is full.

In this way water is passing continuously from top to bottom of the wash tank while the film rotates in it. These features can be seen in the illustration Plate 18.4. In their absence, the reel in a plain dish or tank can simply be placed under a running tap, but the system is bound to be less efficient as water then enters and leaves it at the same level, that is from the top of the tank.

The spiral drier. This has a fan and in most cases a heater as well so that the air which is blown through the film spiral is warm. The reel is placed on a central spindle, upon which the current of air causes it to rotate. Water is flung off the surface of the film by centrifugal force as well as being evaporated by the passage of the warmed air.

The period required for drying may vary considerably and tends to be longer than that which sheets of cut film usually need in a conventional cabinet drier. This is partly due to the quantity of film involved at one time but mainly to some difference in the standard of dryness which is acceptable. Fluorographic film must be absolutely dry before any attempt is made to remove it from the reel or to rewind it on to another spool for projection. On the other hand conventional radiographs are often removed from the drier when 'finger dry', although the occasional spot of water may linger in corners sheltered by the clips of the processing hanger: these may be trimmed in any case and their presence usually is not materially damaging to the quality of the radiographic image. This is manifestly not true of roll film containing miniature fluorograms. In this case even a small water blister can create a very large defect on projection.

It can be said that drying time averages about 1 hour. Its actual duration will depend on a number of factors which are significant whether fluorograms, radiographs, or indeed any category of photographic film are considered. These have been discussed in Chapter VIII and are restated briefly at this point.

(1) The water-absorbing properties of the particular emulsion.

(2) The degree to which the film was hardened in the fixer.

31

(3) The length of time it was washed.

(4) The ambient temperature and humidity of the atmosphere.

The interval required for complete drying will be minimized if the following points are observed.

(1) The fixing solution is fresh, so as to ensure optimum hardening.

(2) Washing is not unnecessarily prolonged nor the temperature of the water too high. Both these conditions result in increased swelling of the gelatin and consequently prolong the period of drying.

(3) Efficient removal of excess water from the film surface before drying is begun. This means the use of a wetting agent as a final rinse. Immersion for about 1 minute in such a solution not only shortens drying time but prevents the formation of drops and consequently drying marks on the films.

(4) The film is dried in a well ventilated room.

(5) The drying apparatus both circulates and warms the air in the vicinity of the film. Most modern driers do this but some models may have a fan only.

Careful inspection of the edges of the film on the spool is the best means of verifying that a roll film is completely dry. An adjustment of the turn-table to allow the spool to rotate independently, withdrawal of the film guide and removal of the upper flange of the reel permit the Hansen apparatus to be used to rewind the film on to its original or another suitable spool.

While it has been described in some detail in order to illustrate certain points of processing procedure, the Hansen unit differs only in various practical refinements from other simple and convenient equipment. This may be hand operated and is suitable usually for a particular width of film.

GRAININESS IN FLUOROGRAMS

It has been seen in Chapter 11 that the photographic image is a grainy structure. This formation is not normally apparent to the eye but it may become so when the image is magnified.

In relation to most medical radiography the possibility of graininess in the radiographic image is not a problem. However, with the exception of the 100 mm category, all other fluorograms are viewed enlarged. In some cases the degree of magnification may not be high; for example, 70 mm pictures of the chest viewed by one person in a reporting office. Other types of work can require much greater enlargement. We have only to think of 16 mm cine fluorograms projected in a lecture hall to appreciate how different the criteria may be. The point at issue is that the graininess of the fluorographic image is a practical entity which must be considered.

A number of factors, as was stated in Chapter II, affect graininess. One of these is the grain size of the emulsion and it is easy to appreciate that when the average grain size is large then the particulate structure of the emulsion will become apparent more readily than when the grains are small.

However, this is not the only significant factor. Other important influences are found in the developing solution and the degree of development. It is easier to understand the effect of these if we keep in mind that when we complain of a certain film that it is grainy it is not the individual particles of emulsion which are troubling the eye. These in fact are much too small and even at magnifications of 100 diameters would not become intrusive or perhaps even visible.

Graininess is due to the tendency of silver particles during development to cluster. These aggregates, since they are bigger than the individuals which compose them, can often be detected at quite low levels of magnification. They become perceptible because light percolates unequally through the groups and creates on the film areas of uneven density which are interpreted by the eye as a granular appearance. The student should understand that *grain* and *graininess* are not synonymous terms. Grain size is an important factor in the production of graininess, since materials which have a large average grain size generally show greater graininess.

In the processing of miniature films, attention must be given to reducing as far as possible the tendency of silver particles to form these aggregates. For this purpose certain developers known as *fine grain* are available.

CHOICE OF DEVELOPER

The reasons why variations in graininess are obtained in different developing environments are perhaps not fully understood, nor need they concern us closely in the present context. We can accept as a practical fact that aggregation of the silver particles occurs more easily when the process of development is rapid; this implies an active, highly alkaline developer. It follows that fine grain developers are solutions of low energy. There are a number of types of such developer but those in most general photographic use are normal Metol-hydroquinone or Phenidone-hydroquinone developers in which the sodium carbonate has been replaced by an alkali of lower activity, for example borax. They have a pH value between 8 and 9. Usually their content of sodium sulphite (the preservative) is much increased.

One of the characteristics of sodium sulphite is that it is a weak solvent of silver bromide and during the relatively long period of development, which the lowered activity of the solution requires, this substance may dissolve a proportion of small, less sensitive halide grains. It has been thought that the solvent action of sodium sulphite on silver bromide may take part in inhibiting the production of graininess, perhaps by preventing the intermingling of developing centres in different crystals of the emulsion. However, the mechanism and facts of this are not known with certainty.

While it may seem desirable in principle to process fluorograms, particularly cinefluorograms, in fine grain developers, the following aspects of their use must be remembered.

(1) They are generally, although not invariably associated with some loss of emulsion speed.

(2) They produce images of comparatively low contrast. This is to the advantage of decreased graininess as the latter is more apparent when contrast is high, but it is to the disadvantage of detail perception in the fluorogram and of its suitability for projection.

(3) The development time required to produce a given gamma may prove inconveniently long in the X-ray department.

(4) The preparation and maintenance of separate baths of developer in a general radiographic darkroom inevitably complicate the work and are to be avoided for practical reasons, unless there are strong arguments of another kind in their favour.

These considerations amount to the result that fluorographic roll film of the 70 mm category generally is processed in a standard X-ray developer. Development times depend on the degree of density and contrast which may be considered desirable but are of the order of 6–9 minutes. However, in the matter of cinefluorograms practice tends to vary. This was discussed briefly in the last section of Chapter xvi and reference was made to the difficulties of balancing acceptable levels of radiation input with the requirements of optimum image quality in terms of resolution, contrast and freedom from grain.

The graininess inherent in a faster emulsion might be combated successfully if the material were processed in a fine grain developer. However, this could entail a loss of emulsion speed sufficient to cancel the original advantage for which the emulsion was chosen. In these circumstances the combination would offer no improvement in effective speed over a slower film of finer grain in association with a standard X-ray developer; indeed the latter might be the preferable partnership since the resolution obtained with the finer grained material would be superior and its contrast would be higher.

Differences in contrast increase the difficulty of comparing such film/developer combinations. Processing to a high degree of contrast in an X-ray developer may permit visualization of details which are not apparent when a fine grain, low contrast developer is used; but there is equal likelihood of this treatment's producing a grainy pattern in the image, particularly in the case of 16 mm film of which magnification must necessarily be higher for comparable viewing.

It is very clear that there is not an ideal 'right' answer to the problem created by these opposing forces. In order to summarize the matter we can high-light the pinnacles of the argument as follows.

A fast film processed in high contrast, X-ray developer results in:
(1) maximum speed, therefore diminished dose to the patient and least electrical load on the X-ray tube;
(2) maximum image contrast;
(3) maximum graininess.

A slow film processed in a fine grain developer results in:
(1) maximum detail but high radiation dosage and severe electrical load;
(2) lower contrast in the image;
(3) minimum graininess.

Depending upon the camera available, the characteristics of its lens and shutter speeds and the type of work which it is intended to undertake, practical cinefluorographic techniques are likely to be found with some intermediate combination of these materials. It must be recognized that the ultimate choice can hardly be made theoretically but only from experiment and experience in the conditions obtaining and with the equipment at hand.

VIEWING OF FLUOROGRAMS

Reference has been made elsewhere in this book (Chapter xii) to the influence of correct viewing conditions on the quality of the radiographic image. A radiograph held fortuitously to the light from the ward or consulting room window has to contend with factors which are unpredictable and should not—indeed cannot—comprise any part of its correct assessment.

Fluorograms fortunately are spared such hazards as a rule, since in the majority of them detail can be properly appreciated only if the image is first enlarged. This means that they are viewed by controlled illumination, usually in a room in the design and equipment of which some attention has been given to the function of radiological reporting.

Still Fluorograms

Many 100 mm fluorograms are viewed without magnification. In this case, if a standard X-ray illuminator is used it is better if a mask can be provided in order to prevent dazzle from the large brightly lit area behind the film. This mask can be a very simple device; perhaps a 14 × 17 in. sheet of opaque card or thin plywood in which an aperture 4 × 4 in. has been cut. Built-in masking devices no longer appear to be a feature of illuminators designed for medical radiography, although they are usual in industrial models which must provide a high intensity light source for viewing much greater densities.

Equipment for enlarging 100 mm cut film is available and its use may be desirable in some cases, particularly when the observer is long sighted. Two types of enlarger are shown in Plates 18.5 and 18.6, following p. 414.

In Plate 18.5, the 100 mm image is projected on to the back of a fine grain opal glass screen to the dimensions of a full sized 14 × 17 in. radiograph. It can easily be viewed by several people simultaneously. In a double model of this kind two 100 mm fluorograms can be analyzed side by side, or one miniature can be compared with a direct radiograph placed on the companion screen. This facility is obviously helpful when progress of a case must be assessed.

Smaller models give magnification of the order of 1·5 to 1·9. Plate 18.6 shows a typical example in which three 100 mm films can be examined together; alternatively the slide at each side can be used to cover one or two thirds of the illuminated area if these are not required. The magnifying glass can be moved into position over any one of the films or moved away from the field altogether if the operator has no need of it. This device includes an 'In' and an 'Out' tray for films that are waiting to be read and those on which the report has been completed.

Other small viewers may accept either a single 100 mm radiograph or a roll of 70 mm film. Plate 18.7, following p. 414 shows one suitable for reading 70 mm film on either 3 metre or 30 metre spools.

In this model the film transporter can be turned through 90 deg. in order to accommodate the lengthways format of the serial cassette or the sideways disposal of the image in the case of the M.C.S. cassette. The illumination is by means of two fluorescent tubes.

Projectors are available for 70 mm film which can satisfactorily enlarge the image either up to about 6 inches square or, if preferred, up to full size. A typical model accommodates the 450-exposure spool of the M.C.S. cassette and is illuminated by a 750 watt projector lamp which is cooled by a fan. The lens has a focal length of 6 inches and a maximum aperture of f/2·8.

When the intention is to read miniature radiographs by projection rather than directly from a viewer, it is necessary to provide a suitable screen in the reporting room. This need not be elaborate or expensive. For example a sheet of white card of an appropriate size could be fixed to an empty area of wall and the reader seated at a table some convenient distance away, with the projector beside him. However, viewing screens apart from this do-it-yourself variety are of course available and in some cases may be supplied with the projector.

Cinefluorograms

The equipment necessary for viewing cinefluorograms is not essentially different from that used for other forms of cinematography.

A useful addition is the facility to project a loop of film. This means that a length of film which shows a self-contained sequence of events —for example the cardiac cycle as it is demonstrated in angiography—is joined end to end and may be continuously projected, the finish of each cycle being immediately followed by its beginning through as many repetitions as the observer wishes. This type of study is an obvious aid when interpretation is difficult and in all teaching.

The projection of 35 mm cine film presents some problems. Properly it requires bulky equipment of the kind suitable for cinemas. Apart from the difficulty of handling this in the X-ray department, the use of such projectors is controlled in some countries by legislation. Because of these features the viewing of 35 mm cinefluorograms is usually by means of an apparatus intended for editing such film.

Unlike the upright arrangement of the conventional projector, in this machine the film travels *horizontally* between two spools. As normally the vertical axis of each frame runs lengthwise on cine film, the optical system of the editor turns the image through 90 deg. It thus appears in correct aspect to an observer seated in front of it; he is spared the necessity of himself adopting a horizontal position.

Films can be run in either direction through the editor at any speed from zero to 24 f.p.s. The motion can be halted or reversed as the observer wishes. A counting device makes it possible to give to any interesting frame or sequence a numerical index, by means of which, once noticed, its position on the reel can readily be found again.

In some 16 mm projectors the minimum rate of projection is 16 f.p.s. This means that the camera's speed of taking must be at least this, and if a slow-motion analysis is to be made it will in fact have to be higher, with concomitant problems of radiation dose and electrical load. The possibility of operating the film editor at very low running speeds offers some advantage in making the production of slow motion studies technically easier. For example, a film exposed at no more than 16 f.p.s. might be shown at 5 f.p.s. with the effect of slowing down the motion by 70 per cent. This machine undoubtedly possesses increased tendency to flicker compared with conventional types of projector, although perhaps it is not unduly obtrusive in radiographic subjects and consequently of little importance.

The image is projected by the editor on to a metal screen, painted white, which is about 8 in. × 10 in. in size and is a self-contained part of the unit. It is not easy for more than one or at most two persons to look at this screen together, since the best position for viewing is to be seated directly behind the editor at 90 deg. to the projection area. However, this screen can be removed and thus a longer throw and a bigger image obtained if examination by a larger group or more prominent demonstration of detail becomes necessary. In this event a conventional cine screen at some appropriate distance would be used; the screen might be, for example, about 40 in. (101 cms.) square.

The editor is normally powered by a 12 volt, 100 watt lamp and in a darkened room this gives adequate illumination of the small screen. However, when the intention is to enlarge the image to some further extent the strength of the lighting is insufficient: 250–300 watts at least would be required. The lamp housing is cooled by a small fan beneath the unit: cooling is likely to become a problem if a much higher power of lighting is sought.

Paramount in maintaining their efficiency is regular cleaning of all viewing instruments, whether projectors and illuminators or screens. Perhaps particular emphasis of this is required for the X-ray department where only occasional use may be made of such equipment. Once apparatus has become very dusty its restoration to freshness is much more difficult. For glass, other than front-surfaced mirrors, a lint-free cloth and methylated spirit are effective. A soft-haired brush is also useful for this work.

PRINTING CINEFLUOROGRAMS

The advantage of making duplicates of many cinefluorograms is mentioned in an earlier section of this chapter. To have this done professionally some knowledge of the terms used in the cinema industry is likely to be of value to the radiographer. A few of these are given with their meanings below.

COPY. This results in an exact duplicate of what has been taken, i.e. it is a negative if the original was negative.

REDUCED COPY means that the copy will be in the same tone but will be made on 16 mm film if the original was 35 mm.

PRINT implies reversal to a positive image. Projection in the positive image has some advantage if the subject (for example, a coned-down study of the duodenal cap) does not occupy the full area of the frame. Positive projection in this case avoids a large amount of light surrounding the image which creates dazzle and reduces appreciation of detail. If processing of the original is done professionally, blacking-out of the unwanted areas can be undertaken for the negative image and this undoubtedly is to its enhancement and usefulness.

STRETCH PRINTING is repeat printing of one frame. This is an effective means of providing for improved study of an instantaneous movement since it makes it appear slower. Some jerkiness may become apparent but usually this is of little detriment in the nature of the subjects examined.

SKIP PRINTING means the removal of frames. Its cinematic effect is to accelerate movement.

FROZEN FRAME PRINTING results in a still picture without halting the projector.

SPLIT PRINTING means that half of the frame appears still, while the other half is in motion. The moving section shows the sequence of events either immediately prior to or immediately after the arrested situation.

Some intensifiers linked to cine cameras are provided with the means to magnify the image during cinefluorography. Enlargement of the image during the examination requires higher intensities of current and therefore limits the camera's run if the X-ray tube is not to be overloaded. For this reason or following viewing of a particular sequence it may be found advantageous to magnify some parts of a film at a later stage. It can be done during printing if it is desired.

CHAPTER XIX

Some Special Processes

SUBTRACTION APPLIED TO RADIOGRAPHY

In some angiographic examinations, radiographs taken after the injection of a contrast agent may be unhelpful because other structures are superimposed on blood vessels outlined by the contrast agent. For example, certain parts of the cerebral vascular pattern may be difficult to see because bony structures in the base of the skull obscure them; parts of the vessels arising from the arch of the aorta can be obscured by the bony skeleton and soft tissues of the neck and upper thorax.

Subtraction is a technique to remove the obstructive parts of the image and to give a radiographic record in which the bones and soft tissues are not shown, and the vessels outlined with contrast agent remain clear of intrusive shadows. The name subtraction indicates that the process takes away certain radiographic shadows. This removal is achieved by using a positive and a negative image to cancel each other.

To consider an example from cerebral angiography; an antero-posterior projection of the skull made before injection of the contrast agent (Film I) is used to make a copy in the positive image (Film II). Film II is a positive transparency and the tones in it are the reverse of those in Film I; Film I has 'white-grey bones' on a black ground and Film II has 'black-grey bones' on a light ground. These are shown in Plates 19.1(a) and (b), following p. 414.

After the contrast agent has been injected a radiograph (Film III) is taken. This is identical to Film I as regards (a) the projection, (b) the position of the patient, the film and the X-ray tube and (c) the exposure factors; the only difference is that in Film III the blood vessels are outlined with contrast agent and in Film I they are not. Film III is shown in Plate 19.1(c), facing p. 415.

Film III and Film II are used together to make another transparency (Film IV) which shows the subtracted image. The positive image of Film II and the negative image of Film III are made to cancel each other by superimposing the two images; on printing through the two super-imposed images, Film IV is made and this shows the parts of the radio-graphic image which were not common to Film II and Film III. These are the blood vessels outlined with contrast agent and shown clearly free of other structures. Film IV is seen in Plate 19.1(d), facing p. 415.

By way of summary the four films are listed below.

Film I is the preliminary radiograph taken before injection of the contrast agent. It is the control radiograph in the angiographic series and it will be taken in any case whether subtraction is or is not to be done.

Film II is a positive transparency or positive image copy made from Film I.

Film III is a radiograph identical with Film I except for the fact that an opaque agent has been introduced into the blood vessels. It is one of the angiographic series.

Film IV is the subtracted image made by superimposing Film II and Film III. Its image tones are reversed from those of Film III and it shows the vascular pattern as dark on a light ground. The blood vessels outlined with contrast agent have no intrusive shadows around them.

Photographic Subtraction

There is more than one way of obtaining a subtracted image. It can be done by X-ray methods which need no special equipment but have dis-advantages arising from unsharpness in the detail, excessive contrast and fog from the use of direct X rays. It can be done electronically by means of sophisticated equipment which is expensive to buy and to maintain, takes up space and may not be very quickly used except by the practised. It can be done photographically, and this is probably the method most widely used by X-ray departments in the United Kingdom. On this account the technique commends itself for description here.

Equipment Needed

The equipment needed is very simple.

(i) Film material to be used for making the positive image transparency which is Film II and the subtracted transparency which is Film IV. This is a fine-grain low-contrast material with the emulsion coated on one side only of the base. It is used to make the positive transparency (Film II) because its low contrast gives easier control of the range of tones in the positive transparency and because the fine-grain emulsion on one side only of the base results in a sharper image. This film is somewhat more expensive than X-ray film.

If it is wished, the subtracted transparency (Film IV) can be made on X-ray film. This saves the more expensive material and allows the subtracted transparency to be processed in X-ray solutions, either manually or in an automatic processor. The fine-grain single-coated film used for the positive transparency is developed in a photographic rather than a radiographic developer and is manually processed.

(ii) A photographic frame for contact printing. This is a simple piece of apparatus. It consists of a frame with a glass front similar in form to an ordinary picture frame and its glass. The back is hinged. When two pieces of film are put into the frame, one on top of the other, they are kept in perfect contact by pressure from the closed back of the frame; this is specially designed to maintain firm even pressure over the whole surface. The glass front allows light to reach films in the frame.

As an alternative to a photographic printing frame, a home-made device may be used with satisfaction. It consists of a piece of firm hardboard of appropriate size (i.e. as large as the largest radiograph to be subtracted), one surface of which is covered with a thin layer of polyfoam. A piece of heavy plate glass of the same size as the hardboard is used as the front for this improvised frame. The glass should be heavy because its weight is necessary to keep two films, one on top of the other, in perfect contact with each other when they are placed on the polyfoam surface with the glass laid on top of them.

THE PROCEDURE

First stage

(a) The first stage makes the positive image copy (Film II) from the preliminary radiograph (Film I) after it has been processed. This preliminary radiograph must be of high quality with a long range of tones; if it is lacking in sharpness and/or has contrast which is too low or too high, it cannot be used to make a satisfactory positive image copy.

Under safe-light conditions, Film I is put into the printing frame with one aspect against the glass. A sheet of fine-grain low-contrast single-sided photographic film of the same size is put on top of it, with the emulsion aspect of the photographic film in contact with the radiograph and with the two films in registration. The printing frame is then closed.

If the polyfoam-covered piece of hardboard is being used, it is put on the darkroom bench with the polyfoam surface uppermost. The photographic film is placed on the polyfoam with its emulsion surface uppermost and the radiograph is placed on top. The piece of glass is then placed to cover both films.

(b) The printing frame (or the hardboard assembly) is then exposed to white light with the glass front towards the light source. The light passes through the glass and through the radiograph (Film I) to produce an image in the photographic film. This is the procedure known as contact printing and it results in a positive image being produced in the photographic film (in accordance with the explanation given on page 2 in Chapter 1 of this book).

A suggested exposure is 10 seconds to a 15 watt pearl lamp with the printing frame or hardboard at a distance of 4 feet (122 cm) from the lamp, if the radiograph (Film I) is of average density and Kodak Commercial Fine Grain Film CF7 is being used to make the positive transparency (Film II). This suggestion is a guide only and the correct exposure can be determined by experiment. Later in this chapter (p. 431) there is a description of how to make a series of test exposures when using a printing frame (or the hardboard and glass). When the positive transparency (Film II) has been developed, its tonal range should match in reverse that of the radiograph (Film I).

(c) The fine-grain photographic film (Film II) is then processed by hand in a photographic developer recommended for it; for example, if it is Kodak CF7 a recommended developer is Kodak D163 diluted 1 + 3. Development time is about 1 minute at 20°C (68°F) if the positive image copy is being made from an average radiograph. The time of immersion should certainly be not less than 45 seconds if even development over the whole film is to be obtained. The film should be continuously agitated while it is being developed.

Film II is fixed, washed and dried according to recommendations for the particular material being used. When it is dry it is used in the second stage of the procedure for obtaining a subtracted film (Film IV) as a permanent record.

To make the one-sided photographic film easier to handle, it should perhaps be said here that the emulsion side of this film has a pale matt surface and the other aspect of it is dark and shiny. So it is easy to distinguish the two surfaces even under safelighting.

Second stage
The second stage makes the subtraction film (Film IV).
(a) The radiograph in the angiographic series which is selected for subtraction (Film III) is now carefully superimposed on the positive

transparency (Film II). The two must be placed in exact registration and held together with adhesive tape. If the films are not exactly superimposed the final result in the subtracted film will be a sculptured effect (*bas relief*) which is not wanted and does not aid diagnosis. If the tonal range of Film II does not match in reverse that of Film III, a ghost image of the bony parts will show in the subtracted image (Film IV); this may not be a disadvantage if it is not too obtrusive. An X-ray illuminator used for the purpose of superimposing Film II and Film III is more helpful if it is placed horizontally; this saves a battle with the force of gravity!

(b) Film II and Film III, superimposed and taped together, are put into the printing frame in contact with the glass front. If fine-grain single-sided photographic film is to be used to make Film IV, it is put into the printing frame with its emulsion aspect downwards (i.e. in contact with the taped-together Film II and Film III). If X-ray film is to be used for Film IV, it can be put into the printing frame with either aspect downwards since it has emulsion on both sides. The printing frame is closed and its glass front is exposed to a source of white light.

If the polyfoam-covered hardboard is being used, it is put on the darkroom bench with the polyfoam surface uppermost. The photographic film is placed on the polyfoam with its emulsion side uppermost; or X-ray film is placed on the polyfoam with either one of its surfaces uppermost. Film II and Film III taped together are put on top, and the piece of plate glass is put on top of the complete series. The front of the glass is then exposed to white light.

(c) If Kodak CF7 is being used for Film IV as well as for Film II, then a similar exposure technique, as given under *First stage* (b) (p. 427), will serve with some increase in the exposure time. If X-ray film is being used the exposure can be determined experimentally.

(d) Film IV is removed from the printing frame or the hardboard device and is processed. If it is Kodak CF7 it can be developed as before with the development time lengthened to 3 minutes; it can also be developed by hand in an X-ray developer (Kodak DX80) for 4 minutes at 20°C (68° F). If it is X-ray film it can be given normal standard development by manual or automatic methods.

If subtraction is to be a valuable procedure the subtracted film should be available to the radiologist with all the films in the angiographic examination at the time he makes his report. Techniques for successful subtraction which are quick and easy to apply are therefore the only ones of real use.

COPYING RADIOGRAPHS

To copy a radiograph is to produce a second from the first. If the second is smaller in size it is a reduced copy; if the second is larger in size it is an enlarged copy; if the second is identical to the first it is a facsimile.

At the present time manufacturers produce a special film which can be used to make facsimiles by a simple one-stage technique. This special film has been treated so that its reaction on being developed (without exposure to light previously) is to become uniformly black. Exposure to light and subsequent development reduce this blackening, so the photographic response of this film is the opposite of the usual one.

If this special film is put into perfect contact with an ordinary radiograph and is exposed to light through the radiograph, the result on development is a facsimile of the original. The black areas of the original radiograph let no light through to the film which therefore has identical black areas after it is processed. The translucent 'white' areas of the original let light through to the copying film which on development has lightened in response. It therefore finally has translucent areas identical with those of the original and the result is a facsimile of the radiograph.

The availability of this film to make copies directly from radiographs as a one-stage process has encouraged X-ray departments to undertake copying. There are various indications for making copies. Radiographs which show particular appearances may be wanted for teaching or for interest and for collections in medical film libraries and other purposes. If a patient is to be transferred to another hospital or centre for treatment, he can take radiographs with him which are copies and the original hospital does not lose from its files radiographic records which have been made.

Additional radiographs wanted for academic or transfer purposes should not be obtained by submitting the patient to extra radiographic exposures. This is to give him a dose of radiation beyond what is necessary for his own benefit. So a simple method of making copies in the X-ray department with a minimum of special equipment, material and skill is very useful.

Making a Contact Copy

EQUIPMENT NEEDED
The equipment needed consists of:
(i) the special film used for copying;

(ii) a means to hold the radiograph and the copying film in perfect contact with each other and to allow light to reach the copying film through the radiograph. A simple way of achieving this is to use the photographic frame for contact printing or the hardboard and sheet of plate glass which have already been described (p. 426).

A manufacturer states explicitly what safelight conditions are suitable for the copying film which he makes, and it is common for the film to be handled safely in the safelighting of the X-ray darkroom. It can be exposed to tungsten or fluorescent lighting (i.e. to the normal 'white lights' of the darkroom) and it can be processed in X-ray solutions. Some of the copying film available has been designed for automatic processing, but not for automatic processors with very quick processing cycles.

There are two important points to be remembered about the copying film. (i) These materials must be handled with care for they are sensitive to handling marks, much more so than are unprocessed medical X-ray films. (ii) Unlike X-ray films, the copying film has emulsion on one side only of its base.

The emulsion side of the copying film must be in contact with the radiograph to be copied and must face the light source being used for the exposure. With the darkroom lit by safelighting the radiographer can identify the emulsion side of the copying film very easily. It is a pale matt surface, whereas the other side is dark and shiny, reflecting the light.

After the copy is processed, the matt nature of the emulsion surface and the shiny reflecting nature of the other surface are still apparent. If one wants to spare a radiologist the slight shock of viewing an unusually glossy radiograph, it is easy to arrange for the copy to be viewed always from its matt aspect; this is explained below.

THE PROCEDURE

The steps in the procedure are given below.

(a) The radiograph to be copied is put into the photographic printing frame with its conventional viewing aspect against the glass. This ensures that the copy will eventually be viewed from its non-glossy side so that to the radiological eye it looks more familiar and like the original.

(b) A sheet of the special copying film of the same size as the radiograph to be copied is put into the printing frame. Its emulsion aspect must be in perfect contact with the radiograph and the two films must be in registration.

(c) The printing frame is closed and turned over so that its glass is facing the light source to be used.

(d) The copying film is exposed by turning on the white light for the required period of time (see below under *The Exposure*).

(e) The white lights are turned off at the end of the exposure, and under safelight conditions the copy is processed (see p. 432).

If the polyfoam-covered hardboard is being used instead of the printing frame, it should be placed on the darkroom bench with the polyfoam surface uppermost. The sheet of copying film is then put on top of it, with the emulsion surface uppermost, and the radiograph to be copied is put on top of the copying film. The viewing aspect of the radiograph should be uppermost, i.e. towards the light source and next to the sheet of glass when that is put on top.

The Exposure
The time of exposure to light which is required to make a good copy depends on:
(i) the density of the original radiograph;
(ii) the brightness of the light source used;
(iii) the distance between the light source and the film which is being exposed;
(iv) characteristics of the material which is being used to make the copy.

If the light source is a 100 watt (pearl) tungsten lamp 4 feet (122 cms) above the printing frame, and the radiograph to be copied is a normally exposed chest radiograph, a suggested exposure for Kodak Radiograph Duplicating Film is 16 seconds.

A test exposure. The exposure time can be determined by trial in this way.

(1) Take a piece of card large enough to cover the radiograph which is to be copied.

(2) When the radiograph and the copying film have been put into the printing frame and the frame turned towards the light source, place the card over the glass front of the frame so that a narrow strip (say 2 ins. or 5 cms deep) across the top is left uncovered. Begin the exposure with the card in this position.

(3) At the end of 4 seconds withdraw the card so that another strip 2 ins. or 5 cms deep is left uncovered; now there are 4 ins. or 10 cms of film left exposed by the card.

(4) At the end of a further 4 seconds withdraw the card another 2 ins. or 5 cms, leaving uncovered a total of 6 ins. or 15 cms.

(5) Continue in this way moving the card every 4 seconds until the lowermost strip is uncovered and has received 4 seconds exposure.

32

(6) Switch off the light source used for the exposures and process the copying film.

The strip at the uppermost edge of the film has received the full exposure, the duration of which depends on the number of moves made and the length of the interval between each move. The strip at the lowermost edge of the film has received 4 seconds exposure. In between are strips which have received exposures that increase by 4 seconds in progression up the film. Fig. 19.1 makes this clear.

It must be remembered that *increased density* in the copy is the result of *less* exposure; and *decreased* density in the copy is the result of *more* exposure. So the radiograph which results from the test exposure shown here will have increasing density from its upper edge down. Where the image is very dark and lacking in contrast, there is marked under-exposure. Where the image is somewhat lacking in contrast but is reasonably good in detail, there is some under-exposure. Where the contrast is fairly good but the image is somewhat 'thin', there is some over-exposure.

The exposure which gives the best result can be selected from the test film and used to make the final copy. Even a good copy should be expected to be somewhat less in contrast than the original radiograph, for this special film does not attain such a high maximum density as X-ray films do. This will be especially noticeable in the 'backgrounds'—that is the regions of the radiograph which have not been covered by the patient and have received full exposure to the X-ray beam. Nevertheless a good copy will show clearly all the structures seen in the original. In some cases where the original was of very high contrast, the copy may show some structures to better advantage.

Processing the copy

Kodak Radiograph Duplicating Film may be processed in a Kodak X-Omat so long as it is not of the Rapid Process type. The copying film of other manufacturers also can be processed automatically. For manual processing X-ray solutions and the deep-tank units which are standard features in X-ray darkrooms equipped for manual processing can be used. The manufacturers give full instructions as to processing and supply tables of development times and temperatures—for example 4 minutes development at 68°F (20°C) from Kodak Ltd for their material.

When development is complete, the film is rinsed in clean running water for 30 seconds; it should be agitated vigorously for the first

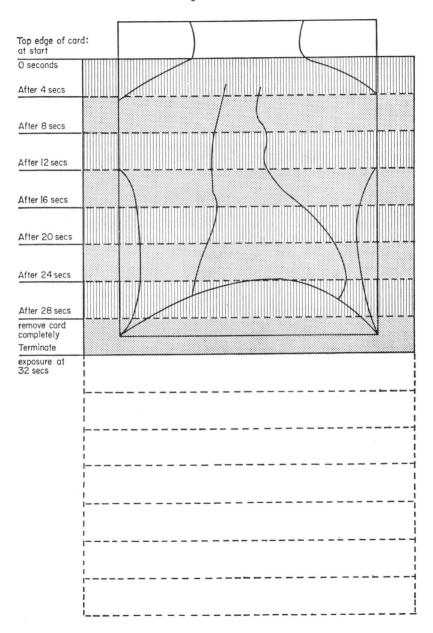

Top edge of card: at start

0 seconds

After 4 secs

After 8 secs

After 12 secs

After 16 secs

After 20 secs

After 24 secs

After 28 secs
remove card completely
Terminate
exposure at
32 secs

FIG. 19.1.

10 seconds in the rinse. The film is then fixed in X-ray fixer for 5–10 minutes, being agitated continuously for the first 10 seconds and often thereafter. It is washed for 30 minutes in a flow of clean water sufficient to give at least two complete changes of water in that time. The manufacturers recommend that the temperature of the rinse, the fixer and the washing bath should be within the range 60°F–75°F (16°C–24°C), and should be close to the temperature of the developing solution.

PHOTOGRAPHIC REDUCERS

The term *photographic reducer* means an application which can be used to remove silver from a developed image and thus diminish or reduce its photographic density. The action in which the silver is involved is *not* one of *chemical reduction*; it is oxidation of the silver to silver compounds. These may be water soluble or soluble in hypo according to the agents used.

To add to the confusion, there is yet another use of the word reduction in photography. This is *optical reduction* by means of a lens to reduce an image in size—as for example in reproducing radiographs for illustrative purposes.

Photographic reducers may be used in X-ray departments to treat radiographs which are too dense; they thus provide an escape route when films have been over-exposed or over-developed. They are seldom used in modern departments. Nevertheless from time to time to save repeating an examination it may be useful to have a technique for reducing density.

Various specific formulae are in use and can be found in photographic reference books. It is unreasonable to be dogmatic about them, for choice rests mainly on personal selection. Those in the following paragraphs are from data by Kodak Ltd. It is probably true to say that this after-treatment is not used to make the difference between a film which is not diagnostic and one which is; by the aid of bright illumination the diagnosis could in fact be made on the existing film. Photographic reducing with chemicals is used simply to provide a better-looking and more readily viewed result.

A Subtractive Reducer

This type of reducer (known also as a cutting reducer) removes the same amount of silver from all parts of the image. It thus lessens overall density, and theoretically leaves the contrast of the image unaltered. This means that it should be used to treat radiographs in which the gradation of densities is correct, but all the densities are too high. This follows from some degree of over-exposure, the fault radiographers are most likely to be seeking to correct.

The subtractive reducer encountered in X-ray departments is Farmer's reducer; it was originated by Howard Farmer. Potassium ferricyanide and sodium thiosulphate are mixed in one solution, and the chemical action which takes place is that the potassium ferricyanide oxidizes silver to silver ferrocyanide, which being readily soluble in sodium thiosulphate solution dissolves as soon as it is formed.

Two points are important when using these solutions. The first is that potassium ferricyanide is a Scheduled Poison, and therefore must be kept and used with care. The second is that acid fixing baths are unsuitable for this use; a plain sodium thiosulphate solution must be used.

This reducer is often used in X-ray departments after being prepared in a haphazard manner. An unknown quantity of potassium ferricyanide crystals is dissolved in a volume of water which is recognizably small but is not measured. Some drops of this are added to a solution of hypo which has been similarly made up with unstated quantities, and when the result is a pale lemon colour it is used to treat the film.

This very simple method works, which is doubtless why it continues to be practised. In fact the action of the reducer is modified by the relative concentrations of the constituents, so this is hardly the way to achieve accurately predictable results. For those wanting a more precise approach, the following technique is given.

THE FERRICYANIDE SOLUTION

	Metric	Avoirdupois
Potassium ferricyanide (crystals)	75 g	6 ounces
Water to make	1000 ml	80 ounces

If this solution is to be kept prepared it should be stored in the dark. If used infrequently, it is better prepared just before use.

THE HYPO SOLUTION

	Metric	Avoirdupois
Sodium thiosulphate (hypo crystals)	240 g	19 ounces
Water to make	1000 ml	80 ounces

THE METHOD

The radiograph to be reduced should be fixed and washed in the usual way, but not dried. If it has been allowed to go through the drier, it must be soaked in water for 30 minutes or so before any attempt at reduction is made. The film is then placed in a photographic dish. The ferricyanide solution and the hypo solution are combined in the proportions of 1 part of the first to 4 parts of the second, adding 27 parts of water, the resultant mixture being pale yellow. This is poured at once into the dish from one corner so that it covers the film quickly. The dish is rocked continuously to avoid uneven results, and the process is carefully watched to assess progress.

The film can be removed, rinsed in water, inspected, and then again immersed for further reduction if necessary. If it takes longer than 5 minutes to reach the desired result, it is probably advisable to discard the used solution and begin again with a fresh one. This helps to avoid yellow staining in the radiograph which it is virtually impossible to remove.

This one-solution reducer can be used as a local application if it is not desired to reduce the whole radiograph. The method is to apply it to particular areas by means of a cotton wool swab soaked in the hypo-ferricyanide combination, the excess fluid being squeezed out.

After reduction, films are refixed and are well washed before drying.

A Proportional Reducer

This type of reducer removes silver proportionally and takes most from the areas where there is most silver. It therefore removes more from the heavily exposed than from the lightly exposed regions of the film. It thus decreases contrast in the result. Radiographers seeking proportional reduction to correct for over-development by lowering contrast turn to Farmer's reducer again. This can give a proportional result if it is used with a two-solution technique instead of a one-solution method. The radiograph is placed first in a solution of potassium ferricyanide and then in a hypo solution after being rinsed in water.

THE FERRICYANIDE SOLUTION

	Metric	Avoirdupois
Potassium ferricyanide (crystals)	7·5 g	260 grains
Water	1000 ml	80 ounces

THE HYPO SOLUTION

	Metric	Avoirdupois
Sodium thiosulphate (hypo crystals)	200 g	16 ounces
Water	1000 ml	80 ounces

THE METHOD

The fixed and washed wet radiograph is put in a photographic dish holding the first solution. It should be slid in quickly so that the whole film is rapidly covered with the solution. It is immersed for 1–4 minutes depending on the degree of reduction needed, and is continuously agitated. It is then rinsed in water and transferred to another dish containing the hypo solution, in which it is immersed for 5 minutes, again with continuous agitation. The film is then rinsed in water before being examined, and the whole process can be repeated if necessary. Afterwards the radiograph is refixed and is washed before drying.

Any film which has been given after-treatment, and perhaps particularly if local applications have been made, should be clearly marked to this effect. Films which have been reduced by the use of chemicals in the way described acquire as a result a characteristic 'glazed' look which makes them different from those which have received normal processing.

Maintenance of Automatic Processors

Chapter x of this book included a very short section on the care of automatic processors of the roller type (p. 231). For superintendent radiographers and senior radiographers in charge of departments and thus responsible for processing rooms and the quality of their output, the information in Chapter x is much too brief to be helpful. In response to a reader's suggestion we have expanded the subject here in the hope of providing a little guidance to:

(a) the maintenance of roller processors;

(b) troubleshooting in respect of film faults which are produced in the processor.

In regard to (a) it is proper to make a distinction between the maintenance of processors and their servicing. Automatic processors should be serviced at regular intervals by technical staff who preferably are instructed and employed by the manufacturer of the equipment. Superintendent radiographers have a duty at the time that a unit is installed to see that supplies officers are advised of the need for routine expert inspection once the period of warranty is expired. A suitable contract for such maintenance can then be agreed between the hospital and the manufacturer which will ensure that the processor is examined, say, every three months.

It is not within the scope of this textbook to describe in detail the fault-finding checks which an engineer might make in the course of such an inspection. By *maintenance* we mean in the present context the daily and weekly routines to be followed by the operator in keeping the processor in clean working order throughout its life. However, reference will be made to mechanical defects which may result in spoiled films. In attempting to elucidate troubles attributable to the processor it is necessary to remember that what appears to be merely a mechanical fault—for example, failure of films to be transported through the drier or to become dry—may have a chemical cause, such as incorrect replenishment. The equipment should not immediately be assumed to be the culprit in all circumstances. Examination of the solution-mixing techniques employed by darkroom staff may show that the chain reaction of disaster was begun outside the processor.

Though the purpose of this appendix is to provide some information on the management of automatic processors, the best work of reference on the subject is not this book but the manual published on the processor concerned by its manufacturer. The following paragraphs can be helpful only in a general way. In them we shall consider the subject under three headings:

(i) cleaning and operational routines;
(ii) solutions;
(iii) faults.

CLEANING AND OPERATIONAL ROUTINES

The principles of care of an automatic processing machine are similar to those which relate to manual processors. Regular cleaning routines are more than advisable: they are essential if the equipment is to work satisfactorily. Whether it is well-used or ill-used in this respect a manual processor may continue to process radiographs but a dirty automatic processor is liable to break down: for instance, sticky crossover rollers can halt the transport of films through the processing section.

Below are given some general notes on the cleaning routines which should be applied to automatic processors of the deep-tank, vertical-transport variety. Summarizing their construction, we can say that inherent in this type of processor are some or all of the following roller assemblies:

(i) a vertical rack of rollers in each of the developing, fixing and washing sections;

(ii) a single rack of crossover rollers between each processing section (replaced in some instances by a crossover plate);

(iii) a similar rack of turnaround rollers at the bottom of each section (replaced in some instances by guide plates);

(iv) a rack or series of rollers in the drying section, depending on the variety of processor;

(v) a squeegee crossover group of rollers between the wet and dry sections (not a feature of every processor).

Because of their differing detailed construction all processors are not exactly alike in their maintenance needs, so reservations are necessary in reading these notes: they are not intended to replace the particular recommendations of the manufacturer regarding the care of his product.

Daily Routines

Manufacturers' instructions on starting up and shutting down the processor each day vary in detail but they follow similar patterns of 'good housekeeping', designed to keep roller assemblies clean and free of encrusted chemical deposits. The following is a recommended daily procedure which is included in either the starting-up or shut-down routine of many processors.

(i) Remove the crossover roller assemblies or plates. Rinse under warm running water. Wipe dry.

(ii) Wipe down the entrance rollers.

(iii) Wipe off all chemical deposits in the processing section.

(iv) Wipe all top rollers above solution level.

STARTING-UP

Starting-up routines necessarily vary and it is not helpful to give here any account of the steps by which particular machinery is put into operation. However, the following observations should normally be made before radiographic processing is begun:

(i) solution levels in the processing tanks;

(ii) solution levels in the replenisher tanks;

(iii) operation of the replenisher flow-meters;

(iv) water flow-rate and temperature;

(v) developer temperature;

(vi) temperature of the drier;

(vii) two or three test sheets of film to be put through the processor to clean those rollers which are above solution level and may have accumulated particles of foreign material during the shut-down period.

SHUTTING-DOWN

Shutting-down routines usually include an instruction to leave the processor covers slightly open in order to allow chemical fumes to escape which might otherwise cause rust or corrosion in the processing tanks.

Many manufacturers advise emptying the wash tank each night in order to inhibit bacterial growth. This can be done easily if the drain valve is always kept open to a very little extent, enough to permit the tank to empty slowly over a period of time but not to prevent its being filled from its normal supply tap when work is resumed. Alternatively a small permanent hole may be drilled in the drain pipe to provide a similar outlet.

Weekly Routines

The procedures listed below are recommended usually as a weekly but sometimes as a fortnightly routine. The latter is perhaps the maximum interval advisable.

(i) Remove crossover rollers or guide plates. Rinse under warm running water (38°C). Work on obstinate chemical stains with a soft brush and the recommended proprietary solution (e.g. Kodak Developer System Cleaner) or the recommended abrasive (proprietary examples are Scotch-brite and Pako-pad). Rinse thoroughly and wipe dry. The use of chemical cleaners is a matter for caution always: note the warning on page 444 of this appendix.

(ii) Remove solution racks and similarly clean these rollers. Rollers in the washing section may normally darken with use: the stain is not harmful but bacterial growth *is*. Drier rollers also may darken in time. Manipulations of the solution racks require care in order to prevent splashing of the developer and fixer solutions into each other's tank. A movable splash guard to protect each tank in turn as the other rack is lifted may be provided and should be used.

(iii) Operate each rack manually to make sure that the rollers rotate freely, that gears engage as they should and that there are no missing teeth, broken springs, loose chains or screws or any other evidence of trouble.

(iv) While the racks are out of the tanks inspect the developer and fixer solutions for foreign material.

(v) Clean the drier rollers with a damp cloth, removing hard deposits with the recommended abrasive material (Scotch-brite is one example).

(vi) Remove the drier air tubes and clean them by vigorous agitation in warm water; do not allow them to soak in water for a prolonged period.

(vii) Inspect filters and change them as necessary, a supply being kept available in the department. There may be filters present in all or some of the following systems:

(a) developer recirculation;

(b) hot water supply;

(c) cold water supply;

(d) air-intake of the drier.

There is some further information about the use of water-filters on p. 446 of this appendix.

It is beyond the scope of this book to give itemized instructions of a how-to-do-it type for the performance of the above: obviously manufacturers' manuals should be consulted in relation to each processor and operators made familiar with the necessary dismantling and reassembly of the specified parts. These tasks are simpler in practice than in print but should be done carefully.

SOLUTIONS

Preparation of Solutions

The preparation of solutions for automatic processors and their use are important matters which can affect the correct operation of the equipment in ways not always at once recognized. For instance, when developer replenisher is mixed and the solution is stirred, rather than effectively agitated with an up-and-down motion by means of a plunger, the chemicals can form layers which may result in the solution entirely failing to develop exposed film. Sheets of cleared base are delivered at the output end of the processor in place of radiographs with startling effect.

Developer and fixer solutions which are mixed too dilute may initiate mechanical troubles in the processor which do not necessarily become immediately apparent and of course are *not* specifically mechanical. This is because such weakened solutions cannot sufficiently harden an emulsion in the time available.

Softened gelatin may accumulate on rollers and thus halt the transport of films through the processing section; or films may fail to dry because the emulsion is soft and has absorbed too much water during the wet stage of processing.

On the other hand, such troubles may have origins which truly are due to physical unsoundness within the processor, such as transport rollers not being correctly seated in their holders or a fuse having blown in the drier's heating circuit. Radiographers confronted with these situations can more quickly solve their problems if the techniques of the darkroom staff are known to be above suspicion; otherwise, the question of chemical unbalance as the cause of a fault must often be present.

Changing Solutions

The frequency with which solutions in automatic processors are changed seems usually to be decided by the user's experience. Rapid-cycle machines, especially those operating on a high temperature chemistry, need a solution change rather more often than those with a dry-to-dry interval of 3½ minutes or longer. This applies particularly to the developer solution if fewer than about 150 films are processed for every 24 of the processor's working hours. Any specific instructions in this respect issued by chemical or equipment manufacturers should be followed.

In the absence of such protocol it is usual to change solutions not less often than the following:

every 12 weeks	half-cycle and full-cycle machines;
every 8–10 weeks	rapid-cycle machines;
every 5 weeks	rapid-cycle with low throughput.

It is convenient to combine a change of chemicals with a service inspection of the equipment and in practice this factor often has the deciding influence in determining when solution changes are actually made.

When the processing tanks are drained in order to renew chemicals there is an opportunity to clean them. A manufacturer may supply a proprietary solution for the purpose of cleaning tanks and racks and in this event the appropriate one may be used. The instructions relating to it should be conscientiously obeyed. Not all manufacturers recommend the use of such cleaners as in certain instances the cleansing substance has penetrated the laminations of rollers constructed in this manner and has caused them to warp.

With reference to the cleaning of tanks, some manufacturers publish advice on the general care of stainless steel and the section on p. 197 of Chapter IX is also relevant here.

FAULTS

As equipment becomes more intricate the possibilities of its malfunction also increase. So long as there is someone to work in the darkroom, manual processors usually operate. Artefacts on radiographs attributable to manual processing are fewer and generally well recognized (or *are* they, now that so little manual processing is done?). However, when the occupant of the darkroom is an automatic machine a dual potential for trouble exists:

(i) the processor may fail to transport films;

(ii) the processor may function but the films carry artefacts or be otherwise unacceptable by reason of a processing fault.

The second situation has perhaps the greater difficulty, but the more generally automatic processors are used the more familiar are practising radiographers likely to become with the artefacts and defects which may result from their mal-operation or may be initiated by faulty techniques in the darkroom.

Manufacturers' service manuals usually contain a 'trouble-shooting' section which is intended to be a guide to the processor's operator and as a helpful source of reference cannot be replaced by such general observations as must be made here. The reader of the following pages should bear in mind that a transport fault or a film artefact may occur because of a particular mechanical defect in a particular processor. For instance if we take a heading such as **cocking or twisting of film in the processing section** here are three different diagnoses from three service manuals:

guide vane bowed or out of place;

worn crossover roller studs;

burrs on the guide plates in the racks.

All this book can hope to do as a problem-solving aid is to cover the common ground between a number of processors and provide a few general indications of possible sources of trouble. In the following pages difficulties are listed alphabetically.

Artefacts on the Film Surface

Artefacts produced by an automatic processor on the surfaces of a film may have a cause which is simple but remains obscure. The following paragraphs have no pretension to providing a complete reference library of detection: the most they can hope to do is to give a little guidance to the events most likely to have occurred.

LENGTHWISE SCRATCHES

(i) If on the undersurface of the film these are probably scratches from the feed-tray and are caused by too heavy finger-pressure as the film is fed into the processor. Check also the possibility of grit on the tray.

(ii) Any roller held stationary can produce fine dark scratches. Carefully check for any hesitation in the drive system and inspect all racks and gears, including the detector rollers.

Other possible causes are:

(iii) encrusted chemicals on the racks, especially at the levels of solutions;

(iv) roughnesses or uneven spacing of guide plates;

(v) air tubes in the drier out of position.

PRESSURE MARKS

Possible causes of pressure marks on the emulsion are:

(i) torsion springs too tight (if the rollers are spring-held);

(ii) foreign material on the rollers;

(iii) any defective roller.

STREAKS AND MOTTLES

Streaks and spots on the film may occur in the drying section as a result of any of the following conditions:

(i) dirty slots in the air tubes;

(ii) slots incorrectly adjusted for width;

(iii) faulty positioning of the air tubes;

(iv) too high a temperature in the drier;

(v) dirty filter in the air intake;

(vi) squeegee rollers not properly adjusted.

Streaks and mottles can be produced chemically as well. They occur in:

(i) a developing solution which is too weak;

(ii) a developing solution which has too high a concentration of developer.

Dirt on the film surface is very probably due to dirty water. In areas where the water is excessively dirty, frequent changes of the water-filter or filters in the processor become necessary. So long as this is done all remains well. Unfortunately the practical situation is sometimes one in which—from pressure of work on the darkroom or other cause—the filters are forgotten for a while. They may then become so blocked with dirt that too little water is in circulation and consequently films are not properly washed and are sticky and do not dry. Faced with a recurrent trouble of this kind, a manufacturer may paradoxically recommend that if the water is very dirty no filter should be fitted, as—misused—it can cause more trouble than it is worth.

Stripping of the Emulsion

The reasons for emulsion peeling may be:

(i) mechanical rollers too tight,
               defective rollers;
(ii) chemical   developer temperature too high,
               fixer not properly replenished,
               fixer/hardener concentration not correct.

Density Incorrect Overall

The reasons for radiographs emerging from the processor either too light or too heavy in overall density—assuming the exposure of each to have been properly made in the X-ray room—are inevitably numerous. They include:

incorrect replenishment rate of the developer;
contamination of the developer (for instance by the fixer);
exhausted developer;
incorrect developer temperature;
incorrect techniques of solution preparation;
no circulation of the developer solution.

Each of the above situations has several potential causes. Examples are:

electrical failure in a pump;
microswitch out of adjustment;
blocked filter;
disconnected hose;
kinked or otherwise obstructed pipe.

Such defects, though possibly simple in origin, are not necessarily quick to elucidate. Radiographers who are required to solve them appear to need a variety of talents which range from a penchant for plumbing to interviewing skills (darkroom technicians' accounts of what they do).

If the fault is not with some mechanical part or system of the processor but is due to an incorrectly prepared developing solution, trouble sometimes arises because the role of the developer-starter is not fully understood. In Chapters VI and X it is explained that the function of the starter is not to start but to brake: that is, it decreases the initial energy of the developer when solutions are changed and the developer is fresh. If too much is used the developer will be lethargic and the processed radiographs too light in density; if too little starter is used the restraint on the reducing action of the developer is not strong enough and radiographic densities consequently are too high overall. It is most important that the proportions of developer to starter should be correct.

Drying Difficulties

FILMS NOT DRY

Many of the troubles listed in the next section as the causes of films not being transported through the drier may also be agents which prevent it from becoming dry in the interval before it is ejected from the processor. The reader is referred to the conditions which affect transport but the following factors should be eliminated as well:
(i) drier tubes dirty;
(ii) drier tubes improperly located;
(iii) air inlet filter dirty;
(iv) squeegee roller not tight;
(v) squeegee roller wet—because for any reason water level in the washing section is too high;
(vi) insufficient water circulation.

FILMS NOT TRANSPORTED THROUGH DRIER
The following conditions are among those which may prevent films from moving through the drier.
(i) Mechanical defects. Examples: warped rollers; incorrectly seated rollers; hesitation in the drive because the rollers are too tightly or too loosely engaged.
(ii) Film surfaces tacky for any reason, such as the following:
emulsion inappropriate to the processing cycle;
improperly replenished solutions;
improperly mixed solutions;
solution temperatures too high;
wash-water temperature too high;
drier temperature setting too low;
a fault in the drier's heating circuit.

Fogging of Films

Films which appear to have been fogged in the processor suggest the following situations:

(i) covers not tight on the processing section;

(ii) processor not sealed against the darkroom wall;

(iii) safelight over the feed-tray not safe (check particularly the wattage of the lamp);

(iv) developer contaminated by fixer.

Jammed Films

When a number of films jam, the one which began the trouble is fairly obviously the film nearest the exit of the processor. This is not to say that the fault which originates the pile-up is necessarily at the same site: it could be further back in the system. For instance, too high a developer temperature may cause the surfaces of a film to be tacky and prevent its travel through the fixing or the drying section. It is consequently essential when dealing with a film jam both to inspect the immediate site for evidence of trouble and to think of the possible causes which might be found at any earlier processing stage.

Clearing a Film Jam

(i) Unless the film being processed is a roll, do not turn off the power.

(ii) Remove a crossover ahead of the pile-up.

(iii) Remove the jammed films and put them in a dish of water to avoid them sticking together.

(iv) Carefully remove the rack where the jam occurred—if it is a solution rack turn off the circulation pump for that particular solution.

(v) Examine the rack and tank for a possible cause of the trouble, such as sheared gear teeth, warped rollers, stretched or missing springs.

(vi) Replace the rack if it is satisfactory.

(vii) Re-introduce the films lengthwise into the processor as near as possible to the jamming point.

In the case of roll film the power must be switched off and the film cut at the feed-tray before the jammed section can be cleared.

Afterwards the following possibilities should be considered and eliminated in turn.

(i) Two films overlapped or fed one on top of the other.

(ii) Too short a film (less than 10 cm) fed without a leader.

(iii) A damaged or folded leading edge on a film.

(iv) Detector rollers unevenly set.

(v) Warped rollers.

(vi) The feed-tray out of alignment.

(vii) Any crossover, roller or solution rack out of alignment.

(viii) Solutions not up to level; recirculating pumps not operating.

(ix) Solution improperly mixed.

(x) Solution temperature too high.

(xi) Incoming water temperature too high.

(xii) Drier temperature too low—if the failure occurred in the drier.

(xiii) Rollers and racks dirty.

Twisting of Films in the Processing Section

The following conditions are among those which cause films to cock or turn in the processing section.

(i) Any mechanical factor which causes uneven roller pressure at any point. Examples: gear teeth broken; gears not fully meshed but riding on top of each other; warped rollers.

(ii) Chemical deposits on solution rollers which impede or alter their motion.

(iii) Algae or bacterial growth on the wash rack which results in slimy rollers.

(iv) Roughnesses on guide plates or crossovers.

(v) Feed-tray or detector rollers out of alignment.

Transport difficulties obviously are ascribable either directly or indirectly to the automatic processor involved; they do not occur in the course of manual processing. However, when radiographic artefacts are under investigation there is a tendency to put the blame on a complicated component of the darkroom and thus on the automatic processor. It is important at the same time to exclude simple extrinsic causes, for the processor is not necessarily the agent of every trouble. Fogging may be due to defective safelights or lightleaks in the darkroom as a whole; rough handling of film can occur elsewhere than in the equipment itself.

Tabulated Factors in the Radiographic Image

Contrast here refers to *objective contrast*—that is difference between densities in different parts of the image.

Detail means *sharpness of outline* in the image. U_g means unsharpness arising from the geometry of image formation—i.e. geometric unsharpness. U_m means unsharpness arising from movement of the subject. U_s means the unsharpness arising from the use of intensifying screens.

Factor in image production	Any effect on image contrast?	Any effect on image detail?
Anode film distance (A.F.D.)	**No effect.**	**Yes.** (i) Alters U_g for given focal spot size and patient-film distance. (ii) Also an **indirect effect** since U_m may increase with A.F.D. because longer exposure times may be necessary.
Beam-limiting cone or diaphragm.	**Yes.** Reduces the volume of tissue irradiated and thus the amount of scattered radiation is less and contrast is improved.	**No direct effect.** An **indirect effect** because when very small fields are used it may be necessary to increase the exposures times and hence U_m may increase.
Compression of body part.	**Yes.** (i) The volume of tissue irradiated is less and thus the amount of scattered radiation is less. Contrast is improved. (ii) Lower kilovoltages can be used and hence there is increased differential absorption in different tissues. Contrast is improved.	**No direct effect.** An **indirect effect** as compression aids immobilization and thus lessens risk of U_m.

Factor in image production	Any effect on image contrast?	Any effect on image detail?
Developer Constitution Exhaustion Temperature Time.	**Yes.** These processing factors can increase or diminish contrast.	**No effect.** It is the **visibility** of detail which the developer alters and not the sharpness of shadow borders.
Exposure time.	**No direct effect.**	**No direct effect.** An **indirect effect** because longer times may increase U_m.
Film contrast.	**Yes.** Image contrast is enhanced if the contrast of the film material is high.	**No effect.**
Focal spot size.	**No effect.**	**Yes.** (i) U_g increases with focal spot size for a given A.F.D. and patient-film distance; (ii) Also an **indirect effect** as *small* focal spots may mean the use of low milliamperes and longer exposure times; hence U_m may increase. So in focal spot size what makes U_g small can make U_m very big. Larger U_g accepted to keep U_m small.
Intensifying screens.	**Yes.** (i) Increase contrast between low densities in the image. (ii) Absorb soft scattered radiation. (iii) Intensify the primary beam more than the long wavelength scattered radiation. (iv) Allow the use of lower kilvoltages. All these improve contrast.	**Yes.** (i) Very greatly reduce U_m by allowing the use of short exposure times; (ii) Add U_s but this is accepted in order to obtain the great reduction in U_m.
Kilovoltages used.	**Yes.** (i) Alters differential absorption in the tissues so that contrast increases as kilovoltage is lowered. (ii) Alters the amount of scattered radiation reaching the film; this increases as kilovoltage is raised and contrast is lowered.	**No direct effect.** An **indirect effect** because intensity increases with raised kilovoltage and hence shorter times may be used, resulting in less U_m.
Milliamperes.	**No direct effect.**	**No direct effect.** An **indirect effect** as high milliamperage (i) implies short exposure times which reduce U_m and (ii) implies larger focal spots which increase U_g for a given A.F.D. and patient-film distance. Increase in U_g accepted to lessen U_m.

Factor in image production	Any effect on image contrast?	Any effect on image detail?
Patient–film distance.	**No direct effect. An indirect effect.** When the patient is a long way from the film (air-gap technique) less scattered radiation falls on the film and contrast is improved.	**Yes.** U_g increases with patient-film distance for a given focal spot size and A.F.D.
Radiation contrast in the subject.	**Yes.** Image contrast increases with radiation contrast in the subject.	**No effect.** It is the *visibility* of detail which is altered by radiation contrasts in the subject and not the sharpness of shadow borders.
Secondary radiation grid.	**Yes.** Prevents scattered radiation from reaching the film and hence markedly improves contrast.	**No appreciable direct effect.** An **indirect effect.** (i) It may increase patient-film distance and hence also increase U_g; (ii) It may increase U_m as longer exposure times may be necessary.

Bibliography

The following publications were consulted by the authors of this book:

ARDRAN G.M. and CROOKS H.E. (1963) Silver recovery. *Radiography* **XXIX**, 256.

ARDRAN G.M. and CROOKS H.E. (1965) Detection and recording of the radiological image. *Proceedings of the XIth International Congress of Radiology, Excerpta Medica International Congress Series, No. 105.*

ASHWORTH W.J. (1958) Electrolytic silver recovery in practice. *Radiography* **XXIV**, 314.

ASHWORTH W.J. (1960) Gas agitation in silver recovery. *Radiography* **XXVI**, 11.

BAINES H. (1958) *The Science of Photography.* Fountain Press, London.

BRAY J.K. and JOHN D.H.O. (1957) The replenishment of radiographic developers. *Radiography* **XXIII**, 149.

BRAY J.K. and JOHN D.H.O. (1959) The replenishment of radiographic developers. *Radiography* **XXV**, 133.

BRITISH STANDARDS INSTITUTION; Specification No. 4304; 1968.

BROWNBILL D. (1958) The eletrolytic recovery of silver from fixing baths. *X-ray Focus* **II** (No. 1) 15.

BROWNBILL D. (1963) The theory and practice of radiographic processing, *X-ray Focus* **IV** (No. 1) 15, **IV** (No. 2) 27, **IV** (No. 3) 18.

FRANK M. (1963) Silver recovery by steel wool. *Radiography* **XXIX**, 351.

GOODES H.G. (1952) Silver recovery and fixer regeneration. *Radiography* **XVIII**, 252.

HERCOCK R.J. (1963) X-ray sensitometry. *X-ray Focus* **IV** (No. 2), 2; **IV** (No. 3), 27.

JOHN D.H.O. (1961) The darkroom—yesterday, today, and tomorrow. *Radiography* **XXVII**, 2.

JOHN D.H.O. and FIELD G.T.J. (1963) *A Textbook of Photographic Chemistry*. Chapman and Hall, London.

JOHN D.H.O. and STAFF C. (1961) Radiographic processing. *Radiography* **XXVII**, 399.

JOHN D.H.O. and STAFF C. (1962) Radiographic processing. *Radiography* **XXVIII**, 219.

JOHN D.H.O. and STAFF C. (1963) Radiographic processing. *Radiography* **XXIX**, 4 and 346.

LEVENSON G.I.P. (1963) Silver recovery by steel wool. *Radiography* **XXIX**, 256.

Manual of Photography (1958). Ilford Ltd., Ilford, Essex.

Manufacturers' Technical Literature.

Index

Page numbers in bold type are important references. Italicized page numbers indicate pages which have relevant illustrations.

457

35